MINERS' LUNG

Miners' Lung
A History of Dust Disease in British Coal Mining

ARTHUR MCIVOR
University of Strathclyde, UK

and

RONALD JOHNSTON
Glasgow Caledonian University, UK

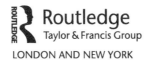

LONDON AND NEW YORK

First published 2007 by Ashgate Publishing

Published 2016 by Routledge
2 Park Square, Milton Park, Abingdon, Oxfordshire OX14 4RN
711 Third Avenue, New York, NY 10017, USA

First issued in paperback 2016

Routledge is an imprint of the Taylor & Francis Group, an informa business

British Library Cataloguing in Publication Data
Miners' lung: a history of dust disease in British coal
   mining. – (Studies in labour history)
   1. Coal miners – Health and hygiene – Great Britain – History 2. Coal mines and mining
   – Great Britain – Safety meaures – History 3. Miners' phthisis – Great Britain – History
   I. McIvor, Arthur II.Johnston, Ronald
   363.1'19622334'0941

Library of Congress Cataloging-in-Publication Data
Miners' lung: a history of dust disease in British coal mining / Arthur McIvor and Ronald Johnston.
      p. cm. – (Studies in labour history)
   Includes bibliographical references and index.
   ISBN-13: 978-0-7546-3673-1 (alk. paper)
   ISBN-10: 0-7546-3673-9 (alk. paper)
   1. Lungs–Dust diseases–Great Britain–History. 2. Coal miners–Diseases–Great Britain–History. I. McIvor, Arthur. II. Johnston, Ronald. III. Series: Studies in labour history (Ashgate)

 RC773.M56 2007
 616.2'4400941–dc22

                                                                                    2006016621

ISBN 13: 978-1-138-27374-0 (pbk)
ISBN 13: 978-0-7546-3673-1 (hbk)

Contents

List of Figures

List of Tables

Studies in Labour History
General Editor's Preface

This series of books provides reassessments of broad themes in labour history, along with more detailed studies arising from the latest research in the field. Most books are single-authored but there are also volumes of essays, centred on key themes and issues, usually emerging from major conferences organized by the British Society for the Study of Labour History. Every author approaches their task with the needs of both specialist and non-specialist readerships in mind, for labour history is a fertile area of historical scholarship, stimulating wide-ranging interest, debate and further research, within both social and political history and beyond.

When this series was first launched (with Chris Wrigley as its general editor) in 1998, labour history was emerging, reinvigorated, from a period of considerable introspection and external criticism. The assumptions and ideologies underpinning much labour history had been challenged by postmodernist, anti-Marxist and, especially, feminist thinking. There was also a strong feeling that often it had emphasized institutional histories of organized labour, at the expense of histories of work generally, and of workers' social relations beyond their workplaces – especially gender and wider familial relationships. The Society for the Study of Labour History was concerned to consolidate and build upon this process of review and renewal through the publication of more substantial works than its journal *Labour History Review* could accommodate, and also to emphasize that though it was a British body, its focus and remit extended to international, transnational and comparative perspectives.

Arguably, the extent to which labour history was narrowly institutionalized has been exaggerated. This series therefore includes studies of labour organizations, including international ones, where there is a need for modern reassessment. However, it is also its objective to maintain the breadth of labour history's gaze beyond conventionally organized workers, sometimes to workplace experiences in general, sometimes to industrial relations, and naturally to workers' lives beyond the immediate realm of work.

Malcolm Chase
Society for the Study of Labour History
University of Leeds

Acknowledgements

We would like to acknowledge our thanks to a considerable number of people and to some organisations who have provided invaluable assistance during the preparation and writing of this book. Our most significant debt is to all those who agreed to allow us to interview them and record their memories, including the many miners we spoke to in South Wales, Scotland and the North East of England. Many of our respondents suffered from varying degrees of respiratory impairment, so for them to give up their time to tell us their stories and to answer our sometimes intrusive and occasionally naïve questions was really appreciated. The hospitality and support we received from the mining communities we visited was truly incredible, deeply humbling and very inspiring. The full list of the interviewees is provided in the Appendix. This book, we believe, is all the more enriched by the inclusion of this testimony. We are also indebted to a number of individuals and organisations who assisted in initially putting us in contact with a number of respondents, including Susan Rayfield (the Coal Industry Social Welfare Organisation) and Wayne Thomas (NUM South Wales), Nicky Wilson, Tommy Coulter and Alec Mills (NUM Scotland) and David Guy (NUM Northumberland and Durham). Our thanks also go to Neil Rafeek for undertaking a number of the oral interviews and for archive work in the North East of England, to Sue Morrison for conducting initial archival research and a pilot interview in South Wales, and to Hilary Young, who assisted with the interviewing and transcribing process in the latter stage of the project.

We also owe a great debt to a number of scholars, specialists and students of occupational health who provided information, commented on our work and with whom we exchanged ideas. Michael Jacobsen – former Director of the Institute of Occupational Medicine – provided constructive critical feedback on the book, helping us to better understand some of the complex medical aetiology of miners' respiratory diseases and the role of key players. Robin Howie – an independent occupational hygienist and lung disease specialist – also provided invaluable feedback and many useful research leads. We have also benefited considerably from Joseph Melling's erudite comments on our research project. Joe provided much-appreciated encouragement and a frequent forum over the past five years or so through the occupational health history and dust-related disease conferences and seminars organised at the Medical History Centre, University of Exeter. We have also benefited enormously from the interchange of ideas with specialists in this field, and here our particular thanks go to Chris Sellers, Geoff Tweedale, Mark Bufton, Anne Borsay, Chris Wrigley, Callum Brown, Alan Campbell, Eileen Yeo and Elaine MacFarland, as well as our energetic and dedicated postgraduate students working in labour history and the history of health, including Andy Perchard, Sue Morrison, Andy Higgison, David Walker and Angela Turner. Many of the above-named also attended and gave papers at the Symposium on Dust at Work which we organised at Glasgow Caledonian University in May 2005, and contributed to the formation of our ideas on the history of miners' respiratory disease (other contributors to the symposium were Geoff Tweedale, Robin Howie, Catherine Mills, Andrew Watterson, Chris Williams and Jock McCulloch).

Invaluable financial assistance for our research, interviewing and transcription was provided by several sources: the Nuffield Foundation, the British Academy and from Glasgow Caledonian University and Strathclyde University. Without this, the book would certainly have taken much longer to produce and may well have been much narrower in scope. We also benefited from the expertise of a number of archivists up and down the country who located sources and answered our incessant queries. Sian Reynolds and Sara Brady of the South Wales Coal Collection deserve a special mention in this respect.

Lastly – but by no means least – Arthur wishes to express his thanks and appreciation to his partner Margot and to his sons Kieran and Tom for all their inspiration and support. Ronnie would like to dedicate the book to his granddaughter Carina.

List of Abbreviations

AEU	Amalgamated Engineering Union
CISWO	Coal Industry Social and Welfare Organisation
COAD	Chronic Obstructive Airways Disease
CWP	Coal Workers' Pneumoconiosis
ECSC	European Coal and Steel Community
FEV1	Forced Expiratory Volume over 1 second
HMWC	Health of Munitions Workers' Committee
HSE	Health and Safety Executive
IPDC	Industrial Pulmonary Diseases Committee
IHRB	Industrial Health Research Board
IIAC	Industrial Injuries Advisory Council
ILO	International Labour Office
IOM	Institute of Occupational Medicine
ISS	Interim Standards Study (of the PFR)
LRTP	Long Running Thermal Precipitator
MFGB	Miners' Federation of Great Britain
MFP	Ministry of Fuel and Power
MNI	Ministry of National Insurance
MOH	Ministry of Health
MRC	Medical Research Council
MSWCOA	Monmouthshire and South Wales Coal Owners' Association
NACODS	National Association of Colliery Overmen, Deputies and Shotfirers
NCB	National Coal Board
NJPC	National Joint Pneumoconiosis Committee
NUM	National Union of Mineworkers
PFR	Pneumoconiosis Field Research
PMF	Progressive Massive Fibrosis
PPCC	Particles Per Cubic Centimetre
PRU	Pneumoconiosis Research Unit
PSI	Pounds per Square Inch
RDR	Coal Mines Respirable Dust Regulations (1975)
ROLF	Remotely Operated Longwall Face
SMA	Socialist Medical Association
SMB	Silicosis Medical Board
SMRAB	Safety in Mines Research Advisory Board

SMRE	Safety in Mines Research Establishment
SPTP	Standard Period Thermal Precipitator
STUC	Scottish Trades Union Congress
SWCOA	South Wales Coal Owners' Association
SWMF	South Wales Miners' Federation
TB	Tuberculosis
TUC	Trades Union Congress
WCA	Workmen's Compensation Act
WRHB	Welsh Regional Hospital Board

Glossary of Medical Terms

Alveoli: The air sacs in the lungs where oxygen is exchanged for carbon dioxide.

Anthracosis: A nineteenth-century term for coal workers' respiratory disease, named after anthracite coal.

Asbestosis: A debilitating lung condition caused by inhaled asbestos fibres scarring the lungs.

Asthma: Disease characterised by a narrowing of the bronchi – the lung passageways – and the production of extra mucus, making breathing difficult.

Beat Disease (Bursitis): In mining, this is normally inflammation of the elbows or knees, due to working in cramped conditions.

Bronchitis: Inflammation of the mucous membrane of the bronchial tubes.

Byssinosis: Lung disease caused by inhaling dust from textile fibres, resulting in increased breathlessness.

Caplan's Syndrome: A form of rheumatoid arthritis showing up as fibrosis of the lung.

Centriacinar Emphysema: A form of emphysema affecting mostly the central bronchioles of the lung.

Coal Workers' Pneumoconiosis (CWP): A chronic lung disease which develops after prolonged exposure to coal dust. The disease can progress from simple pneumoconiosis to the most advanced form: Progressive Massive Fibrosis.

Chronic Obstructive Airways Disease (COAD): Lung damage due in varying degrees to chronic bronchitis and emphysema. The main symptoms are cough, sputum and breathlessness.

Dermatitis: Inflammation of the skin.

Dyspnoea: Difficult or laboured breathing.

Emphysema: Disorder of the lungs in which the air sacs (alveoli) become enlarged and lose flexibility.

Epidemiology: The scientific and medical study of the cause and transmission of disease within a population.

Fibrosis: The formation of fibrous tissue.

Glaucoma: A group of eye diseases characterised by a build-up of pressure within the eye causing defects in the field of vision.

Hypertension: Persistently high blood pressure.

Melanoptysis: The production of black sputum; a symptom of Progressive Massive Fibrosis.

Mesothelioma: Cancer of the lining of the lung caused by inhalation of asbestos fibres.

Nystagmus: An eye condition once common amongst miners, caused by working in poor light.

Panacinar Emphysema: A form of emphysema which usually affects all of the lung.

Phthisis: A nineteenth-century term for Tuberculosis (TB).

Pneumoconiosis: Fibrosis and scarring of the lungs due to inhalation of dust – for example, silica dust, asbestos dust and coal dust.

Progressive Massive Fibrosis (PMF): The most advanced stage of Coal Workers' Pneumoconiosis, characterised by severe fibrosis of the lungs.

Pulmonary Fibrosis: Scarring of the lung in which the air sacs become replaced by fibrotic tissue. This reduces the lung's ability to transfer oxygen into the bloodstream.

Rheumatism: A disease characterised by inflammation of the joints and muscles, which can extend to the heart.

Silicosis: Lung disease caused by the inhalation of silica dust.

Streptomycin: An antibiotic introduced in 1947 which became the most important drug in the treatment and prevention of tuberculosis.

Tuberculosis (TB): A disease caused by an infection with the bacterium *Mycobacterium tuberculosis*. Up to 25% of deaths in Europe in the nineteenth century were caused by TB. Effective medicines were developed in the 1940s.

Vibration White Finger: Numbness of fingers caused by using power tools, also known as Raynaud's Phenomenon.

Weil's Disease (Leptospirosis): An infectious disease carried in rats' urine, causing flu-like symptoms. The disease can be serious if untreated.

Introduction

In the nineteenth and twentieth centuries, dust inhaled at work was a major killer in Britain, and responsible for substantial levels of disability. 'Uncontrolled dust in industry', the Socialist Medical Association observed in 1954, 'is killing and maiming large numbers of people employed.'[1] A few years later, the eminent radiologist and Labour MP Dr Barnett Stross estimated that about two million workers in British industry were suffering from respiratory disability as a result of inhaling dust from their employment.[2] Stross and the Socialist Medical Association were amongst those medical professionals campaigning in the 1950s to raise awareness about the health hazards of inhaling industrial dust and to attack the prevailing widespread stoical acceptance by workers of coughing and breathlessness. As another doctor commented: 'a cough had come to be regarded as normal'.[3] Breathlessness and persistent coughing were common ailments within working-class communities up to the middle of the twentieth century, as was the ubiquitous spitting. As a consequence of industrialisation, Britain had the worst rates of pneumoconiosis and bronchitis in Europe in the middle of the twentieth century, and a key cause was the inhalation of dust at work, especially in the heavy industries, including coal mining, iron and steel manufacture, shipbuilding, engineering and textiles.[4]

---

1   Letter from Socialist Medical Association (Edinburgh and South East Scotland Branch) to Secretary of State for Scotland, 18 November 1954; Scottish Home and Health Department Records; Department of Health for Scotland, NAS/HH104/29.

2   *Hansard*, 30 July 1958, pp. 1,540–51, cited in Scottish Home and Health Department Records; Department of Health for Scotland, NAS/HH104/29.

3   Dr Horace Joules, in *Report of a Conference Organized by the Edinburgh Branch of the SMA, in Co-operation with the NUM (Scottish Area)* (6 November 1954); Scottish Home and Health Department Records; Department of Health for Scotland, NAS/ HH104/29.

4   See *Report of a Conference Organized by the Edinburgh Branch of the SMA, in Co-operation with the NUM (Scottish Area)* (6 November 1954); Scottish Home and Health Department Records; Department of Health for Scotland, NAS/HH104/29. See also the SMA pamphlets *Dust at Work* (*c.* 1953), *The Fight Against Bronchitis* (*c.* 1953) and *Industrial Dust Diseases* (*c.* 1954). According to one estimate in 1960, Britain's death rates from bronchitis were more than thirty times higher than the USA, France and Norway. See I.T.T. Higgins, 'Bronchitis', paper given at the Annual Provincial Meeting of the MRC, 8 September 1960, *Pneumoconiosis Research Paper* 243, p. 124. Mortality from bronchitis in the UK was six times higher than in West Germany. See SMA, 'Action Required', *Record*, vol. 36 (February 1957), p. 231.

Coal mining, however, stood out as being exceptional, as nowhere was respiratory disease more prevalent or more deadly. For miners, breathing impairment was a normal part of day-to-day existence, caused by inhaling large volumes of stone and coal dust in the course of their employment. Miners' respiratory illnesses were designated with different names in different parts of the country at different times – 'miners' asthma'; 'miners' lung'; 'black lung'; black spit'; 'the dust'; '*diffug anal*' (Welsh: shortness of breath). Their impact was devastating, with more than a thousand miners officially recorded as dying each year from pneumoconiosis alone in Britain in the 1950s and 1960s. Indeed, measured by the cumulative morbidity and mortality figures, there is no doubt that occupation-induced respiratory disease (primarily pneumoconiosis, bronchitis and emphysema) in coal mining represented the largest occupational health disaster in British history. The recent British Coal Respiratory Disease Litigation, for example, generated over half a million claims for compensation for bronchitis and emphysema (by closure in March 2004), making it the largest single class action against an employer in Europe to date. This book tells the story of this public health catastrophe, providing a rather different social history of miners – one that places their bodies at centre stage.

The book is divided into four parts. It is not a conventionally structured chronological narrative, but rather analyses the subject under review thematically, focusing in turn upon advancing medical knowledge, the industrial politics of respiratory disease, and finally, on the personal experience of the miners, both in terms of their exposure to dust in the workplace and their experience of disability.

Part I provides some background and context, to enhance understanding of the respiratory disease catastrophe and to locate this within prevailing interpretations in the limited but expanding historiography of occupational health. Chapter 1 also includes a comment on our methodology, including our integration of a systematic oral history project into our research design. Chapter 2 outlines the changing nature of work in British coal mining, and evaluates how work environments, labour processes and techniques impacted upon the body, both in terms of traumatic injury and longer-term, chronic industrial disease.

Part II investigates the contested nature of medical knowledge on miners' respiratory disease, from the early discovery of 'anthracosis' through to the somewhat belated recognition of Coal Workers' Pneumoconiosis by the British government for industrial compensation purposes in 1943. Also analysed here are the contributions that medical professionals working in the coal industry made to epidemiology, especially in relation to the pioneering Rhondda Fach studies in the 1950s and the National Coal Board's comprehensive 25-pit epidemiological study. Chapter 5 explores the evolving medical knowledge on bronchitis and emphysema up to the breakthrough studies in the 1980s which unequivocally demonstrated that these diseases were associated with industrial dust inhalation, and were not just the product of general environmental pollution and cigarette smoking. Bronchitis and emphysema were officially scheduled as occupational diseases of coal miners in 1993.

Part III evaluates the role of the state, the mine owners, the National Coal Board and the trade unions in the respiratory disease disaster. The main focus of Chapter 6 is the efficacy of the NCB's dust control strategies in the workplace. Here we address the question of whether the NCB was an enlightened or a negligent employer. Chapter 7 analyses the collective responses of miners to the dust problem, exploring the role of the Trades Union Congress, the Miners' Federation of Great Britain, the National Union of Mineworkers (from 1946) and the regional miners' federations, with a particular emphasis on South Wales, the epicentre of the pneumoconiosis crisis in the UK.

Part IV assesses the problems of respiratory disease from the perspective of the workers themselves, drawing heavily upon the oral testimonies of miners. Chapter 8 provides a view from the workplace, where the evidence suggests that dust control measures were far less effective than the regulators anticipated. The oral evidence also sheds significant insights into the damage accrued to workers' bodies from the interface between a productionist managerial ethos in a period of contraction for deep coal mining and the persistence of a *machismo*, high-risk work culture. The final chapter investigates what it meant to be disabled by respiratory disease, exploring the impact pneumoconiosis, bronchitis and emphysema had upon miners' lives, as well as the attitudes, responses and coping strategies of individuals and the mining community to this modern-day 'black death'.

PART I
Interpretations and Context

Chapter 1

Methodology and Historiography

Methodology: The Oral History Project

This study of miners' lung disease in the UK combines archival research with oral history interviewing, a methodology similar to that used in our previous study which explored the causes, consequences and social impact of asbestos-related disease in Scotland.[1] A wide range of sources have been consulted in the research for this book, including the medical literature (especially for Part II), the papers of government agencies (such as the Mines Inspectors), and the records of the NCB and the trade unions (notably for Part III). However, we believe that the hidden history of the work process of coal mining, the culture of work and risk, and the impact of occupational disease are areas of experience that can only be fully understood when experiential testimony is utilised. The work environment in mining consisted of a wide variety of functional spaces within which – as one commentator has noted – bodies constituted the biological core of an ecological system.[2] Autobiographical accounts by miners sometimes provide an insightful window into this neglected area, though unfortunately they are not plentiful and tend to focus more on miners' trade union and political activities, rather than health and the workplace – although one outstanding exception is Bert Coombes' evocative *These Poor Hands*.[3] The history of the body is not well covered in the extant literature, and consequently the importance – and timeliness – of gathering oral history evidence of work and health in coal mining is underscored. This, then, is the main rationale for our use of a comprehensive oral history project.

---

1   See R. Johnston and A. McIvor, *Lethal Work: A History of The Asbestos Tragedy in Scotland* (East Linton, 2000); R. Johnston and A. McIvor, 'Dust to Dust: Oral Testimonies of Asbestos-related Disease on Clydeside, c. 1930 to the Present', *Oral History*, vol. 29, no. 2, Autumn 2001, pp. 35–48; R. Johnston and A. McIvor, 'Oral History, Subjectivity and Environmental Reality: Occupational Health Histories in Twentieth Century Scotland', in G. Mitman, M. Murphy and C. Sellers, (eds), *Landscapes of Exposure: Knowledge and Illness in Modern Environments*, *Osiris*, vol. 19, (Washington, DC, 2004), pp. 234–50.

2   Arthur F. McEvoy, 'Working Environments: An Ecological Approach to Industrial Health and Safety', in Roger Cooter and Bill Luckin (eds), *Accidents in History: Injuries, Fatalities and Social Relations* (Amsterdam, 1997), p. 62.

3   B.L. Coombes, *These Poor Hands: The Autobiography of a Miner Working in South Wales* (London, 1939). For an excellent worker's account of mining in the USA, see R. Armstead, *Black Days, Black Dust: The Memoirs of an African American Coal Miner* (Knoxville, TN, 2002), and for a workers' account of a recent US mining disaster, J. Goodell, *Our Story: 77 Hours Underground – by the Outcreek Miners* (London, 2003).

The discipline of oral history has developed significantly over recent years, largely under the influence of post-structuralist ideas, with practitioners now tending to be more sensitive towards the complexities of memory construction, the inter-relationship between the present and the past, dominant discourses (narratives and 'messages') embedded within testimonies and the inter-subjective nature of the interview itself. Summerfield and Thomson have made vital contributions here in what one writer has described as a transition of oral history from a 'reconstructive' to an 'interpretive' mode.[4] Oral history has been enriched by these new approaches, and exponents of oral history have enhanced our knowledge and understanding of a wide range of issues previously 'hidden from history', including women's perceptions of work during both world wars, the nature of family life, gender identities, social protest and militancy, migrant communities, and the role of religion in people's lives, to name just a few.[5] Oral history has also deepened our understanding of the impact of several health-related agendas, including disability, the ageing process, the role of community pharmacies and district nurses, the impact of birth control, and the testimonies of HIV sufferers.[6] In addition, medical researchers have begun to see the benefits of utilising such a methodology to explore doctor–patient relationships.[7] However, there has been very little use of oral testimony in the field of occupational health history, and – related to our own subject of investigation – only Bloor has used a combination of oral/life history techniques and primary source analysis to highlight the conflict between lay and professional knowledge with respect to the medicalization of coal dust disease in the UK in the first half of the twentieth century.[8] In Scotland, MacDougall has collected valuable oral history testimony of

---

4   M. Roper, 'Oral History', in B. Brivati, J. Buxton and A. Seldon (eds), *The Contemporary History Handbook* (Manchester, 1996), pp. 346–7; P. Summerfield, *Reconstructing Women's Wartime Lives* (Manchester, 1998); A. Thomson, *Anzac Memories: Living with the Legend* (Oxford, 1994).

5   See R. Perks and A. Thomson (eds), *The Oral History Reader* (London, 1998); Summerfield, *Reconstructing Women's Wartime Lives*; L. Abrams, *The Orphan Country* (Edinburgh, 1998); C. Brown, *The Death of Christian Britain* (London, 2001); M. Glucksmann, *Women Assemble* (London, 1990); E. Roberts, *Women and Families: An Oral History 1940–1970* (Blackwell, 1995); Caroline Daley, '"He Would Know, But I Just Have a Feeling": Gender and Oral History', *Women's History Review*, vol. 7, no. 3 (1998), pp. 343–59.

6   J. Bornat (ed.), *Oral History, Health and Welfare* (London, 2000).

7   G. Smith et al., 'Treatment of Homosexuality in Britain since the 1950s – an Oral History: The Experience of Patients', *BMJ*, 328:427 (21 February 2004), http://bmj.bmjjournals.com/cgi/reprint/bmj.37984.442419.EEv1; M. King et al., 'Treatment of Homosexuality in Britain since the 1950s – An Oral History: The Experience of Professionals', *BMJ*, 328:429 (21 February 2004), http://bmj.bmjjournals.com/cgi/reprint/bmj.37984.496725.EE.

8   M. Bloor, 'The South Wales Miners' Federation, Miners' Lung and the Instrumental Use of Expertise, 1900–1950', *Social Studies of Science*, vol. 30, no. 1 (February 2000), pp. 125–40. See also F. Cappelletto and E. Merler, 'Perceptions of Health Hazards in the Narratives of Italian Migrant Workers at an Australian Asbestos Mine, 1943–1966, *Social Science and Medicine*, vol. 56, no. 5 (March 2003), pp. 1,047–59.

coal miners' working lives, though unfortunately health and disease do not feature significantly in this material.[9]

From the outset of this study we were interested in getting under the skin of the coal dust problem in British coal mining, and this involved analysing the causation of the problem in the workplace and reconstructing how it felt to be disabled by lung disease caused by dust inhalation at work; how individuals, families and communities were affected by the blight of dust-induced respiratory disease, and how miners' attitudes towards their work impacted upon their bodies. We were also interested in the construction of lay knowledge as much as professional medical expertise and wanted to explore workplace culture, including how working in one of the classic 'heavy industries' forged masculinity and in turn how manly identities impinged upon the body. Whilst aware of prevailing competitive pressures, the profit motive and power structures within the workplace, we wished to also probe the parameters of choice and individual agency. Oral testimony offered the potential to reconstruct something of the personal experience of disabled workers, as well as the mentalities and identities within the community on the dust that wrecked so many lives.

Therefore, to complement our primary source research at several archives throughout the UK, we undertook 45 interviews with 55 individuals, drawn from three geographical areas – South Wales, Scotland and Durham. The full list of our interviews is provided at the end of the book (see Appendix). We aimed to talk to a cross-section of mineworkers from several different coalfields which included representation of all the main occupational groups. We also targeted ex-miners who were impaired to some degree or other with dust-induced respiratory disease. In the event, our interview cohort did include a wide range of mining operations and different levels of employment, including coal face workers, haulage workers, surface workers, mine craftsmen, and different categories of supervisors (such as firemen and dust suppression officers) and lower/middle management. The oldest of our respondents was born in 1909, and the youngest in 1959. Their personal experience of working in coal mining thus stretched from the 1920s through to the 1990s. However, mine managers and the professions were not targeted, nor were company/NCB medical officers and top trade union officials, nor did we interview any Area or Central NCB personnel. We justified these choices on the grounds that there existed considerable documentary evidence for the policy makers through institutional records such as the NCB Reports and Archives, the papers of the National Joint Pneumoconiosis Committee and the archives of the NUM and its constituent regional branches (such as NUM South Wales). Coal mining is probably the most documented of all British industries in the twentieth century, but within this considerable body of evidence, the voices of ordinary miners are hard to come

---

9 See interviews with miners who worked at Lady Victoria Colliery, Newtongrange and other pits of the Lothian Coal Company, National Archives Scotland (NAS) Acc 10801/37; I. MacDougall, *Mungo McKay and the Green Table* (East Linton, 1981); I. MacDougall, *Voices from Work and Home* (Edinburgh, 2000). See also W. Maurice, *A Pitman's Anthology* (London, 2004).

by. Our oral history project was explicitly designed to elucidate the experience and feelings of working miners and of the disabled mining community – to privilege the accounts and memories of those immediately and directly affected by respiratory disease. As the interviewing progressed, we expanded our cohort to include several of the wives and widows of pneumoconiotics, as well as three specialist 'experts' involved in respiratory disease litigation and occupational hygiene research. The latter group included Robin Howie, who worked for the Institute of Occupational Medicine in Edinburgh, and two lawyers, Roger Maddocks from Durham and Mick Antoniw from Cardiff.

The interviewees were told beforehand of our interest and the project's aims, with a written 'informed consent' statement presented to each potential respondent. This is vital in any oral history project so that the potential respondent can make an informed decision about whether or not he or she agrees to being interviewed, and to the subsequent deposition of their testimony in an archive (in our case, the Scottish Oral History Centre Archive and the South Wales Miners' Library). Several of the cohort of 55 wished to remain anonymous, whilst the others expressed the desire that their names be made known. Most completed a pre-interview questionnaire which told us something about their work experience and enabled us to go to the interview prepared. The respondents were recruited in a number of ways, though primarily through contacting the National Union of Mineworkers and the Coal Industry Social and Welfare Organization in Scotland, Durham and South Wales. These organisations did tireless work as advocates for the disabled in mining communities. Indeed, this welfare and pastoral service now remains the primary role of the mining trade unions in some areas, such as Scotland, where employment in deep mining has now completely ceased (the last Scottish deep mine, Longannet, closed in 2002). Some of our respondents had been or were involved in compensation litigation (either as claimants and/or as NUM 'volunteers' assisting other miners with claims), especially claims under the recently settled bronchitis/emphysema (or Chronic Obstructive Airways Disease) scheme. This undoubtedly had significant effects upon the discourses embedded in the narratives. We will return to this later.

Several people were involved in the interviewing process. The bulk of the interviews in Scotland and South Wales were conducted by the authors. The ones in Durham and several in Scotland were undertaken by a colleague, Neil Rafeek (Research Fellow in the Scottish Oral History Centre), assisted in Scotland by Hilary Young (then a history postgraduate at Strathclyde University).[10] In the majority of cases, the interviews took place on a one-to-one basis in the homes of respondents (with Ronnie Johnston conducting most of these individual interviews, notably those in Lanarkshire and Ayrshire). However, there were six 'group' interviews where several miners shared their memories with us simultaneously, and on a number of occasions we (that is, Ronnie and Arthur) conducted interviews together, taking turns to ask questions (this was the predominant pattern in the interviews in South

---

10 Sue Morrison, a history postgraduate working on silicosis at Glasgow Caledonian University, also undertook a pilot interview in South Wales.

Wales and several in Scotland). In four interviews the wives or other relatives of respondents were also present, and in several in Scotland our contact in Ayrshire, an ex-miner Alec Mills, also sat in. Recently, oral historians have identified and elucidated the inter-subjective nature of the oral interview, and how the resultant testimony can be affected. Clearly, there were different dynamics operating in our 'group' interviews than the single ones. In the former, a 'dominant' individual could influence the testimony of the others. On the other hand, memories were 'triggered' and sometimes contradicted within the group interview, leading on occasions to more in-depth and insightful recollections.

Undoubtedly the interviewer also had an influence, however subtly, upon the process of recollection. Now an academic, Ronnie is an educated (mature student), working-class male Glaswegian aged in his late forties. He was born and brought up in a shipyard community (Govan, Glasgow), where his father was a joiner who worked in both the shipyards and in construction. Arthur's background and age is similar (born in Coventry; father a docker from Liverpool, then car assembly line worker), and he has been a full-time academic for more than twenty years. Our age, background and gender may well have had further effects, in that respondents felt comfortable (rather than threatened) with their largely 'traditional' male identities and expressed this more openly than they otherwise might have. The dynamics of this relationship were indicated starkly in another recent oral history project on masculinity in Glasgow by Hilary Young, where several elderly male respondents 'reconfigured' their male identities because the interviewer was young (early twenties), female, educated, and perceived to be 'feminist', and to some extent were influenced by their interview situation, with different results, for example, when a spouse was present, and when the interview was conducted in the pub.[11] Our other interviewer, Neil Rafeek, was in his mid-thirties and was one of the most experienced oral historians in Scotland, having worked on a wide range of projects. Whilst his family background was middle-class (father a town planner; mother a teacher), Neil was brought up in a heavy industry community (Sunderland) and had been actively involved in trade union (building trade) and labour politics (Labour Party). Neil had developed an informed, well-honed, non-patronising interview technique, drawing upon his experience and background to empathise and 'bond' with his subjects, creating a comfort zone that facilitates the free flow of recollections.

The interviews were both interpretive and informative. The testimonies tell us much about the experience, culture and attitudes of workers, facilitating the reconstruction of male identities in mining communities at this time, and of the rather neglected interaction between the workplace and the body. Reflecting in these interviews, miners were trying to make sense of their working lives; to review and in some cases to come to terms with the processes that damaged their bodies and those of their close friends and relatives. This was especially evident, for example, where respondents were disabled and where the testimony constituted something akin to a

---

11 H. Young, 'New Men, Hard Men: An Oral History of Masculinity in Glasgow, from 1950–2000' (Honours Dissertation, History Department, University of Strathclyde, 2001).

trauma narrative (in one case, a seriously bronchial respondent struggled to tell us his story between gulping on his oxygen supply). Some respondents had particular agendas they wished to pursue, such as attaching unqualified responsibility for diseased and damaged bodies upon the employers, management and the government. Such a discourse was evident amongst some of those we spoke to who were or had been affiliated to the Communist Party. Surprisingly, perhaps, some respondents also had an identifiable anti-trade union discourse, and were especially critical of the union leadership for 'failing' the workers and contributing to the respiratory disease disaster. Only rarely was any individual culpability directly conceded, though the oral testimony does shed much light on the existence of a high-risk work culture and helps us to understand the productionist context in which miners' bodies were damaged.

A consistent theme in the oral evidence is the enjoyment and satisfaction that miners extracted from their work experience. For some respondents, paid employment was looked back upon in a nostalgic and positive light. Perhaps most emphasised in this 'optimistic' reconstruction was the camaraderie of work mates, the banter and black humour, and the rewarding experience of the labour process itself. The skilled craftsmen, supervisors and hewers were most likely to represent this positive vision of work, though in some cases this was tinged with regret at the erosion of craft skill and discretion with technological change and the reorganization of work. Such oral testimonies undoubtedly elucidate work spaces that have all but disappeared, illustrating labour processes, describing work environments and conditions, and shedding insights into relationships, attitudes and rituals that characterised the now defunct heavy industries which once dominated the British economy. The rites of passage of on-the-job training, where youths were socialised into a dangerous and macho environment, would be a good example. The way that workplace camaraderie dissected and negated sectarianism in the pits also comes across strongly. Oral history provides rich, 'thick' description which helps us to evoke the workplace, providing a conduit to the past which places us shoulder to shoulder with the hewer, coal-cutting machine man, the heading driver, conveyor operator and ostler (horse attendant) working deep underground.

However, a critical scepticism needs to be applied to some of the testimony, as to some extent the present undoubtedly contaminates these memories of the past and nostalgia can unconsciously distort the picture. Many of our respondents interpreted a primary 'task' in the interview as 'educating' us about how grim work was a half century or so ago. In the process, there may well have been an element of marking their own manliness in contrast to the 'easy life' of today (and, perhaps indirectly, of the 'academic'). In some cases, the interpretation would be offered that there was absolutely no state presence, no union involvement and no protection at all at work. At its extreme, this unequivocal negative and 'pessimistic' evaluation seems hardly plausible, given the weight of evidence to the contrary. However, what is important here is how such workers, reflecting back, *perceived* their working lives. This propensity, evident in some testimonies, to paint the work experience as universally grim, was indicated, for example, in the recurrent use of the 'hell' metaphor in describing the work environment. Some of the rank-and-file union activists fall into this category, presenting a kind of heroic and solidaristic discourse of workers uniting to struggle against inhumane work conditions dictated by the profit motive, and ultimately succeeding in ameliorating the worst excesses of the private mine owners and a state-controlled corporation.

Being critically reflexive about such oral testimony is important. Undoubtedly, the perspective of these men about their own work has been influenced to some degree by the improvement they have seen and experienced over time in work conditions. Views expressed *at the time* may well have been markedly less critical. In the process of recalling past work experience, respondents were informing us about material circumstances and prevailing attitudes, whilst also re-interpreting their working lives, not least in the light of what has happened since the events being recalled. Some respondents also subtly and unconsciously blended into their personal narratives other stories, anecdotes and interpretations drawn from their reading or from discussions with colleagues. Evident here is what Thomson has referred to as the 'cultural circuit', where the actual experience being recalled (sometimes several decades ago) is confused by or conflated with media, literary or collective representations constructed up to the present.[12]

Awareness of the complex processes of memory reconstruction and reconfiguration does not, however, invalidate oral evidence or, in our view, fundamentally challenge the veracity of oral testimony. We have argued elsewhere that where it is used sensitively and carefully, oral evidence has the potential to shed many important insights into areas of experience that are inadequately documented, including the occupational health experience of British workers.[13] Several points might be briefly highlighted. Firstly, the oral testimony illuminates the intimate relationship between employment and the body, and, connected to this, the many and varied ways that those holding power in the workplace, the employers, managers and supervisors, exploited those lacking such power. This was invariably so even where statutory provision existed to 'protect' workers' rights, such as the Mines Acts. Cutting corners on managerial instruction, connivance or implicit sanction was endemic in British industry, including coal mining, where production frequently took precedence over health and well-being. The most insecure workers were most vulnerable, and as the mining industry contracted from the 1920s this insecurity was everywhere evident, especially as the pit closure programme intensified from the 1950s. Secondly, the interviews indicate the persistence in the pits of a vibrant popular workplace culture which could in itself act as a drag anchor, slowing the pace of improved occupational health and safety standards. Whilst the collectivist, solidaristic culture of mining communities have been emphasised in many accounts, the oral testimony exposes another dimension – that of the individualistic, competitive, *machismo* work culture

---

12 Thomson, *Anzac Memories*, p. 215.

13 R. Johnston and A. McIvor, 'Oral History, Subjectivity and Environmental Reality'; A. McIvor and R. Johnston, 'Voices from the Pits: Health and Safety in Scottish Coal Mining since 1945', *Scottish Economic and Social History*, vol. 22, no. 2 (2002), pp. 111–33.

in the pits, where risks were taken, especially if the trade-off was higher wages or a shorter work shift. There was conflict and contradiction evident here. Peer pressure – in part linked to male identity – operated to induce workers to eschew safety measures, whilst the increasing age-profile of the workforce led to the fossilisation of attitudes and stagnation in occupational health and safety standards. Thus oral testimony provides a view from the point of production which tells us much about the influence and the limitations of state regulation of the workplace. The twentieth century has been characterised by a revolution in government intervention in mining employment, with legislation affecting most areas of working life, from wages, hours, union recognition and rights to health and safety on the job.[14] However, what comes strongly through the oral testimony is the existence of a considerable gulf between statutory control and the reality of actual workplace practice. In short, legislation continued to be widely ignored or subverted. Moreover, the oral evidence facilitates engagement with debates on the role of the trade unions on occupational health and safety. In this case, the oral testimony, together with other evidence, tends to affirm a positive role for the mining trade unions in relation to occupational health, somewhat against the grain of 'orthodox' views within the historiography. We will return to this later.

For several reasons, then, we believe that our methodology – integrating primary source evidence and systematic oral history interviewing – will make a valuable contribution to the historiography of occupational health, and it is to an overview of this historiography that we now turn.

Occupational Health History in the UK and the USA: Concepts, Theories and Themes

After years of virtual neglect there is now a steadily growing literature on the history of occupational health. However, within this the balance is still heavily weighted towards the USA, where a vibrant strand of research emerged in the 1970s and 1980s and has continued unabated ever since. Within the growing corpus of work by American historians, the work–health interaction has been explored in its widest sense, with several infamous work processes receiving special attention, including working with phosphorus, lead and radioactive material.[15]

---

14 See A. McIvor, *A History of Work in Britain, 1880–1950* (London, 2001), pp. 148–73.

15 See, for example, G. Rosen, *A History of Public Health* (Baltimore, MD, 1993); M. Aldrich, *Safety First: Technology, Labor, and Business in the Building of American Work Safety, 1870–1939* (Baltimore, MD, 1997); C. Sellers, *Hazards of the Job: From Industrial Science to Environmental Health Science* (Chapel Hill, NC, 1997); C. Levenstein et al. (eds), *Work, Health and Environment: Old Problems, New Solutions* (New York, 1997); A. Dembe, *Occupation and Disease: How Social Factors Affect the Conception of Work–related Disorders* (New Haven, CT, 1996); J.K. Corn, *Responses to Occupational Health Hazards: A Historical Perspective* (New York, 1992); R. Bayer (ed.), *The Health and Safety*

The situation in the UK, though, has until fairly recently fallen far short of the high volume of work produced in America. Several sociologists and commentators on the politics of industrial ill health have done important research on the twentieth-century workplace, with Nichols, Bellaby and Dalton standing out for special mention.[16] However, although historians have scrutinised the evolution of general health care and public health in the UK, the impact of work on health has not been given the attention it deserves. Weindling's important edited volume *The Social History of Occupational Health*, published in 1985, stimulated some interest, though it is really only over the past decade that published material on the history of occupational health has proliferated. Bartrip, Burman and Harrison have done important work on the 'dangerous trades' in the late nineteenth/early twentieth century and on state policy, including workmen's compensation.[17] Some work has been done on occupational health in Britain in the inter-war slump and during the Second World War.[18] Moreover,

---

of Workers: Case Studies in the Politics of Professional Responsibility (New York, 1998); D. Rosner and G. Markowitz (eds), *Dying For Work: Workers' Safety and Health in Twentieth Century America* (Bloomington, IN, 1987). For lead, see C. Warren, *Brush With Death: A Social History of Lead Poisoning* (Baltimore, MD, 2001). For phosphorus, J. Emsley, *The Shocking History of Phosphorus: A Biography of the Devil's Element* (London, 2001); For radiation, see C. Clark, *Radium Girls: Women and Industrial Health Reform, 1910–1935* (Toronto, 1997); C. Caufield, *Multiple Exposures: Chronicles of the Radiation Age* (Chicago, IL, 1989). Byssinosis has also been studied in some depth: see C. Levenstein, Gregory DeLaurier and M. Dunn, *The Cotton Dust Papers* (New York, 2002); J.K. Corn, *Responses to Occupational Health Hazards*, pp. 147–74; B.M Judkins, *We Offer Ourselves as Evidence*, Part 3, 'The Brown Lung Movement', pp. 111–53. For byssinosis in the UK, see S. Bowden and G. Tweedale, 'Poisoned by the Fluff: Compensation and Litigation for Byssinosis in the Lancashire Cotton Industry', *Journal of Law and Society*, vol. 29, no. 4 (December 2002), pp. 560–79; S. Bowden and G. Tweedale, 'Mondays without Dread: the Trade Union Response to Byssinosis in the Lancashire Cotton Industry in the Twentieth Century', *Social History of Medicine*, vol. 16, no. 1 (2003), pp. 79–95.

16 See T. Nichols, *The Sociology of Industrial Injury* (London, 1997); P. Bellaby, *Sick From Work: The Body in Employment* (Aldershot, 1999). A. Dalton, *Safety, Health and Environmental Hazards at the Workplace* (London, 1998); G.K. Wilson, *The Politics of Safety and Health: Occupational Safety and Health in the United States and Britain* (Oxford, 1985). See also A. Watterson, 'Occupational Health and Illness: The Politics of Hazard Education', in S. Rodmell and A. Watt (eds), *The Politics of Health Education* (London, 1986).

17 P. Bartrip and S. Burman, *The Wounded Soldiers of Industry: Industrial Compensation Policy* (Oxford, 1983); P. Bartrip, *Workmen's Compensation in Twentieth Century Britain* (Aldershot, 1987); P. Bartrip, *The Home Office and the Dangerous Trades: Regulating Occupational Disease in Victorian and Edwardian Britain* (Amsterdam, 2002); B. Harrison, *'Not Only the 'Dangerous Trades': Women's Work and Health in Britain, 1880–1914* (London, 1996). See also A. McIvor, 'Employers, the Government and Industrial Fatigue in Britain, 1890–1918', *British Journal of Industrial Medicine*, 44 (1987), pp. 724–32.

18 A. McIvor, 'Manual Work, Technology and Health 1918–39', *Medical History*, 31 (1987), pp. 160–89; H. Jones 'Employers' Welfare Schemes and Industrial Relations in Inter-war Britain', *Business History* (1983), pp. 61–73; H.A. Waldron, 'Occupational Health During the Second World War: Hope Deferred or Hope Abandoned?', *Medical History*, 41 (1997),

there have been a number of seminal studies on specific occupational diseases, the politics of occupational health and the struggles over medical knowledge – including the work of Melling and Bufton.[19] None the less, Bartrip draws attention to the relative barrenness in a historiography of occupational health in his recent appraisal of the interaction of the British Home Office and the 'dangerous trades' in the late nineteenth and early twentieth century, noting that, although there have been several important articles, monograph chapters and chapters in edited collections, much more work needs to be done.[20] Certainly, significant gaps persist. For example, we have no systematic exploration of the role of the trade unions in occupational health, and as far as occupational health and safety in the nationalised industries goes, we still only have Hutter's work on the railways.[21]

Although lacking in mass, occupational health history has – like all good history – stimulated intense debate, and much of this has been provoked by British and American writers of the left. With exploitation at its core, the traditional Marxist model of occupational health depicts workers suffering occupational diseases and work-related injuries through the domineering and profit-maximising policies of their employers.[22] Such accounts fly in the face of more optimistic depictions of the

---

pp. 197–212; R. Johnston and A. McIvor, 'The War and the Body at Work: Occupational Health and Safety in Scottish Industry, 1939–1945', *Journal of Scottish Historical Studies*, vol. 24, no. 2 (2005), pp. 113–36.

19 M. Bufton and J. Melling, '"A Mere Matter of Rock": Organized Labour, Scientific Evidence and British Government Schemes for Compensation of Silicosis and Pneumoconosis among Coalminers, 1926–1940', *Medical History*, vol. 49, no. 2 (April 2005), pp. 155–78; M. Bufton and J. Melling, '"Coming Up for Air": Experts, Employers and Workers in Campaigns to Compensate Silicosis Sufferers in Britain, 1918–39', *Social History of Medicine*, vol. 18, no. 1 (2005), pp. 63–86. See also A. McIvor and R. Johnston, 'Medical Knowledge and the Worker: Occupational Lung Disease in the United Kingdom, c. 1920–1975', *Labor: Studies in the Working Class History of the Americas*, vol. 2, no. 4 (Winter 2005), pp. 46–72.

20 Bartrip, *The Home Office and the Dangerous Trades*, pp. 29–35. See also V. Berridge, *Health and Society in Britain since 1939* (New York, 1999); P. Weindling (ed.), *The Social History of Occupational Health* (London, 1985). See also P. Weindling, *International Health Organisations and Movements, 1918–1939* (Cambridge, 1995); A. McIvor, *A History of Work in Britain* (London, 2001), pp. 111–47; H. Jones, *Health and Society in Twentieth Century Britain* (London, 1994); J. Welshman, *Municipal Medicine: Public Health in Twentieth Century Britain* (Oxford, 2000); J. Lane, *A Social History of Medicine: Health, Healing and Disease in England 1750–1950* (London, 2001); A.S. Wohl, *Endangered Lives: Public Health in Victorian Britain* (London, 1983). The special edition of *Scottish Labour History* (vol. 40, 2005) features recent work on the history of occupational health.

21 B.M. Hutter, *Regulation and Risk: Occupational Health and Safety on the Railways* (Oxford, 2001). For the earlier period, see E. Knox, 'Blood on the Tracks: Railway Employers and Safety in Late-Victorian and Edwardian Britain', *Historical Studies in Industrial Relations*, no. 12 (Autumn 2001).

22 For example, V. Navarro and D. Berman (eds), *Health and Work Under Capitalism: An International Perspective* (Farmington, NY, 1983); C. Gersuny, *Work Hazards and Industrial Conflict* (Hanover, 1981); D. Berman, *Death on the Job: Occupational Health and Safety*

evolution of British industrial capital, and indeed contradict the notion of an upward curve of improvement regarding the successes of workmen's compensation.[23]

One of the most important stimulants to research into the history of occupational health – in the UK and beyond – was the attention devoted to the causes and consequences of the asbestos disaster. The high death toll from what the British Health and Safety Executive classed as the biggest occupational health mistake of the twentieth century inspired research into the history of asbestos from socio-legal perspectives, corporate perspectives, and from the perspective of the workers themselves. Tweedale's seminal *Magic Mineral to Killer Dust* and our own *Lethal Work: A History of the Asbestos Tragedy in Scotland* are two examples of texts which point to corporate negligence and blatant denial, and a prioritisation of profit over workers' health and safety in the face of a growing medical awareness of the dangers of working with one of the world's most dangerous minerals.[24] In contrast, Bartrip's *The Way from Dusty Death* argued that employer awareness of the dangers of working with asbestos was not sufficient to trigger comprehensive action by employers to protect their workers from harm until much later than most commentators have argued. To Bartrip, the asbestos companies did all they reasonably could have been expected to do given the state of knowledge at the time, and he chastises historians who use hindsight to criticise big business and the regulators retrospectively.[25]

The influence of gender on occupational health has also crept into the genre, thanks to the combined efforts of historians and sociologists – with Harrison, Hepler and Messing making important contributions to our understanding of women workers

---

Struggles in the United States (New York 1978); P. Brodeur, *Expendable Americans* (New York, 1974); D. Rosner and G. Markowitz, 'Labor Day and the War on Workers', *American Journal of Public Health*, vol. 89, no. 9 (September 1999), pp. 1,319–21. For an excellent summary from a leftist point of view, see H.K. Abrams, 'A Short History of Occupational Health', *Journal of Public Health Policy*, vol. 22, no. 1 (2001), pp. 34–80.

23 P. Bartrip and S. Burman, *The Wounded Soldiers of Industry: Industrial Compensation Policy* (Oxford, 1983); E.H. Hunt, *British Labour History 1815–1914* (London, 1981).

24 See G. Tweedale, *From Magic Mineral to Killer Dust: Turner and Newall and the Asbestos Hazard*, (Oxford, 1999); Johnston and McIvor, *Lethal Work*; M. Greenberg, 'Knowledge of the Health Hazards of Asbestos Prior to the Merewether and Price Report of 1930, *Social History of Medicine*, 7 (1994), pp. 493–516; D.J. Jeremy, 'Corporate Responses to the Emergent Recognition of a Health Hazard in the UK Asbestos Industry: The Case of Turner and Newall, 1920–1960', *Business and Economic History*, 24 (1995), pp. 254–65; P.W.J. Bartrip, 'Too Little Too Late': The Home Office and the Asbestos Industry Regulations, 1931', *Medical History*, vol. 42 (1998), pp. 421–38; G. Tweedale and P. Hanson, 'Protecting the Workers: The Medical Board and the Asbestos Industry, 1930s–1960s', *Medical History*, vol. 42 (1998), pp. 439–57. For the asbestos disaster in South Africa, see J. McCulloch, *Asbestos Blues: Labour, Capital, Physicians and the State in South Africa* (Oxford, 2002). See also A, Higgison, *Asbestos Politics in the UK: A Critical Examination of Giddens' Thesis* (PhD Thesis, History Department, University of Strathclyde, 2005).

25 This research was partly financed by the asbestos industry; P.W.P. Bartrip, *The Way From Dusty Death: Turner and Newall and the Regulation of Occupational Health in the British Asbestos Industry 1890s–1970* (London, 2001).

and work-related health issues.[26] The impact of gender on occupational health is important in the male-dominated heavy industries too. Masculinity is a concept which has been under-researched, and nowhere is this more evident than in the activities of work and production in the twentieth century. Whilst an increasing body of work addresses this gap, the seminal studies of masculinity by Segal, Connell, and Roper and Tosh all have little to say about the traditional manual workplace, focusing on the family, sexual relations, or on the building blocks of masculinity such as boys' comics, modes of play, education, and within male institutions.[27] Recently, we have developed some reflections on the forging of masculinity in the workplace, explored the role of risk-taking in health behaviour and examined the impact upon masculinity of disability.[28] Throughout our research for this book, and in our previous work on asbestos, we have grown to realise the crucial effect of masculinity on occupational health and safety practices. It could be argued that the generation of men whose lives were ordered by Fordist working conditions spent their health resource on a project of hegemonic masculinity that is now fading with the decline of patriarchy and the advent of the 'new man'. Male-dominated occupations – like coal mining, construction, heavy engineering and shipbuilding – tended to incubate and nurture traditional, hegemonic forms of masculinity. Sociologists have been debating this

---

26 K. Messing, *One Eyed Science: Occupational Health and Women Workers* (Philadelphia, PA, 1998); K. Messing et al., 'Prostitutes and Chimney Sweeps Both Have Problems: Towards Full Integration of Both Sexes in the Study of Occupational Health', *Social Science and Medicine*, vol. 36, no. 1 (1993), pp. 47–55; K. Messing et al., 'Sugar and Spice and Everything Nice: Health Effects of the Sexual Division of Labor Among Train Cleaners', *International Journal of Health Services*, no. 1 (1993), pp. 133–46; Harrison, *Not Only the 'Dangerous Trades'*; B. Harrison, 'Women's Health or Social Control? The Role of the Medical Profession in Relation to Factory Legislation in Late Nineteenth Century Britain', *Sociology of Health and Illness*, vol. 13, no. 4 (1991), pp. 469–91; B. Harrison, 'Some of Them Gets Lead Poisoned: Occupational Lead Exposure in Women, 1880–1914', *The Society for the Social History of Medicine*, vol. 2 (1989), pp. 171–95. See also M. Abendstern, C. Hallett and L. Wade, 'Flouting the Law: Women and the Hazards of Cleaning Moving Machinery in the Cotton Industry, 1930–1970', *Oral History*, vol. 33, no. 2 (Autumn 2005), pp. 69–78.

27 L. Segal, *Slow Motion: Changing Masculinities, Changing Men* (London, 1990); R.W. Connell, *The Men and the Boys* (Oxford, 2000). See also P. Willis, 'Shop Floor Culture, Masculinity and the Wage Form', in J. Clarke, C. Critcher and R. Johnson (eds), *Working Class Culture* (London, 1979); M. Roper, *Masculinity and the British Organization Man Since 1945* (Oxford, 1994); C. Cockburn, *Brothers: Male Dominance and Technological Change* (London, 1983); D. Wight, *Workers not Wasters: Masculinity, Respectability, Consumption and Employment in Central Scotland* (Edinburgh, 1993); R. Evans, *You Questioning My Manhood, Boy? Masculine Identity, Work Performance and Performativity in a Rural Staples Economy*, Arkleton Research Paper no. 4 (University of Aberdeen, 2000). For other partial exceptions, see S. Walby, *Patriarchy at Work* (Oxford, 1986); M. Glucksmann, *Women Assemble* (London, 1990), and Summerfield, *Reconstructing Women's Wartime Lives*.

28 R. Johnston and A. McIvor, 'Dangerous Work, Hard Men and Broken Bodies: Masculinity in the Clydeside Heavy Industries', *Labour History Review*, vol. 69, no. 2 (August 2004), pp. 135–53.

for some time. For example, Cockerman, regarding lifestyles in central Asia, has argued – following Weber – that health lifestyles are 'collective patterns of health related behaviours based on choices from options available to people according to their life chances'.[29] Cockerman has also been utilising the concept of *habitus* as an explanation for health lifestyle behaviour. This implies a certain way of behaving within social groups that is passed on from generation to generation, and through which certain social-cultural practices are maintained and reproduced. A study by Cornwell involving traditional working-class males from the East End of London illustrated how the respondents had a clear conception of the nature and extent of the threats to their health, but saw no point in developing any strategies to counter them. Most worked in traditional male occupations and took the view that because they needed to work, and that the work was inevitably unhealthy, their long-term health was beyond their control.[30] Our miners' study throws up similar stoical acceptance of the inevitability of health risks, as well as substantial collective action to protect the body at work.

Another important theme with which we engage in this book is that surrounding the contested nature of knowledge of diseases and, more centrally, the complexities involved in the process of diseases being classified as occupationally related. The issue of contested knowledge regarding industrial disease is as old as industrialisation itself.[31] Dembe in his *Occupation and Disease* uses three case studies – cumulative trauma disorders of the hands and wrists, back pain, and noise-induced hearing loss – to illustrate the importance of social factors in shaping medical recognition of occupational disorders. For Dembe, Marxist perspectives, medical perspectives, epidemiological perspectives, the perspective of the individual worker, the sociological perspective, and the influence of workers' compensation all need to be factored in to create a comprehensive model regarding the emergence of new occupational diseases.[32] To a significant degree, this holds true regarding the history of dust disease in the coal industry. As far as dust in the mines is concerned, recognition occurred in 1918 with silicosis, 1942 with coal workers' pneumoconiosis, and in 1994 with emphysema and bronchitis. As we will see, such acceptance involved – as Dembe suggests – a complex interplay between medical experts, employers, the state, and the workers and their trade unions.[33]

---

29 W. Cockerman, 'The Sociology of Health Behaviour and Health Lifestyles in Central Asia', in C. Bird et al. (eds), *Handbook of Medical Sociology*, 5th edn (Englewood Cliffs, NJ, 2000); M. Weber, *Economy and Society* (Berkeley, CA, 1978).

30 J. Cornwall, *Hard Earned Lives* (London, 1984).

31 See, for example, Bartrip, *The Home Office and the Dangerous Trades*, *passim*; P.W.J. Bartrip 'Petticoat Pestering': The Women's Trade Union League and Lead Poisoning in the Staffordshire Potteries, 1890–1914', *Historical Studies in Industrial Relations*, no. 2 (September 1996), pp. 3–26.

32 Dembe, *Occupation and Disease*, pp. 3–21 and *passim*.

33 For other examples of the contested nature of occupational disease, see R. Gillespie, 'Accounting for Lead Poisoning: The Medical Politics of Occupational Health', *Social History of Medicine*, vol. 15, no 3 (1990), pp. 303–31; Harrison, *Not Only the Dangerous*

As is the case with the ongoing asbestos tragedy, the high death toll from respiratory diseases in mining can be looked upon as an occupational health disaster. However, this is a disaster which is heavily camouflaged by the incremental nature of the process of death and disablement, and the absence of the headline-grabbing shock of a sudden high death toll. Although coal mining deaths and injuries tend to be associated with mining disasters such as major cave-ins and explosions, in reality there was a constant flow of small accidents which decimated the labour force. We discuss this in some depth in the next chapter. Allen has summed this process up in this way:

> When the deaths and the injuries are spread out over the weeks and months and are scattered among the collieries in various coal-fields they tend to be ignored. It is only when there is a disaster that people suddenly become aware of the hazardous nature of mining, and even then it becomes a ten day wonder until the next time. [34]

Like all accidents and disasters, though, the question of blame is one that cannot be ignored. Interestingly, in the 1930s a study of 'accident proneness' in the British coal industry showed wide variations across the coal fields – South Wales and Kent having the highest level of accidents, and Scotland recording the lowest.[35] Some commentators have noted that industrial accidents and disasters are socially constructed, and some have argued convincingly that in many cases catastrophes, such as Piper Alpha and Bhopal, should be seen more as the consequences of a chain of corporate irresponsibility than 'accidents' in the blameless sense of the word. Indeed, speaking about the UK situation, Nichols argues that the term 'industrial injury' is more appropriate than 'industrial accident'[36] Dwyer has also looked at this in some depth in his *Life and Death at Work: Industrial Accidents as a Case of Socially Produced Error* (1991), and suggests that sociological theory regarding work accidents can be reduced to four simple hypotheses:

1. Social relations of work produce industrial accidents.
2. The greater weight of a level of social relations in the management of workers' relationships to the dangers of their jobs, the greater the proportion of accidents produced at that level.

Trades; Bartrip, *The Home Office and the Dangerous Trades*. See also P. Bellaby, *Sick from Work: The Body in Employment* (Aldershot, 1999).

34 V.L. Allen, *The Militancy of British Miners* (Shipley, 1981), p. 92.

35 W.H. Scott, *Coal and Conflict: A Study of Industrial Relations at Collieries* (Liverpool, 1963), p. 153.

36 See T. Nichols, *The Sociology of Industrial Injury*, Part 1, *passim*; J. Foster and C. Woolfson, *Paying For the Piper: Capital and Labour in Britain's Offshore Oil Industry* (London, 1997); P. Shrivastava, *Bhopal: Anatomy of a Crisis* (London, 1992); R. Cooter and B. Luckin (eds), *Accidents in History: Injuries, Fatalities and Social Relations* (Amsterdam, 1997).

3. The greater the degree of auto-control by workers at a level, the lower the proportion of accidents produced at a level the worker seeks to control.
4. The greater the degree of managerial safety management at a level, the lower the proportion of accidents produced at the level the management seeks to control. [37]

In short, then, what is being suggested here is that the more control over the workplace workers have, the safer their working environment will be, and the fact that modern trade unionised workplaces are statistically safer than non-trade unionised workplaces bears this out.[38]

What needs to be examined, though, is the fact that by the 1920s the coal mining workforce was 90% unionised, but miners worked in the most dangerous of workplaces. Moreover, although this might be a valid set of hypotheses regarding safety at work in some workplaces, the situation becomes even more complex in relation to the longer-term consequences regarding working in unhealthy work processes. The British Health and Safety Executive (HSE) admitted in the 1990s that it had placed too much priority on the immediacy of work safety and not enough on protecting workers' health. Moreover, several of our oral history interviews of men who had been exposed to asbestos clearly illustrated that in many cases workers ignored – or rationalised – the longer-term health risks for the sake of economic factors.[39]

The notion of acceptance of risk, then, is a very important one, and ties in with sociological arguments from the early 1990s regarding risk in modern society. Beck, for example, argued that it was not class struggle which provided the motor of history, but the unintended consequences of industrialism, including large-scale industrial disaster.[40] Within the resultant risk culture there is constant instability and uncertainty, with people's definition of risk being influenced by complex social and cultural factors.[41] Several sociologists also suggest that risks are experienced

---

37 T. Dwyer, *Life and Death at Work, Industrial Accidents as a Case of Socially Produced Error* (New York, 1991), p. 150. This text provides an excellent international comparative historical survey of society and occupational safety.

38 R. O'Neil, 'When it Comes to Health and Safety, Your Life Should be in Union Hands', Labour Education, 2002/1, issue no. 126, ILO Bureau for Workers' Activities. http://www.ilo.org/public/english/dialogue/actrav/new/april28/index/htm; D. Walters, 'Trade Unions and the Effectiveness of Worker Representation in Health and Safety in Britain', *International Journal of Health Services*, vol. 25 (1996), pp. 625–41; A.I. Gordon and R.T. Booth, 'Workers' Participation in Occupational Health and Safety in Britain', *International Labour Review*, vol. 121, no. 4 (July–August 1982), pp. 121–87; A.J.P. Dalton, 'Lessons from the United Kingdom: Fightback on Workplace Hazards, 1979–1992', *International Journal of Health Services*, vol. 22, no. 3 (1992), pp. 489–95.

39 Johnston and McIvor, *Lethal Work, passim.*

40 E. Beck, *Risk Society: Towards a New Modernity* (London, 1992), *passim.*

41 See, for example, J. Cornwall, *Hard Earned Lives* (London, 1984); J. Zinn, 'The Biographical Approach: A Better Way to Understand Behaviour in Health and Illness', *Health*

and assessed individually rather than collectively – which ties in with Beck's highlighting of a process of individualisation within society.[42] A crucial element, then, is the social context in which risks are perceived and understood, with some people being aware of the negative health consequences of their risky behaviour but preferring to prioritise other concerns.[43] We would argue that although an individual approach to risk may be important in some working environments, our study of the way in which coal miners approach the hazards of coal dust suggests that in close-knit working communities a collective acceptance of and response to risk is as important. This notion is supported by Bloor's recent work on South Wales mining communities, in which he illustrates the importance of miners' collectivist approaches to occupational safety in the 1900–1947 period. This process of miners securing control of vital areas of pit safety – which Bloor refers to as *conscientization* – led to significant improvements in their working environment, including the introduction of workmen's inspectors in 1911 to police safety in the mines.[44]

This leads us on to the notion of lay knowledge of occupational health, in which workers are frequently aware of the health hazards of their working environments. Once again it is sociologists who have done most of the work regarding this, and there is a general consensus that lay epidemiology plays an important role in how people make sense of health risks, and how they make decisions based on professional knowledge.[45] Workers do not make choices regarding risky work based solely on decisions made for them by medical professionals. Therefore, although the dynamic of contested professional medical knowledge in relation to miners' respiratory diseases is illustrated throughout this book, we also hope to highlight – through our oral history interviews – the importance of lay knowledge regarding industrial hazards in the productionist environment of twentieth-century British coal mining.

We also examine in some depth the involvement of the miners' trade unions with occupational health and safety. This is another area of occupational health history which needs to be given more attention. Once again, it is American scholars who have been more to the fore regarding the important interaction of trade unions and workers' health.[46] Some historians have argued that trade unions in the UK

Risk and Society, vol. 7 (2005), pp. 1–9.

    42 A. Furlong and F. Cartmel, *Young People and Social Change: Individualism and Risk in Late Modernity* (Buckingham, 1997); Beck, *Risk Society*.

    43 J. Cornwall, *Hard Earned Lives* (London, 1984).

    44 M. Bloor, 'No Longer Dying for a Living: Collective Responses to Injury Risks in South Wales Mining Communities, 1900–47', *Sociology*, vol. 36, no. 1 (2002), pp. 89–105.

    45 C. Davidson et al., 'Lay Epidemiology and the Prevention Paradox: the Implication of Coronary Candidacy for Health Education', *Sociology of Health and Illness*, vol. 13 (1991), pp. 1–19; G. Williams and J. Popay, 'Lay Knowledge and the Privilege of Experience', in J. Gabe (ed.), *Challenging Medicine* (Oxford, 1994); P. Brown, 'Popular Epidemiology, Toxic Waste and Social Movements', in J. Gabe (ed.), *Medicine, Health and Risk: Sociological Approaches* (Oxford, 1987).

    46 See, for example, A. Derickson, *Workers' Health, Workers' Democracy: The Western Miners' Struggle, 1981–1925* (London, 1988); A. Derickson, 'Part of the Yellow Dog: US

marginalised health and safety for the sake of increased wages, and that they failed as a countervailing force.[47] However, although this is countered to some degree by the work of industrial relations writers on the modern workplace, we still await a comprehensive historical study of trade unions and health and safety. Recent studies – of coal mining in South Wales in the first half of the twentieth century by Bloor and Melling and Bufton, and of cotton workers' unions and byssinosis by Bowden and Tweedale – suggest that the 'orthodox' negative portrayal of the trade unions and occupational health needs to be revised.[48] We also argued for a more complex relationship and mixed picture in our study of the trade unions and the asbestos tragedy.[49] In these reappraisals, the unions emerge as much more proactive and progressive in their occupational health strategies.

Workers' Health in UK Mining History

The history of British coal mining has been extensively researched, with the three in-depth studies by Church, Supple and Ashworth standing out as high-calibre examples of work taking in the wide chronological sweep of the industry from early industrialisation to decline.[50] The history of the industry in Scotland – although also covered by Church, Supple and Ashworth – is given particularly close attention, notably by Campbell in his two-volume study *The Scottish Miners 1874–1939* and *The Lanarkshire Miners: A Social History of their Trade Unions 1775–1874*. South Wales has also attracted much attention from historians, not least in the work of Francis and Smith, and Williams.[51] However, despite the extent of historical research on the industry, very little has been done regarding the history of occupational health and safety in British coal mining. Again, this is in contrast to the situation in the USA,

---

Coal Miners' Opposition to the Company Doctor System, 1936–1946', *International Journal of Health Services*, vol. 19 (1989), pp. 709–20; P. Landsbergis and J. Cahill, 'Labor Union Programs to Reduce or Prevent Occupational Stress in the United States', *International Journal of Health Services*, vol. 24, no. 1 (1994), pp. 105–29.

47 Bartrip, *The Home Office and the Dangerous Trades*; J. Melling, 'The Risks of Working Versus the Risks of Not Working: Trade Unions, Employers and Responses to the Risk of Occupational Illness in British Industry, c. 1890–1940s', ESRC Centre for Analysis of Risk and Regulation, Discussion Paper no. 12 (December 2003); Tweedale, *From Magic Mineral to Killer Dust*.

48 Bloor, 'The South Wales Miners' Federation'; Bufton and Melling, 'Coming Up for Air'; Bowden and Tweedale, 'Mondays without Dread'.

49 Johnston and McIvor, *Lethal Work*.

50 R. Church, *The History of the British Coal Industry, Volume 3: 1830–1913* (Oxford, 1986) p. 758.

51 H. Francis and D. Smith, *The Fed: A History of the South Wales Miners in the Twentieth Century* (London, 1980); C. Williams, *Capitalism, Community and Conflict: The South Wales Coalfield 1898–1947* (Cardiff, 1998).

where Derickson and other scholars have subjected the topic to close analysis.[52] The subject of silicosis has also been given some attention by American scholars too, in particular by Rosner and Markowitz in their *Deadly Dust* (1994).

Granted, the general histories of British coal mining give health and safety some coverage. Church, for example, in his *History of the British Coal Industry* has a 17-page section on 'Occupational Mortality and Health', while for the twentieth century Ashworth devotes 14 pages in his 700-plus-page text.[53] Interestingly (and tellingly), although the NCB's in-house publication *A Short History of the Scottish Coal-Mining Industry*, published in 1958, has a chapter on 'Mining Hazards and the Development of Safety Precautions', the short sub-section on the dangers of mine dust refers only to the hazard of dust explosions. This to some degree reflects the late acknowledgement of the dangers of respirable dust in the Scottish coal fields.[54] Benson's *British Coalminers in the Nineteenth Century* dedicates eight pages to the dangers miners faced at their work, including the hazards of dust inhalation.[55] For more detailed information regarding the work–health interaction in the pits, and especially for the impact of mining on long-term health, we really have to depend upon specialised accounts (usually written by medical experts or regulators), such as Bryan's *The Evolution of Health and Safety in Mines* and Rogan's *Medicine in the Mining Industries* – the former by a one-time Chief Inspector of Mines, and the latter from a long-serving Chief Medical Officer of the NCB.[56] These detailed accounts, although useful for the historian of occupational health, are nevertheless rather unilinear, 'insider' or 'participant' narratives, tending to focus upon depicting the upward curve of progress in their respective fields.

The reluctance of miners' trade unions to take industrial action over dangerous and unhealthy working conditions is reflected in the almost invisibility of the topic in labour history and trade union history texts. This seeming disinclination for unions to get involved with health and safety at work fits into an acceptance by some scholars that this was something which unions just did not prioritise. Dwyer,

---

52 A. Derickson, *Black Lung: Anatomy of a Public Health Disaster* (Ithaca, NY, 1998); B.M. Judkins, *We Offer Ourselves as Evidence: Toward Workers' Control of Occupational Health* (New York, 1986); B.E. Smith, *Digging Our Own Graves: Coal Miners and the Struggle Over Black Lung Disease* (Philadelphia, PA, 1987); A.F.C. Wallace, *St Clair: A Nineteenth Century Coal Town's Experience with a Disaster-prone Industry* (Ithaca, NY, 1987); for silicosis, see D. Rosner and G. Markowitz, *Deadly Dust: Silicosis and the Politics of Occupational Disease in Twentieth-century America* (Princeton, NJ, 1994).

53 Church, *History of the British Coal Industry, Volume 3*, pp. 582–99; W. Ashworth, *The History of the British Coal Industry, Volume 5: 1946–1982, The Nationalised Industry*, (Oxford, 1986), pp. 558–72; B. Supple, *History of the British Coal Industry: The Political Economy of Decline*, vol. 4 (Oxford, 1987).

54 NCB, *A Short History of the Scottish Coal-mining Industry* (London, 1958), pp. 89–101.

55 J. Benson, *British Coalminers in the Nineteenth Century: A Social History* (London, 1980), pp. 39–48.

56 J.M. Rogan, *Medicine in the Mining Industries* (London, 1972).

for example, for the late twentieth century, suggests that trade unions' integration with state and employer interests can be blamed for this. According to Dwyer, the trade unions' unwillingness to give a high priority to workplace safety and health issues was linked to their bureaucratisation, their acceptance of employer and state models of safety, the effectiveness of compensation, and the embourgeoisement of workers.[57] Certainly, the activities of the miners' trade unions regarding health and safety is hardly considered in some key texts. Most significantly, Taylor's recent monographs on the history of the National Union of Miners (NUM) makes virtually no mention of health and safety in the mines in general, least of all the problem of dust disease.[58] This is also the case with Campbell's two volumes on *The Scottish Miners* and his *Lanarkshire Miners*, whilst McCormack's *Industrial Relations in the Coal Industry* gives scant attention to occupational health too.[59] Allen's *The Militancy of British Miners*, on the other hand, acknowledges the centrality of the harsh working environment in mining, and examines the pneumoconiosis issue in some depth – he also highlights the significance of medical and health facilities as well as the miners' demands for retirement at aged 60.[60]

Although minimising the input of the trade unions, some exploration of occupational health in coal mining has been undertaken by scholars of labour relations, although again, the coverage is patchy. Page Arnot's classics *The Miners in Crisis and War: A History of the Miners' Federation of Great Britain from 1930* (1961) and *The Miners: Years of Struggle. A History of the Miners' Federation of Great Britain from 1910* (1953) have little to say about health and safety.[61] The same can be said of G.D.H. Cole's *Labour in the Coalmining Industry (1914–1921)*.[62] However, in contrast, Francis and Smith's *The Fed: A History of South Wales Miners in the Twentieth Century* devotes some attention to pneumoconiosis, dust suppression and attempts by medical science to deal with the dust problem – primarily because South Wales was the epicentre of coal dust disease for some time.[63] Whilst dust was a recurring motif in some miners' autobiographies and other qualitative testimony such as by Coombes and Orwell, it has not been a central concern of historians to analyse systematically the history of dust disease in mining, despite this being the

---

57 Dwyer, *Life and Death at Work*, pp. 72–7.

58 A. Taylor, *The NUM and British Politics, Volume 1: 1944–1968* (Aldershot, 2003); A. Taylor, *The NUM and British Politics, Volume 2: 1969–1995* (Aldershot, 2005).

59 A. Campbell, *The Scottish Miners 1874–1939* (Aldershot, 2000); A. Campbell, *The Lanarkshire Miners* (Edinburgh, 1979); B.J. McCormack, *Industrial Relations in the Coal Industry* (London 1979). The same is true for A. Campbell et al. (eds), *Miners, Unions and Politics 1910–1947* (Aldershot, 1996).

60 Allen, *The Militancy of British Miners*, pp. 92–100 and 291–300.

61 R. Page Arnot, *The Miners in Crisis and War: A History of the Miners' Federation of Great Britain from 1930 Onwards* (London, 1961); R. Page Arnot, *The Miners: Years of Struggle – A History of the Miners' Federation of Great Britain (from 1910 Onwards)* (London, 1953); Francis and Smith, *The Fed*; Campbell, *Miners, Unions and Politics*.

62 G.D.H. Cole, *Labour in the Coal Mining Industry, 1914–1921* (Oxford, 1923).

63 Francis and Smith, *The Fed*, pp. 424–94.

most deadly occupational tragedy in the UK of the twentieth century.[64] Important contributions have been made, however, by Melling and Bufton on silicosis before the Second World War, Mills' research on metal miners in the nineteenth century, and Perchard's study of mine management and dust in Scotland.[65]

Clearly, therefore, there are significant gaps in the historiography of occupational health in the UK in general, and specifically regarding the history of health and safety in the British mining industry. Our emphasis is focused on the history of miners' respiratory diseases, therefore we anticipate that our book will go some way towards plugging an important gap in what is still a fairly marginalised field. However, as we also hope to illustrate, although respiratory health may appear a narrow area of historical investigation, our study of miners' lung illuminates several important aspects of labour history, including industrial relations and workplace dynamics, social history (including masculinity and the impact of disease on communities) and medical history, notably the contested nature of professional and lay knowledge. We also hope that our study will contribute to the growing reputation of oral history as a methodology in the social history of work and health, and may encourage other researchers to integrate this into their research projects.

---

64 Coombes, *These Poor Hands*; G. Orwell, *The Road to Wigan Pier* (London, 1937).

65 Bufton and Melling, 'Coming Up for Air'; Melling and Bufton, 'A Mere Matter of Rock'; C. Mills, 'A Hazardous Bargain: Occupational Risk in Cornish Mining, 1875–1914', *Labour History Review*, vol. 70, no. 1 (April 2005), pp. 53–73; C. Mills, 'The Kinnaird Commission: Siliceous Dust, the Pitfalls of Cause and Effect Correlations and the Case of the Cornish Miners in the Mid-nineteenth Century', *Scottish Labour History*, vol. 40 (2005), pp. 13–30; A. Perchard, 'The Mine Management Professions and the Dust Problem in the Scottish Coal Mining Industry, c 1930–1966', *Scottish Labour History*, vol. 40 (2005), pp. 13–31. Other aspects of the dust problem outside of mining have also recently been explored, including S. Morrison, 'The Factory Inspectorate and the Silica Dust Problem in UK Foundries, 1930–1970', *Scottish Labour History*, vol. 40 (2005), pp. 31–50; A. Higgison, 'Asbestos and the Trade Unions, 1960s and 1970s', *Scottish Labour History*, vol. 40 (2005), pp. 70–86; D. Walker, '"Working in it, through it and among it every day": Chrome dust at J. & J. White of Rutherglen, 1893–1967', *Scottish Labour History*, vol. 40 (2005), pp. 50–69.

Chapter 2

Work and the Body in Coal Mining

As we noted in Chapter 1, recent studies of employment and social relations in British coal mining have shown this industry to be much more diverse than one might suppose. Within this complex employment structure, the labour processes and environment in which miners worked impacted upon their bodies in a wide variety of ways. Essentially, though, work in the pits reflected the multi-faceted nature of all paid labour, having positive, life-enhancing features as well as negative, health threatening and vitality-sapping characteristics. Whilst young miners frequently exemplified the apogee of fit, sturdy manhood, the heavy toll that mining exacted upon the body could be witnessed in the large numbers of disabled older miners and in the graveyards of many pit communities. British miners toiled in an extremely hazardous workplace in the nineteenth and the twentieth centuries in one of the most dangerous and unhealthy of all occupations in Britain. However, as we noted in the previous chapter, whilst a considerable amount has been written on industrial relations in coal mining, the relationship between occupation and health, well-being and the body has attracted surprisingly little attention from historians. In this chapter, we contextualise our investigation of lung disease in the pits, commenting on the economic and social background, the nature of mining employment, mining labour processes and how they changed over time, and the impact that work (and its changing nature) had upon health – in terms of both trauma and chronic disease – including the extent of the miners' respiratory health problems.

Working in Coal Mining

The British coal industry expanded rapidly through the nineteenth century as industrialisation gathered pace. As Table 2.1 indicates, by the First World War numbers employed had swelled to well over one million, located in over three thousand pits scattered across ten major coal fields up and down the country.[1] The industry reached its historic peak during the second decade of the twentieth century, then contracted sharply. However, in the early 1950s there were still 700,000 employed in coal mining in what remained an extremely labour-intensive industry. Employment

---

1   N.K. Buxton, *The Economic Development of the British Coal Industry* (London, 1978), p. 166. There were 3,179 mines in operation in 1913.

dropped sharply thereafter, and deep coal mining had virtually disappeared in Britain by the 1990s.

Table 2.1   Coal output and numbers employed, 1850–2000

	Output (millions)*	No. employed
1850/55	68.4	218,230
1880/85	156.4	458,600
1900/05	227.4	778,700
1920	229.5	1,248,000
1947	200.0	703,900
1960	193.6	602,100
1980	126.6	229,800
2000	Unknown	8,405

Notes: * tons to 1946; tonnes thereafter; average output per annum over 1850–55; 1880–85 and 1900–1905.

Sources: R. Church, *The History of the British Coal Industry, Volume 3. 1830–1913* (Oxford, 1986), pp. 3, 189; B. Supple, *The History of the British Coal Industry, Volume 4. 1913–1946: The Political Economy of Decline* (Oxford, 1987), p. 119; W. Ashworth, *The History of the British Coal Industry, Volume 5. 1946–1982: The Nationalised Industry* (Oxford, 1986), pp. 672–80; M.P. Jackson, *The Price of Coal* (London, 1974), pp. 190, 194; Health and Safety Executive figures for 2000 from http://www.hse.gov.uk/mining/accident /index.htm.

Britain's miners were a heterogeneous group, scattered throughout the country, mostly located in isolated mining towns and villages across a series of coal fields, each of which developed its own distinctive pattern of employment, unique labour customs and work culture. Table 2.2 gives a sense of the relative importance of the main coal fields and the spatial distribution of the mining workforce on the eve of the First World War.

The coal mining labour force included those who worked below ground and those who worked on the surface. Above ground were those responsible for screening, grading and cleaning the coal in preparation for transport from the pit head to customers. They included many older miners who were too unfit and physically incapable of working underground, up to the Second World War, in some districts (such as South Wales, Lancashire and East Scotland), these included several thousand female workers (women working underground had been banned by legislation in 1842).[2] Howard Jones, who worked on the surface of a South Wales pit as a young miner from 1937 to 1942, recalled:

---

2   See A. John, *By the Sweat of their Brow* (London, 1984), pp. 69–93, for a discussion of the work of women at the surface of coal mines.

On the screens I would estimate there was about the best part of two dozen youngsters. One or two older men. For instance, there was one man picking next to me who was eh in my, well as a youngster I thought he was very very old and shouldn't have been working … If a man had an accident and he came back, he would be compensated then under Workmen's Compensation Act, and they were subject to examination by the company doctor, and if the doctor said he was fit for light work then they didn't have to pay comp' he had to come back to work in a suitable light job, and picking stones was considered to be a suitable light job … It was just throwing stones off all day. Very, very tedious job.[3]

Table 2.2   Numbers employed in coal mining by region, 1913

South Wales	233,100
North East	226,800
Yorkshire	161,200
North Midlands	130,500
Lancs. and Cheshire	109,000
West Scotland	79,100
East Scotland	68,500
West Midlands	66,800
North Wales	15,900
South West	15,500
Cumberland	11,000
Kent	1,100
N. Ireland	800
Total GB	**1,127,900**

Source: J. Benson, *British Coalminers in the Nineteenth Century* (London, 1980), p. 217.

A miner who had worked at the Auchengeigh pit in Lanarkshire recalled the intensity of the work at the surface:

My first experiences of the pit was the pit across there, Auchengeigh. That was my pit. And I started there when I was just coming up for 16. I worked in the pit head and it was really hard work separating dirt and coal and breaking dirt up and stuff like that. It was hard, hard work.[4]

Surface workers also included the pivotal winding-enginemen and various grades of craftsmen essential for colliery operations, such as working the engine(s), building and equipment maintenance, such as blacksmiths, wheelwrights, masons, joiners,

---

3   Howard Jones, Interview C25 (SOHC).
4   Carl Martin, Interview C8 (SOHC).

fitters, bricklayers, and storemen and labourers. Many of the larger collieries had an office, with clerical and managerial staff, and later, the colliery medical centres and the pithead baths also required personnel. On average, around 20–25% of the total mining labour force was employed above ground (see Table 2.3), though this proportion varied somewhat across the different coal fields and its composition changed considerably over time.

Table 2.3   Mining workforce, 1945

	Collieries	*Employees underground*	*Employees above ground*
Scotland	384	63,591	20,901
Northumberland and Cumberland	117	33,833	11,797
Durham	227	82,084	23,249
Yorkshire	220	106,246	29,086
North Midlands	170	75,083	25,733
North West	141	44,184	15,395
Cardiff	255	64,223	15,532
Swansea	167	29,091	8,242
Midland and Southern	205	49,716	17,843
Total	**1,886**	**548,051**	**167,778**

Source: W. Taylor, *The Forgotten Conscript: A History of the Bevin Boy* (Durham, 1995), pp. 117–20; see also *Report of Chief Inspector of Mines for Years 1939–46* (London, 1948), p. 5.

Underground work comprised three main operations: hewing, haulage, and development and maintenance. In the hand-getting, pre-mechanisation era, the hewing of coal was widely regarded as the most physically difficult and exhausting job. Various techniques prevailed at different pits and coal fields, depending upon a range of factors, including the geology of the rock and coal deposits, the size of the seam (which could range from 40 cm to 500 cm and beyond) and the type of coal being worked (ranging from 'soft' bituminous to 'hard' anthracite coal). However, invariably the coal had initially to be undercut, or 'holed', with the miner frequently working lying down on his side, or on his knees using a pick to dig a thin but deep cut at the bottom of the seam, through or underneath the coal or rock, perhaps to a depth of 100–800 cm. This could necessitate working right underneath the seam in a hole barely 150–200 cm in height. In the latter case, small wooden props would be used to support the coal while the miner lay underneath the seam, 'bottom-holing'. Once the miner judged he had cut in far enough, he would proceed to remove his props and rip down the coal above the undercut, using a combination of pick and wedge, supplemented, increasingly as the nineteenth century wore on, with explosives, or 'shots', drilled into the seam. The ownership of tools marked the hewer as an independent artisan. A South Wales miner, Bert Coombes, commented about a hewer he worked with:

> John had a pile of tools, and they were all needed. Shovels, mandrils of different sizes, prising bars, hatchet, powder-tin and coal boxes, boring machine and drills and several other things. He valued them at eight pounds' worth, and he was forced to buy them himself ... Nearly every week he had to buy a new handle of some sort and fit it into the tool at his home, so that his wages were not all clear benefit, and his work was not always finished when he left the colliery.[5]

The loosened coal would be loaded onto tubs for transportation from the working face to the pit shaft and thence to the surface. These operations – especially hewing, ripping and shot-firing – inevitably generated considerable quantities of dust and dirt.

Haulage workers ('putters' and 'drawers') were usually responsible for the transportation of coal from the face to the surface, using a combination of muscle power, horse-drawn and mechanical haulage. They were usually a separate category of workers, lesser paid and lacking the status of the hewers within the coal mining occupational hierarchy. However, in some coal fields (such as South Wales) hewers also did some haulage and maintenance work (such as propping) and there was less of a distinctive division of labour. Other work undertaken underground included development, maintenance and 'servicing' operations (for example, transporting materials such as wooden props). Tunnelling was fundamental to pit operations, to access the coal and to transport it to the surface. Tunnels and roadways had to be constantly driven, invariably through rock (known as cutting 'headings'), which once created, had to be maintained. Specialist teams of workers usually did this job. This is how a worker employed by the German sub-contracting firm Tison described this work in the South Wales pits in the 1950s and 1960s:

> You were putting the arches up, you were sheeting, packing tight, making sure that everything was packed tight because of the squeeze and then you carry on again putting the roads down behind you and you'd have belt men then extending the belt on, that you didn't travel far with the enco but you used to have the deputy then to charge holes. He'd be there to charge, make sure that he was in charge of the powder and the 'dets'. You couldn't handle them, he was handling them, and that's what it's like, you know. You used to come in then on the weekends to extend the water pipes, the blast pipes, the air pipes ... There was a team, four men in a heading you see ... you were boring, you had the borers, on legs they were. There were three men boring and they would bore a pattern of holes and you would charge it up and you would put nought to blow the first bit out; you had numbers on your 'dets' and you used to bore them so far apart that you'd make sure

---

5   Bert Coombes, *These Poor Hands: The Autobiography of a Miner Working in South Wales* (London, 1939), p. 38.

that you'd bring it all out, you were firing about eight feet out at a time like, you know, forward eight feet at a time.[6]

The roofs of roadways and the working coal face also had to be supported (propped) to prevent collapse. Larger pits also had coal storage areas and stables for the horses underground which had to be maintained. All these complex operations were planned, co-ordinated and controlled by a small army of managerial and supervisory staff, assisted by the mine professionals – mechanical and electrical engineers, geologists, chemists and the like. The hierarchy of control in the private ownership era depended upon the scale of the enterprise. In the larger collieries, power flowed downwards from the colliery owner to the pit manager, and hence to the workplace, where sub-contractors, overmen, leading hands, the deputies (responsible for statutory safety regulations underground) and firemen (responsible for approving atmospheric conditions underground) all performed some supervisory functions. Such managerial and supervisory employees have tended to be neglected in mining historiography, though work in this area is growing.[7]

What is important to emphasise, however, is that the labour process and the work environment varied considerably from coal field to coal field and from pit to pit. The geological conditions, seam width and distance from shaft to working place (which could be as far away as 8 km in the largest pits) fundamentally affected hewers' ability to win the coal, and hence their workloads. The long walk from shaft to the face meant that miners had to be physically fit. As Walter Greenwood put it in the 1930s: 'An athlete in the prime of condition might easily find himself unable to walk those miles.'[8] Hewers' wages were almost universally determined by the amount of coal they produced, and this was a primary reason why there was so much conflict between management and the men over the working of so-called 'abnormal places' where it was difficult to make a decent wage. Temperature, air quality (ventilation), dampness and levels of illumination were other important factors which impinged upon the labour process, the body and capacity to work. Some pits were notoriously wet. The wife of a South Wales miner recalled: 'he used to come home *soaking wet*, this is before the baths were built and we were always drying clothes in front of the fire you know; soaking wet they'd be, as if he'd been out in the rain (laughs)'.[9] Other pits (especially the deep pits) were unbearably hot. Pits sunk to a depth of 1,000 feet were not unusual by the twentieth century, and here temperatures at the coal face could reach up to 30° Centigrade on a normal warm day in the summer months. Given this diversity of experience, and the ever-changing physical conditions of

---

6   Malcolm Davies, Interview C29 (SOHC).

7   See J. Melling, 'Safety, supervision and the politics of productivity in the British coalmining industry, 1900–1960', in J. Melling and A. McKinlay (eds), *Management, Labour and Industrial Politics in Modern Europe* (Cheltenham, 1996), pp. 145–73; A. Perchard, 'The Mine Management Professions in the Scottish Coal Industry, 1930–1966' (PhD Thesis, University of Strathclyde, 2005).

8   W. Greenwood, *How the Other Man Lives* (1939), p. 31.

9   Anonymous, Interview C34 (SOHC).

many pits, traditionally hewers were left with a great deal of autonomy and discretion at the point of production.[10]

The nature of mining work changed radically with mechanisation and associated alterations in coal-getting and transporting techniques in the late nineteenth and the twentieth centuries. The main changes were the shift from bord and pillar (sometimes called 'room and stoop' or 'pillar and stall') to longwall methods of coal extraction, the application of mechanical power to hewing, drilling and tunnelling, haulage mechanisation with conveyor-belt coal transportation systems, integrated 'power-loading' coal face machinery, power-driven moving hydraulic props, and improved lighting and ventilation methods, not least with electrification of the pits. These developments have been explored in depth by other scholars, but a brief summary of the key changes is crucial here to contextualise our analysis of the respiratory diseases of coal miners.

In the nineteenth century, a common method of extracting coal was to work through a seam leaving pillars of coal to support the roof. Once the seam was worked through, the miners would work back, extracting the mineral from all or most of the pillars. This bord and pillar method was superseded by the longwall technique, whereby a length of seam (perhaps 100 yards) was worked simultaneously by a team of miners, with the roof supported by wooden props as they went along (and allowed to collapse behind them). By the 1940s, 75% of the coal seams being worked in the UK were longwall.[11] Bord and pillar working persisted, though, especially in irregular and thin seams, in parts of the North East coal field, and the western part of the South Wales coal field, until well into the second half of the twentieth century.

The mechanisation of coal production was a long, uneven and incremental process. The first machines designed to undercut the coal were developed in the middle of the nineteenth century. They were powered by compressed air which drove a toothed chain cutter rotating around an arm, or a disc cutter (similar to a circular saw) that could be directed against the bottom of the seam. These machines were developed and adapted to electricity. However, their diffusion was relatively slow in most coal fields before the inter-war years. In 1925, just 20% of all the coal produced in the UK was undercut mechanically.[12] Scotland was rather exceptional in the more rapid pace of technological diffusion, with over 50% of its total output of coal cut mechanically by the mid-1920s.[13] At the same time, coal transportation methods underground were changing, with coal wagons running on rail systems being replaced by power-driven conveyor belts taking the newly cut coal from the face to the main roadways. By 1920, 38% of all coal produced was being conveyed mechanically. These systems spread rapidly in the inter-war years, and by 1945

10 See, for example, A. Campbell, *The Scottish Miners, 1874–1939, Volume 1. Industry, Work and Community* (Aldershot, 2000), pp. 73–108.

11 W. Ashworth, *The History of the British Coal Industry, Volume 5. 1946–1982: The Nationalised Industry* (Oxford, 1986), p. 72.

12 Buxton, *The Economic Development of the British Coal Industry*, p. 179.

13 Campbell, *The Scottish Miners, 1874–1939*, vol. 1, pp. 109–113.

just over 70% of all coal produced in Britain was being undercut and conveyed by mechanical means.[14] However, there remained massive differences in levels of mechanisation between different coal fields. In 1939, when 61% of British coal was cut mechanically, the proportions were 92% in Northumberland, 80% in Scotland, 43% in Durham and only 26% in South Wales.[15] Other important developments were the application of mechanical power to drilling – replacing hand-drilling of rock and coal strata (for shot firing), and the development of hydraulic picks – which were widely used in some seams, for example in South Wales. These innovations increased coal output considerably, and enabled the working of deeper, thinner and more inaccessible seams. However, the pace of diffusion remained uneven, and there continued to be many seams deemed unsuitable for mechanisation. Thus, well into the second half of the twentieth century there co-existed a 'modernised' and 'traditional' coal mining sector. As late as 1951, around a third of all coal hewers in the UK were still producing coal using the hand-held pick.[16]

Concurrent with changes at the coal face and in transporting the product were other important innovations in the industry. Development work was also revolutionised with new technology, particularly the application of power to drilling and tunnelling techniques. Gradually, large-scale electrically-driven heading machines capable of shearing through solid rock at high speeds replaced the traditional tunnelling and road-building methods based upon hand-drilling bore holes and the use of controlled explosions. The dark and dirty mine environment was also transformed with the construction of larger roadways and, crucially, with more sophisticated and more powerful electric fan-driven ventilation systems (replacing the older furnace-driven systems) and the extension of underground electric lighting to the main roadways underground. The improvements in ventilation methods meant that better-quality air could be circulated more effectively around even the largest of mines, hence reducing the risk of a methane-ignition explosion. This became a key area of mining operations regulated by the state (stung into action by public outrage after major mine explosions), and this was one reason why the South Wales anthracite mines had such an acute problem with respiratory disease compared to other coal fields. Because there was only a negligible methane risk in the anthracite pits, they tended to be much more poorly ventilated than the norm. Getting the ventilation engineering right was later shown to be critical in the causation and control of pneumoconiosis. The increase in air current velocity could have adverse effects in that dust generated at the coal face could be carried further and expose more mine workers to inhaling contaminated air, especially along what was known as the return end (along the flow of the ventilation air current, beyond the face). Miners working on the intake side usually experienced much purer air quality. We also discuss in Chapter 6 how the air current could be used to diffuse and remove harmful dust.

----

14 Ashworth, *The History of the British Coal Industry*, vol. 5, p. 75.

15 B. Supple, *The History of the British Coal Industry, Volume 4. 1913–1946: The Political Economy of Decline* (Oxford, 1987), pp. 31, 382–3.

16 Supple, *The History of the British Coal Industry*, vol. 4, pp. 437–8.

Another development which impacted very favourably upon the work conditions of miners was the extension of underground transport (for example, by electric or diesel locomotive) to get the miners from the shaft to the face, hence saving the long, arduous walk (often up significant inclines) which was typical of the early twentieth-century miners' experience. Above ground, the spread of pit head baths from the 1920s and medical and welfare centres (from the 1940s) also played an important role in the health, hygiene and well-being of the miners. The newest pits from the 1940s were also constructed with modern, integrated and automated screening and washing machinery, whilst the better layout of plant and transportation methods at the surface (and later computerisation) led to significant efficiencies and the need for substantially less physical labour.

A further fundamental change took place in coal face production methods in the two decades from the Second World War with the development of power-loading. Rather than undercutting the coal seam and then ripping the coal down, machines were developed which combined these processes, quite literally shearing away a substantial portion of the coal face in one operation and depositing the cut coal on to a loader and thence to the conveyor. The earliest power-loading machines appeared during and immediately after the war, and included the Meco-Moore combined cutter-conveyor (1943–), the trepanner (1952–) and the 'coal plough' and combined armoured flexible face conveyors pioneered in Germany during the war. Several hundred of these machines were being used on UK coal faces by the early 1960s. However, what was undoubtedly the pivotal machine in this second coal face technological revolution was the Anderton shearer-loader. This machine, patented in 1953, had a large circular drum cutter up to five feet in circumference which ran along the face, dropping the cut coal onto the integrated loader. It was developed and adapted over subsequent years (for example, with larger drums), and in 1969 the first ranging drum shearer was developed, capable of traversing from the top to the bottom of the seam, thus providing more flexible adaptation to different and changing seam thicknesses. The Anderton machines diffused rapidly throughout the coal fields, and became the dominant power-loader technology by the late 1960s. By 1966 the Anderton shearer produced over 50% of all mechanised coal output in the UK, and by 1977 over 80%. With the working coal face advancing far more rapidly than before, it was essential to have more flexible and efficient methods to prevent roof collapse. The transformation in hewing techniques with power-loading was only made possible, therefore, with technical improvements in roof support associated with hydraulically powered steel props which first appeared in 1946 and spread rapidly in the 1950s and 1960s. The power-loading revolution was achieved relatively rapidly, with the main changes coming in the 1960s. In 1957 just 25% of all coal produced in the UK was continuously cut and loaded mechanically. By 1962 this figure stood at 50%, and by 1970 at over 90%.[17]

---

17 This section is based on Ashworth, *The History of the British Coal Industry*, vol. 5, pp. 75–6, 82–4.

The extent to which these changes in work organisation and technology in the pits transformed the labour process of coal miners has been the subject of much contentious debate.[18] Undoubtedly, the modernisation of coal production created opportunities for more highly skilled and technical work, necessitating more careful planning of production cycles and sophisticated knowledge of mechanical engineering. This required more skilled artisans in the pit and more technical staff at the surface. Supervision, planning and monitoring of all stages of the production process intensified. The duties of deputies expanded from safety regulation underground to supervisory functions from the 1920s, with these mine officials evolving increasingly into the role of the traditional 'foreman'. These changes were reflected in the increased proportion of supervisors, professionals and managerial staff, which rose from around 4% of the total mining workforce in the 1900s to around 7% by *c.* 1950.[19] With advancing mechanisation there was also an increasing tendency for the employment of craftsmen underground, for example constructing, fitting and maintaining roads, water pipes and electrical equipment and cabling. The machinery also took away some of the physically exhausting hard graft from mine work – such as undercutting the seam and transporting men and product from face to shaft. Inevitably, mechanisation required less labour. A 74-year-old Lanarkshire miner recalled changes being made to staffing levels as the power-loading machines were brought in:

> The main difference was … you had maybe 20 or 30 strippers with 40 feet each, and the next thing is when they took out the men and they brought in the machinery … you only needed maybe about six men – two on each of the machines, and four men shifting the props in behind the machine as they were taking the coal out.[20]

And an Ayrshire miner commented about mechanisation in the 1960s:

> It changed the whole composition of coal getting. A conveyor with a pan 6 feet wide that weighed approximately two hundredweight, that could be handled by two men. Either that height or that height. You only handled them once. You didnae need to handle them again.[21]

A Durham miner recalled:

> It was a lot easier because the machines did the work. You see the last machine I was on, all I did was crawl up and down the face at the side of it as it was going up taking coal off. And when I got to the far end, 120 yards, that's what they used to be, we'd come back

18 See Campbell, *The Scottish Miners, 1874–1939*, vol. 1, pp. 113–22; Supple, *The History of the British Coal Industry*, vol. 4, pp. 435–39.

19 Ashworth, *The History of the British Coal Industry*, vol. 5, p. 442.

20 Harry Steel, Interview C9 (SOHC).

21 Alec Mills, Interview C1 (SOHC).

over, putting the coal on to the belts, and that's all it was. Whereas before, everything was manhandled.[22]

And a Welsh miner had similar recollections:

This I can tell you, when the conveyor system came in there were riots in Tŷ Mawr, and the first conveyor that came in was down on the north level … And there was murder, there was murder because, first thing the men were saying, "Right, half of us will be on the dole now, this conveyor's going to take half of us on the dole and we'll lose our jobs." But as time went on the men were beginning to realise than it was better than heading and stalling, and it was safer too. [23]

Work underground changed irrevocably with these developments, which tended towards the deskilling of the hewer, more intensive and regularised working methods, closer control and supervision, and the increasing specialisation of work. The all-round skills of the hewer, with much autonomy at the point of production, were replaced by the more specialised skills of the machine minder and conveyor operator. The new capital-intensive methods also facilitated different shift systems. An Ayrshire miner noted his experience of this in the late 1950s:

The long-wall faces … were undercut on the night shift with a coal cutting machine with a big jib on it. The day shift was the stripping shift where they got rid of a' the coal, and the back shift advanced everything, stepped everything forward, withdrew the waste supports and moved a' the belts or scrapers on it. Quite a confined space, but everybody was specialists at certain jobs.[24]

With power-loading mechanisation, more time could be devoted to the cycle of coal cutting during the working day (usually at least two full shifts). In many pits, once development work had been completed, coal cutting became a continuous operation through each shift, each day. This also impacted on those miners still working traditional methods. One Ayrshire miner described the pressures of working in such a conventional pit (Sorn) in the early 1970s:

We had men working with the pick and shovel. And we had to compete. You had to compete with all the other pits in the area with your pick and shovel as against the big machine.[25]

These changes increased coal output and productivity, but were also capable of generating more dust in the workplace for longer periods, with a wider group of craftsmen and workers exposed to dust inhalation. Compared to the action of the pick upon the coal, mechanised cutting tended to *disintegrate* the mineral. Thus, in

---

22 Frederick Hall, Interview C41 (SOHC).

23 Interview with Haydn Mainwaring, 18/3/1980, South Wales Coal Collection (SWCC), AUD/56.

24 Bert Smith, Interview C14 (SOHC).

25 Billy Affleck, Interview C2 (SOHC).

its initial stages the mechanisation of coal mining made environmental conditions considerably worse underground – especially at the coal face and for those workers located at the return side of the ventilation system (where the dust flowed in the air current from the face). This created a major challenge for the mine engineers and for the health and safety regulators in relation to dust control. We return to this in more depth in Chapter 6.

The Body, Health and Safety in the Pits

Miners' bodies were intimately affected by the work they did, and perhaps more so than almost any other occupational group. Walter Greenwood noted of miners in the 1930s: 'You can usually tell a miner a mile away. Short, stocky, muscular, rarely carrying any superfluous flesh, he has to be hard as nails.' He continued: 'Coal getting calls for the use of specially developed muscles.'[26] Similarly, George Orwell famously eulogised on the physical attributes of Northern coal miners in *The Road To Wigan Pier*:

> It is impossible to watch the 'fillers' at work without feeling a pang of envy for their toughness ... the fillers look and work as though they were made of iron ... It is only when you see miners down the mine and naked that you realise what splendid men they are. Most of them are small but nearly all of them have the most noble bodies; wide shoulders tapering to slender supple waists, and small pronounced buttocks and sinewy thighs, with not an ounce of waste flesh anywhere ... No-one could do their work who had not a young man's body, and a figure fit for a guardsman at that; just a few pounds of extra flesh on the waistline, and the constant bending would be impossible.[27]

This was a two-way process. The mentally and physically tough and fittest of men became permanent miners, working underground as hewers. Where other job opportunities were scarce, the physically weaker, frail and nervous might also find themselves having to work in the pit. However, there appears to have been a tendency for such men to work above ground, become craftsmen, or leave the industry for a job elsewhere. As one occupational mortality statistician pointed out in 1902:

> Miners, however, are a picked class of men in a more especial sense than are the toilers in most other industries. Their labour is so arduous that those only who possess exceptional physical endurance are able to continue at it.[28]

---

26 Greenwood, *How the Other Man Lives*, p. 32.

27 George Orwell, *The Road to Wigan Pier* (1937), cited in K. Thomas (ed.), *The Oxford Book of Work* (Oxford, 1999), pp. 385–6.

28 John Tatham, 'Dust-producing Occupations', in T. Oliver (ed.), *Dangerous Trades* (London, 1902), p. 157. See also Henry Louis, 'Mining', in Oliver, *Dangerous Trades*, p. 534.

Miners working underground became inured to danger, whilst the hard physical graft of pit work honed miners' bodies into fit and supple machines, a process complementing and facilitating enthusiasm for physical sports, with football, rugby and boxing popular amongst younger miners within mining communities. As one Durham miner recalled in his autobiography:

> Lads got their first introduction to football there [on the mining village playing field], which led some of them to first class football. They came out of the mine after ten hours down there and then played a hard game of football without flinching. A tough breed that knew no fear or weakness …[29]

It is not surprising that mining communities produced some of the best football and rugby players of the mid-twentieth century – including, for example, Matt Busby, Jim Baxter, Bill Shankly and Jock Stein (who, as well as playing, went on to become perhaps the most famous club manager in Scotland). Shankly's Ayrshire pit village, Glenbuck, produced over fifty professional footballers over a fifty-year period and developed one of the most famous Scottish amateur teams before the Second World War.[30] A retired Scottish miner who started working in the pits in the 1940s (Tommy Coulter) evocatively expressed this cult of physical fitness and toughness:

> TC: … Especially younger guys, then we thought we were the best in the world. We were the elite. When you went tae work in the coal face you, well, we were strong lads, you had tae be. And your lifestyle was such that if you werenae producing coal you were playing football, or boxing or dancing or walking, mainly engaged in physical pursuits. I mean, I used to walk twenty-five miles every Saturday and Sunday and that was, I done that for years and years.
> NR: Did you feel part of a young elite?
> TC: *Oh yes*, very much so.
> NR: Was that because you were a miner as well as your social life, or was it more the social …?
> TC: No, I think it was, well, because of the nature of work and the nature of lifestyle we could at least hold our own in any, if, and I mean if, we wouldnae of, I mean if there was any fisticuffs involved we were quite able tae do the business because we're hardy buggers and, we thought, I dare say, something like soldiers …[31]

Working in the pits thus forged the male body and incubated manly identities which have been associated with a 'hard man' hegemonic mode of masculinity. A Durham miner described his own personal journey in the years before the First World War

---

29 Thomas Jordan, born 1892, cited in J. Burnett (ed.), *Useful Toil* (Harmondsworth, 1974), p. 102.

30 See http://www.shankly.com/glenbuck.htm. This was even more remarkable as the village had a total population of a little over 1,000. Shankly continued his own personal fitness regime late into his life, commenting to a Liverpool FC colleague: 'When I go, son, I'm going to be the fittest man ever to die.'

31 Tommy Coulter, Interview C21 (SOHC).

from a scared, inexperienced boy to full manhood, and how fear had to be concealed because it was associated with effeminate behaviour:

> When we got out of the pit cage and directed our steps the short distance toward home, he [his father] always asked me how I liked the experience. Always I answered him that I liked going into the mine, which I did several times until I was fourteen years old. He was a fearless man and I did not wish to let him know that I was nervous or else he might have thought that I was 'queer' ... With the passing of the years I became indifferent to the many dangers in the mine. When someone was killed I might become apprehensive for a day or two, then the incident was completely forgotten. This training was valuable to me during the First World War when men were yielding their lives on a far larger scale.[32]

Similarly, an Ayrshire miner reflected back to his late teens as a haulage worker in the 1940s, commenting: 'No kidding you, I was like steel. I was a hard man then.'[33] The hardened physical body and the tough mentality led to miners being regarded as having the ideal body form and personality for warfare. As the Minister for National Service during the First World War enthused:

> The younger miner may be regarded as the best class of recruit in this Region [referring to Wales]; hard, well developed and muscular, he strips well ... the colliers as a class [referring to North West England] are well developed and muscular, and strip much better than the cotton operatives ... Of all miners examined 75% were placed in Grade 1 ... As a rule their muscular development was particularly good. What struck one most was their general aspect of mental and physical alertness.[34]

A few years earlier, the mine owners had opposed the legalisation of an eight-hour working day on the grounds that 'the miners' calling is healthy ... their vital statistics are superior to those of every class in the country'.[35] This comment typified an employers' discourse of denial of risk and dismissal of the brutal realities of bodily damage caused by work before the Second World War. What was also common was a propensity to blame the victim, transferring responsibility for health and safety to the workers. This was prevalent, for example, within the coal owners' trade journal, *Colliery Guardian*, in the coal mining posters of the National Safety First Association in the 1920s and 1930s, and to a surprising extent within the Annual Reports of the Mines Inspectors.[36]

---

32 Thomas Jordan, cited in Burnett, *Useful Toil*, pp. 103, 104.

33 Thomas McMurdo, Interview C20 (SOHC).

34 Ministry of National Service, 1917–1919, *Report upon the Physical Examination of Men of Military Age by National Service Medical Boards*, vol. 1 (1919), pp. 17–18, 134.

35 Miners' Federation of Great Britain, *Coal Mines Eight Hours Bill: Transcript of the House of Commons Second Reading, 22 June 1908* (Manchester, 1908), p. 40.

36 For a sample of inter-war National Safety First posters, see International Labour Organisation, *Industrial Safety Survey, 1925–28*; *Safety Education in Industry, 1929–32* (ILO, n.d.). One of the mining posters depicted a horrified miner's wife on the telephone, with the pit head and an ambulance in the background. The caption read: 'He neglected to be careful.' Another graphically depicted a fist of rock falling down upon a miner and his family, with the

Whilst miners were perceived by the state as epitomising the ideal physique for warfare in the first half of the twentieth century, paradoxically coal mining was one of the most dangerous occupations in the country in terms of its serious and disabling injury rates. As the epidemiological studies of Oliver, Liddell and others indicated, although the standardised mortality rates of miners compared relatively well against other occupational groups, they diverged widely from the average in relation to deaths from accidents and from respiratory disease.[37] Thus, working in the pits helped create the masculine body, whilst holding the potential to emasculate, with physical (and hence earning) capacity undermined by traumatic injury and longer-term chronic illness and disability.[38] As Bert Coombes noted, 'getting battered about' was 'part of the job'.[39] In the nineteenth century only shipping surpassed coal mining for its record of occupational mortality, but by the 1910s accident deaths in the pits also outstripped the death toll from working at sea.[40] Whilst injury and death rates declined sharply in coal mining from the 1850s, it was still the case in 1914 that a miner was killed in Britain every six hours, and severely injured every two hours.[41] Whilst the death rate per thousand employed in coal mining fell from 3.9 to 1.33 between the 1850s and the 1900s, the safety record in the factories improved much more dramatically (especially in textiles) over this period.[42] Moreover, the accident death toll fell heaviest upon the younger miners. At the end of the nineteenth century almost half of all deaths of 15–20-year-olds in mining communities were due to injuries sustained in pit work.[43] In total, almost 40,000 miners were officially recorded as having been killed at their work between 1880 and 1914, an average of well over a thousand a year. Large disasters intermittently devastated local communities, as at Gresford in 1934 where the death toll was 265, and at Senghenydd in South Wales in 1913, when 439 lives were lost in the single worse pit disaster in British history. However, most deaths and serious injuries in British coal mining occurred from

---

caption: 'Watch it! Fall of rock. Miner keep your hanging safe. Your family wants you back today. Your employer wants you back tomorrow.'

37 Oliver, *The Dangerous Trades*, pp. 156–9; F.D.K. Liddell, 'Mortality of British Coal Miners in 1961', *British Journal of Industrial Medicine*, vol. 30 (1973), pp. 15–24. This prompted one occupational health expert to comment in 1902: 'mining is a distinctly healthy occupation'. See Louis, 'Mining', in Oliver, *The Dangerous Trades*, p. 533.

38 This is discussed in more detail in Chapters 8 and 9.

39 Coombes, *These Poor Hands*, p. 43.

40 A.J. McIvor, *A History of Work in Britain, 1880–1950* (Basingstoke, 2001), p. 117. Some sections of other occupational groups recorded higher injury death rates than miners, notably dock labourers and some railway workers; see Louis, in Oliver, *The Dangerous Trades*, p. 530.

41 J. Benson, *British Coal Miners in the Nineteenth Century* (London, 1980), p. 43; R. Church, *The History of the British Coal Industry, Volume 3. 1830–1913* (Oxford, 1986), pp. 582–87.

42 A. Bryan, *The Evolution of Health and Safety in Mines* (Hertfordshire, 1975), table 9.1.

43 Oliver, *Dangerous Trades*, p. 158.

individual accidents, especially roof collapses, what John Benson has referred to as 'a steady drip-drip of death' in the pits.[44]

The number of miners disabled at their work before the First World War is not known, though one estimate by Benson suggests that in the nineteenth century there were around 100 non-fatal injuries sustained by miners (necessitating an average loss of 30 working days per injury) to every coal mining accident fatality.[45] Louis's work on the figures provided by Miners' Permanent Relief Funds in the 1890s confirms this ratio of roughly 100 non-fatal injuries to every fatality.[46] Church estimated that perhaps 1 in every 50 of those injured were permanently incapacitated. This calculation gives an estimate of 83,354 miners permanently disabled in the fifty years from 1850 to 1900.[47] Applying the same calculation to the first half of the twentieth century (when there were 51,258 fatalities – see Table 2.4) suggests around 100,000 or so miners permanently incapacitated as a result of an injury sustained at work (not counting industrial disease cases) between 1900 and 1950. In total, then, more than a quarter of a million miners were killed or permanently incapacitated as a result of injuries sustained whilst at their work over the period 1850–1950.

The occupational mortality and disability toll, moreover, varied considerably across different jobs in mining and from coal field to coal field, depending upon a range of factors, including widely different geological conditions.[48] By 1914, the North East, Yorkshire and the Midlands coal fields, for example, had a markedly lower work-related injury incidence, than did South Wales (and especially the Aberdare valley).[49] Age (as we've seen) and occupation were key factors. In the late nineteenth century, underground workers were two to three times more likely to be killed from a work-related injury than surface workers, and hewers were substantially more likely to be injured than haulage workers.[50] The existence of complex machinery and the network of railway lines and sidings at the surface of most coal mines by the end of the nineteenth century accounted for a relatively high injury and death rate – more than double that of surface workers in metal mines. Church has demonstrated that whilst the average mortality of miners compared well with other occupational groups, deaths due to accidents were 2.3 times the UK average at the end of the

---

44 Church, *The History of the British Coal Industry*, vol. 3, p. 587.

45 Benson, *British Coal Miners in the Nineteenth Century*, pp. 39–41.

46 Louis, 'Mining', in Oliver, *The Dangerous Trades,* pp. 530–32. Louis was also very critical of the under-recording of disablement cases in the Mines Inspectors Reports, claiming injuries were 'more than twenty times as numerous' as the 'official' figures (p. 531).

47 Church, *The History of the British Coal Industry*, vol. 3, pp. 303, 306. Louis provided somewhat lower figures for permanent disability (defined as loss of work for more than six months) for Northumberland and Durham, but this was a relatively low-risk coal field. See Louis, 'Mining', in Oliver, *Dangerous Trades*, pp. 532–3.

48 Oliver, *The Dangerous Trades,* p. 159.

49 Church, *The History of the British Coal Industry*, vol. 3, pp. 587–9.

50 Louis, 'Mining', in Oliver, *The Dangerous Trades*, pp. 524–5.

nineteenth century.[51] Miners would speak about their being 'blood on the coal'. The mining community was very aware of the price it paid for producing coal in terms of damaged and destroyed bodies, and it was customary to insure against such risk by making payments to friendly societies or through the pay packet. One South Wales miner, Howard Jones, noted that when he started underground in 1942, his wage deductions were: 'A penny for the hospital, a penny for the ambulance, penny for the doctor, and a penny for the union.'[52] A few years later, a further deduction of 3d. was being made to cover payment for a diagnostic x-ray.

The coal industry contracted sharply in the inter-war years, with the closure of marginal and unprofitable pits and the loss of around 400,000 jobs. Like the other heavy industries, coal mining communities were hit hard by the Depression, with unemployment rates reaching 50% and more in the worst years of the early 1930s. As the Royal Commission on Safety in Coal Mines of 1935–38 reported, in this period of crisis for the industry the safety record of coal mining stagnated, with the death rate through occupational injury actually increasing slightly in the 1920s and 1930s. At a time when about 1 in every 20 British workers was a miner, the industry accounted for roughly 25% of all work-related injuries in the UK.[53] Even the coal owners' trade journal placed a large portion of the responsibility for this upon the shoulders of management, noting in 1925: 'the increase in the number of accidents due to falls of ground and haulage accidents show that the general state of repair of mines and equipment has deteriorated and that safeguarding is not efficiently carried out by management'.[54] Mechanisation brought some health and safety benefits, including less physically exhausting labour and reduction in the dangerous process of 'bottom-holing'. However, electrification brought its own hazards, and where mechanisation levels were greatest, in Scotland in the inter-war years, injuries and deaths by electrocution were highest.[55] In the 1920s and 1930s, miners accounted for a third of all occupation-related injury deaths in the UK (see Table 2.4), and by 1950 miners were twice as likely as seamen to be killed at work.[56] A measure of the extent of this problem in the coal fields was the creation by the MFGB and Miners' Welfare Fund of rehabilitation centres for injured miners. This brought more doctors and nurses into the service of the miners. In Lanarkshire (a coal field with a poor safety record), over 7,000 men were being injured in the pits every year in the early

---

51 Church, *The History of the British Coal Industry*, vol. 3, p. 592. See also McIvor, *A History of Work*, p. 118, for more detailed comparison of mortality by occupational group.

52 Howard Jones, Interview C25 (SOHC).

53 Supple, *The History of the British Coal Industry*, vol. 4, p. 427.

54 Cited in L. Sheffield, 'Working and Living Conditions in Scottish Coalmining in the Interwar Years' (unpublished Honours Dissertation, Glasgow Caledonian University, 2003), p. 23.

55 A. Renfrew, 'Mechanisation and the Miner: Work, Safety and Labour Relations in the Scottish Coal Industry, 1890–1939' (unpublished PhD Thesis, University of Strathclyde, 1997), p. 169.

56 D. Gallie, 'The Labour Force', in A.H. Halsey and J. Webb (eds), *Twentieth Century British Social Trends* (London, 2000), p. 303.

1930s, and to address this the Lanarkshire Orthopaedic Association opened out-patient clinics in Miners' Institutes and public health centres throughout the county in 1935.[57] Bert Coombes described evocatively the room allocated for medical examinations at his pit in South Wales in the 1930s:

> In the room on the left about twenty men are seated on plank forms waiting for the compensation doctors to come and examine them. The signs of injury are plain on most of them, for several have their arms slung, and four are on crutches. It resembles the dressing-station after a battle.[58]

Such a deterioration in working conditions in the pits between the wars, combined with attacks on miners' wage levels and their trade unions, provided the backdrop for a period of embittered relations between capital and labour, and further fuelled the demands of the miners' unions for the reorganisation of ownership, from private to nationalised. In the first two decades of the twentieth century, British coal miners had become the best-organised group of British workers, with over 900,000 miners members of the MFGB – a union density at its highest point in excess of 90% of those employed. In the fifty years from the late 1880s, coal miners were also the most dispute-prone of all British workers, accounting for 47% of all strikers and a staggering 61% of all working days lost through strikes in British industry.[59] For their part, the British coal owners developed a reputation for being particularly draconian in their labour relations policies and autocratic in their opposition to challenges to their authority by the mining unions prior to the Second World War.[60] In reality, this popular public discourse about the mine owners being the most authoritarian in Britain, and the miners the most militant, obscured a considerable range of experience across a heterogeneous industry. None the less, here was a classic example of contested knowledge, where the different and antagonistic groups representing capital and labour created their own interpretations of the past. This is evident in the field of occupational health, with markedly different discourses about health, mortality and morbidity seeping through different types of evidence, such as the NCB papers, trade union reports and oral testimony.[61]

Miners' bodies were affected in many ways by the work they did. Louis noted in his survey of occupational health in the pits at the end of the nineteenth century that 'probably the most unhealthy part of the coal miners' work consists in "kirving" or

---

57 G. Hutton, *Lanarkshire's Mining Legacy* (Cumnock, 1997), p. 20.

58 Coombes, *These Poor Hands*, p. 231.

59 J. Benson, *The Working Class in Britain, 1850–1939* (London, 1989), p. 179; J. Cronin, *Industrial Conflict in Modern Britain* (London, 1979), pp. 206–10.

60 See Q. Outram, 'The Stupidest Men in England? The Industrial Relations Strategy of the Coal Owners between the Lockouts, 1923–1924', *Historical Studies in Industrial Relations*, vol. 4 (September 1997), pp. 65–71.

61 This is evident, for example, in the early twentieth-century debates in the coal industry over the shorter working week in 1908, and nationalisation of the pits, in 1918–20 (Sankey Commission).

Table 2.4   Occupation-related accident deaths in coal mining, 1885–1949

	*Total UK deaths**	*Deaths in coal mining*	*% of total*
1885–89	20,632	5,116	24.8
1890–94	21,670	5,402	24.9
1895–99	21,750	4,821	22.2
1900–1904	22,030	5,264	23.9
1905–1909	21,377	6,307	29.5
1910–14	23,616	7,288	30.9
1915–19	21,942	6,499	29.6
1920–24	16,020	5,462	34.1
1925–29	17,819	4,959	27.8
1930–34	11,954	4,626	38.7
1935–39	13,052	4,151	31.8
1940–44	14,463	4,063	28.1
1945–49	9,782	2,639	27.0

Notes: *These are *recorded* deaths in the occupations monitored by the state agencies (the Factory and Mines Inspectorate).
Source: Department of Employment, *British Labour Statistics, Historical Abstract* (1971), table 200.

undercutting the coal'.[62] He ascribed problems with posture, joints, eye strain and dust inhalation to this part of the hewers' labour process. Zweig claimed in the 1940s that a miner lost an average of four to five pounds in weight per shift from sweating due to the heat and intensity of the work, and that older miners were distinguished by blue scars all over their bodies.[63] The South Wales miner Bert Coombes noted in his autobiography how almost every part of his body was affected by his first day's work:

> My legs became cramped, my arms ached, and the back of my hands had the skin rubbed off by pressing my knee against them to force the shovel under the coal. The dust compelled me to cough and sneeze, while it collected inside my eyes and made them burn and feel sore. My skin was smarting because of the dust and flying bits of coal … How glad I was to drag my aching body towards that circle of daylight. I had sore knees and I was wet from the waist down. The back of my right hand was raw and my back felt the

---

62 Louis, 'Mining', in Oliver, *The Dangerous Trades*, p. 534.
63 F. Zweig, *Men in the Pits* (London, 1948), pp. 5–6.

same. My eyes were half closed because of the dust and my head was aching where I had hit it against the top, but I had been eight hours in a strange, new world.[64]

Reflecting on the 1970s, one miner, who normally worked in the Lanarkshire coal field in Scotland, remembered working for a while in the Fife pits (on the Scottish east coast), where he was struck by the difference in height of the coal seams:

> We went up to Fife. Fucking *8 feet* fucking high, man! You thought, 'What the fucking hell here?' ... The Fifers cried us 'the Jimmies' 'cause we came from Glasgow, well down this side, you know. We wore knee pads. They didnae. They stood and fucking shovelled, man, because it was that high, you know. But we ... We couldnae shovel standing up because the old back was knackered, you know.[65]

Working in the very small seams could be especially difficult. One Durham mining haulage worker related his experience in the 1950s:

> When I was putting, I used to have an Elastoplast the length of my back on here, the scab would be catching the strut, it was that low. I was working the pit, it was only 13 inches high, the seam was only 13 inches high in one part. Well, you know how high a tub is, well, just about high enough to get a tub in and you had to push it in bent like that, and nine times out ... you were catching your back and you used to have scabs on your back and when you got in the bath, oh dear me.[66]

A Lanarkshire doctor commented in the early 1960s on the positive effects of mechanisation and on the impact mining work had upon the physique of the men:

> The more hardworking coalface miner with his twisted frame in old age will disappear. We never see now the twisted frames, the knarled sort of trunks of trees that look as though they grew in caves, and now we are seeing more upright people and the advent of the machine-cut coal is bearing fruit already.[67]

The development of wider and higher roadways underground contributed to this. Recalling his experience in the 1960s, one South Wales miner noted: '... the steel arches came in. Instead of walking in the same shape as a sickle, you could actually stand up and walk to your coal face.'[68] Another Scottish miner recalled something of the range of work cultures, the impact of work upon the body, and differences in work environments in this commentary on his experience in the 1950s:

> I came to the Fife pit [Comrie]. A lot of people didnae like the Fife pit, I don't know why. Different entirely, different type of men, different contracts ... If there was bad ground or

---

64 B.L. Coombes, *These Poor Hands: The Autobiography of a Miner Working in South Wales* (London, 1939), pp. 32, 38.

65 John McKean, Interview C10 (SOHC).

66 Alan Winter, Interview C42 (SOHC).

67 Dr Thomas, Oral Interview, 1961, South Wales Coal Collection, Audio/374.

68 Howard Jones, Interview C25 (SOHC).

anything, you got physical assistance, well, in Comrie you didnae get physical assistance, you got extra money. And a lot of the men made good money in Comrie, and actually, I'll put it this way, it separated the men from the boys. The likes of [name deleted] and quite a few of them, they were found out what they were, because they had to work for their living and they were involved in the co-operative system in the Devon and Glenochil. Okay, we always tended to carry the older men, well, not carry them but help them out sort of thing to make sure they still got a fair day's wage and everything else, but one or two of the younger ones, when they came to Comrie they were actually found out because you were on your own and you got paid everything for extras ... There was one particular chap who is dead and away now, [name deleted] knows him as well, he was absolutely a first-class miner, big [name deleted], absolutely first class, this was a beast of a man for work, he loved Comrie, he thought this was the best thing because he was actually getting paid what was coming out of his own bat, he wasnae carrying anyone else, and ... used to get extra coal and different things, he thought this was great ... I would say near enough the company murdered him, near enough.[69]

A number of elements are evident in this piece of testimony, including references to individualistic and co-operative work cultures, admiration of hard graft, reverence for the 'big hewer' (whose manly identity was exalted) and a 'heroic' discourse in which men and management were at loggerheads. This also tells us much about the variable effects work had upon the body and the men's perceptions of the bodily damage caused by the intensified work regime of 'the company'. Embedded in here is a variant of the afore mentioned 'blood on the coal' discourse, common in miners' personal testimonies.

Much has been written about the intervention of the state in regulating the worse excesses of the mining labour process, with intermittent Coal Mines Acts passed to control work hours, the employment of women and children, and to protect workers' health and well-being.[70] The Mines Inspectorate policed this legislation, and clearly this did make a positive contribution to health and safety standards in the workplace. However, what also needs to be recognised is that there remained a massive gulf between what was legislated for and actual workplace practice. This was a common and persistent problem. One Scottish occupational hygienist recently noted:

Basically, during a pursuit case you look at what the witnesses say. You compare what the witnesses are saying with what the legislation at the time required, and the disparity very often is petrifyingly large ... Very, very often you find the statutory duties have simply not been met.[71]

---

69 David Carruthers, Interview C23 (SOHC).

70 For recent contributions, see P.W.J. Bartrip, *The Home Office and the Dangerous Trades* (Amsterdam, 2002); J. Melling and M. Bufton, '"A Mere Matter of Rock": Organized Labour, Scientific Evidence and British Government Schemes for Compensation of Silicosis and Pneumoconiosis among Coalminers, 1926–1940', *Medical History*, vol. 49, no. 2 (April 2005), pp. 155–78.

71 Robin Howie, Interview C45 (SOHC). Howie argued that a critical reason for this was the failure of the state to effectively police the legislation, which thus failed to act as a deterrent.

The gap between statutory provision and practice was perhaps widest in mining, where men worked in an environment deep underground, far removed from the eyes of the regulators. Miners' own testimonies provide critical insights into the realities of safety provision underground as well as the trade-offs that miners made in order to satisfy managerial demands for production, and in some cases, in order to maximise their own earnings. Some men reflected on the practice – the bane of the Mines Inspectors – of cutting away at the seam an extra couple of feet before putting up supports. A retired Ayrshire miner made no bones about this: 'We were out for the money ... At times we maybe done ourselves that we shouldnae have done, or we wouldnae be allowed to do ... You're cutting corners.'[72] Others, though, stated that such practices were condoned by the management for the sake of productivity, and that it was only when the Mines Inspector paid a visit that the correct number of supports would be put in place. Mines Inspectors were reported to use sticks to judge if supports were put up safely and imposed fines if powder cans were not locked.[73] A Durham miner reported how a small drift mine where he worked in the 1950s was serviced by a diesel locomotive for years in an illegal fashion, and how the inspector eventually forced the colliery to replace it with a rope haulage system:

> The last pit I worked at, the Hole in the Wall, I was driving a loco, little loco that went in the pit and pulled the tubs out. And the health and safety man came round there and I was going in the pit this day and he stopped us with the loco and he says he was the health and safety man. He says 'How long have you been driving this in here?', I says 'Since it opened', it was a drift, it was a little drift. He says 'You know you're breaking the law?', I says 'How's that?', well, 'There should have been a foot clearance to go over the top of the engine', the canopy of the engine, 'and there should have been a foot to either side.' And this car that I was on driving in it was about two or three inches. So he says to me 'You know you're breaking the law?', I says, 'You don't want to tell me that,' I says, 'tell that man there.' And that was the manager, the deputy, the under-manager was standing in the manhole waiting for us coming in.[74]

However, in some cases the management – whether it was in the private mine era or under nationalisation – knew in advance when the Mines Inspector was making a visit:

> They never went anywhere at random. Anywhere they went, we knew ... We knew maybe two days before they were coming, so production would be halted or slowed down, and as near as possible things would get put into perspective, and after they went away it was just back to normal again.[75]

Another miner told us that after a man was killed by a falling roof in an Ayrshire mine, some of the missing pit props were installed before the Mines Inspector

---

72 George Devenne, Interview C6 (SOHC).
73 Andrew Lyndsay, Interview C4 (SOHC).
74 Alan Winter, Interview C42 (SOHC).
75 Carl Martin, Interview C8 (SOHC).

arrived to investigate the accident.[76] A retired machineman from the Ayrshire coal field recalled that the high death toll from falls of roofs was not always due to miners trying to maximise production. For example, he was one of the first on the scene at a cave-in in which a miner was killed, and this is what he remembered:

> I'm no going to say the man didnae put shores up. He put shores up to the best of his ability, but sometimes there was a shortage of materials, and sometimes you'd tae improvise. [77]

This miner also told us that as a machineman, he had to continually duck under the coal face he was undercutting to check the course of the machine. Technically he should have installed supports every time he had to go under the face. However, he explained that this would have slowed down the production process considerably, and would have been frowned upon by the management. Another good example of how pragmatism may have sometimes got in the way of 'textbook' safety procedures was provided by a 90-year-old retired Ayrshire miner:

> The stuff that came into the pit latterly, there was some of it heavy. Even the props they were using were hard tae handle … And, eh, if you could see an easier way to dae it, you done it.

He could also remember that on some occasions when the time came to take supports down, instead of removing them one by one by hand:

> We emptied the girders with a chain. Just tied it round a' the girders and hold it tae a girder and dropped the haulage away and pulled them out. Things like that. There's numerous things you see.[78]

Oral interview testimony illuminates how ineffective statutory regulations could be when applied to workplaces deep underground, how workers rationalised risks and – very importantly – how they balanced their own health and safety against the pressures of productivity as well as pressures from their peers. The damage the job wrought upon miners' bodies was also seared into their consciousness, and emerged frequently when they were interviewed about their work experience. Injury, death and illness were recurring motifs in the oral interviews undertaken for this study. Many of our oral interview respondents had received an injury or had stories to tell of relatives or friends badly injured or killed in the pit. One recalled having to help carry the bodies of nine colleagues up to the surface after the explosion at Lindsay pit in Fife in 1957.[79] Another recounted how his brother was killed in a disaster at

---

76 Dick Easterbrook, Interview C17 (SOHC).

77 William Dunsmore (Arco), Interview C16 (SOHC).

78 Davy McCulloch, Interview C18 (SOHC).

79 William Dunsmore (Arco), Interview C16 (SOHC). This respondent recalled the joke he came up with at the time to mediate this grim experience: 'Maybe you'll laugh, I don't know, but I can remember saying to the men, "We're ca'ing our guts here carrying these men up, and what will they do? They'll bury them." (laughs) It's a'right laughing now.'

an Ayrshire pit in the late 1950s.[80] A Durham miner reflected back on lost comrades much like a soldier remembering a campaign:

> The lads in the 'C' drift where I was in there – there's only one left alive. All of them died *young*. Hank and all them. Hank collapsed and died. Wally Purvis, Clemensey, all *big hitters*. All gone. Them's the empty chair in the club. And they all worked in the same flat.[81]

Alec McNeish had a brother whose back was broken by a fall of roof, and was himself entombed for three days at the Knockshinnoch mine in Ayrshire in 1951 (when there was an inrush of peat/mud) before being rescued. The danger and risk was something that miners lived with and to which they became hardened. Significantly, Alec McNeish's resolve never to return to mining after being trapped at Knockshinnoch (he got a job on the railways) lasted less than two weeks.[82] This provides further evidence of the depth of acculturation to risk and to bodily damage as an outcome of mining work at the middle of the twentieth century.

Chronic Occupational Ill Health and Disease

Together with the high levels of disability and death through injury in the workplace, miners' bodies were also damaged by a cluster of chronic occupation-related diseases. The eye disease nystagmus was rampant in the pits in the nineteenth and early twentieth centuries – the result, it appears, of poor standards of illumination underground and the strain upon eye muscles, especially amongst the pre-mechanised hewers in the operation of bottom-holing. The symptoms were uncontrollable oscillations of the eyeball, severe dizziness and headaches. Those affected were usually forced to give up hewing. One medical expert noted in 1902:

> Treatment consists essentially of a change of the kind of work. In some cases it will suffice if the patient ceases from coal-getting, without altogether stopping work in the mine, but generally it is advisable, especially if the nystagmus be of high degree and of some standing, to recommend cessation altogether from work underground.[83]

It is hard to imagine how difficult it must have been to see adequately using just the safety lamp (which warned the miner of the existence of methane gas) prior to the widespread introduction of the portable electric lamp in the twentieth century. As Louis noted in 1902: 'A really good safety lamp, giving a light all round at least equal to that of an ordinary candle, is a great desideratum at the present moment.'[84]

---

80 Bert Smith, Interview C14 (SOHC).

81 Alan Napier, Interview C43 (SOHC).

82 Alec McNeish, Interview C13 (SOHC).

83 S. Snell, 'Eye Diseases and Eye Accidents', in Oliver, *The Dangerous Trades*, p. 764.

84 H. Louis, 'Mining', in Oliver, *The Dangerous Trades*, p. 528.

Over 10,000 miners in Britain were incapacitated by nystagmus in the 1920s, and on average over 1,000 new cases were reported every year through to the early 1940s.[85] Whilst nystagmus was amongst the earliest of occupational diseases in Britain to be prescribed for compensation purposes under the Workmen's Compensation Acts, the disease was poorly understood before the Second World War. This uncertainty caused much anxiety within mining communities, where it was widely (but erroneously) believed to lead inevitably to blindness.[86] Many miners did end up severely visually impaired, and a Coal Industry Social Welfare Organisation survey in 1953 identified more than 800 totally blind miners.[87] Numbers afflicted fell off from the 1920s with the spread of electric lighting underground (first introduced in 1881) and cap lamps replacing the Davy safety lamp. Newly diagnosed cases of nystagmus were rare by the 1960s.[88]

The working posture and damp environment of many seams induced a range of muscular, bone and tendon problems, including rheumatism, hernias, arthritis and, most commonly, the 'beat' (inflammation) ailments of knee, elbow and hand. Kneeling or lying down at the seam and manipulating the body to hack out coal from narrow seams were the main causes of these potentially incapacitating conditions. There were more than 10,000 new cases of the beat diseases diagnosed each year in the 1940s and the early 1950s. Thereafter, as Ashworth has shown, the condition was ameliorated by the successful design of knee pads in the 1960s, by new medical treatments (including antibiotics) and by advancing mechanisation which eliminated much of the percussive pick and shovel work, as well as reducing the necessity of miners to work kneeling down or in a restricted, cramped posture.[89] Given the dirty and dusty conditions of the mine environment, dermatitis was another endemic problem in the pits, and whilst rarely incapacitating, proved to be particularly difficult to control until the 1960s. As Bryan pointed out, the key changes which helped to control dermatitis were the introduction of medical centres, pithead baths and the improvements in housing and hygiene, especially after the Second World War.[90] Whilst mining mechanisation was the panacea for a number of physical problems, it also brought new chronic health problems in its wake. Two of the more obvious were vibration white finger (a form of Raynaud's Disease) and industrial deafness.[91] A number of our oral history respondents referred to the higher levels of noise which

---

85 *Annual Report of the Chief Inspector of Mines for 1938*, p. 228; Bryan, *Evolution of Health and Safety in Mines,* p. 108. New cases of nystagmus appear to have peaked at over 3,000 per year in the early 1920s.

86 Mines Department, *First Report of the Safety in Mines Research Board, 1921–22* (1926), pp. 20–21.

87 Coal Industry Social and Welfare Organisation, *Annual Report* (1953), p. 22.

88 Ashworth, *The History of the British Coal Industry*, vol. 5, p. 561.

89 Ibid., pp. 561–4.

90 Bryan, *The Evolution of Health and Safety in Mines*, p. 109.

91 British Coal were liable to pay compensation for miners found to have vibration white finger from 1999.

went along with the advancing mechanisation of coal production at the face, as well as the surface – with power-driven screens and conveyors.[92]

Table 2.5 gives some indication of trends in some of the occupational diseases associated with coal mining in the twentieth century.

Table 2.5   Coal miners' occupational diseases: nystagmus, dermatitis and the beat conditions

	Dermatitis	*Beat (joint) conditions**	*Nystagmus*
1908–12**	—	1,974	944
1923–27**	—	4,456	3,097
1938	254	6,137	1,224
1943	1,207	7,478	2,006
1952	3,863	11,525	191
1960	3,201	9,338	58
1965	2,501	5,099	27
1970	1,528	1,618	5

Notes: Table covers new cases arising under the Workmen's Compensation Acts.
* Including beat knee, beat hand, beat elbow and inflammation of the wrist.
** Annual averages.
Source: *Report of the Chief Inspector of Mines and Quarries for 1938 (1940)*, p. 228; *Report of the Chief Inspector of Mines and Quarries for 1947* (1949), p. 40; *Report of the Chief Inspector of Mines and Quarries for 1972* (1973), table 8, p. 69.

Given this array of chronic occupation-related diseases and the high trauma rate in coal mining, it is hardly surprising that mining communities were characterised by the presence of large numbers of disabled men. Recalling his experience as a young pit worker in the middle of the nineteenth century, the MP Thomas Burt commented that he had never seen 'so many crutches, so many empty jacket sleeves, so many wooden legs …'.[93] The disabled would not have been so evident in mining communities by the second half of the twentieth century. None the less, miners continued to be disproportionately damaged by their work compared to other occupations. At the middle of the twentieth century, miners accounted for less than 5% of the total male labour force, but 60% of all Workmen's Compensation claimants in the UK were miners.[94] Liddell's 1961 epidemiological study found British miners to still have relatively high levels of morbidity, and indeed to suffer more incapacity for work

---

92 Tommy Coulter, Interview C21 (SOHC); Alec Mills, Interview C1 (SOHC). See also Orwell, *Wigan Pier*.

93 Cited in Church, *The History of the British Coal Industry*, vol. 3, p. 195.

94 *The Miner* (July/August 1953), p. 5.

than men in any other employment.[95] According to DHSS figures, in the mid-1970s coal miners accounted for an astonishing 85% (29,720 out of a total of 34,870) of all persons in the UK receiving benefit (under the National Insurance Industrial Injuries Act) for occupation-related lung diseases, and still accounted for 60% (683 out of a total of 1,137) of first diagnoses of prescribed occupation-related lung diseases (including byssinosis and asbestosis) made by the Pneumoconiosis Medical Panels.[96] Moreover, coal miners accounted for a massively disproportionate share of incapacity from all other (that is, non-respiratory) prescribed occupational diseases, with 25–30% of all cases in the early 1970s. At this time, coal miners were on average nine times more likely to contract a work-related disease than other manufacturing workers.[97] Further confirmation of the persistence of high levels of disability in coal mining right through to the end of the twentieth century came with the Labour Force Survey. This survey in 1990 had a 'trailer' question designed to assess the prevalence of occupational morbidity across the UK workforce. After the data was tabulated, coal mining topped the resulting league table of self-reported work-related illness, having more than four times the levels of occupational morbidity for construction workers, and more than eight times the average for all occupations.[98] Clearly, the legacy of ill health and disability that working in the pits generated persisted long after the collieries themselves were closed down.

Dust at Work

The most deadly and disabling of coal miners' chronic occupational diseases were undoubtedly the cluster of diseases of the respiratory system, caused by inhaling dust. These included bronchitis and emphysema, where inhaled particles of dust obstructed and inflamed the airways (bronchial tubes and alveoli in the lungs), damaging tissue and adversely affecting the passage of oxygen into the blood stream, and pneumoconiosis – where the inhalation of stone (silica) dust and coal dust clogged up the lungs, causing progressive damage and scarring (fibrosis) and a deterioration in lung function, leading to breathlessness, wheezing and coughing. This impaired physical capacity, reduced the ability of miners to perform their arduous labour, as well as many other physical activities, such as walking. In the most serious cases, death resulted from lung failure, or cardiac failure as the impaired lung capacity put pressure on the heart. Church noted that whilst tuberculosis rates were relatively low within the mining community in the last two decades of the nineteenth century, other

---

95 Liddell, 'Mortality of British Coal Miners in 1961', pp. 1–2.

96 Health and Safety Executive, *Health and Safety Statistics 1975* (1977), p. 52.

97 Ibid., pp. 50–51.These figures are 'spells of certified incapacity resulting from fresh developments of prescribed diseases by industry'.

98 Health and Safety Commission (HSC), *Annual Report, 1992–3* (1993), p. 88; HSC, *Annual Report, Statistical Supplement* (1993), pp. 22, 25. The question posed was whether they had 'in the last 12 months, suffered from any illness, disability or other physical problem that was caused or made worse by (their) work'.

'diseases of the respiratory system' (including bronchitis) were prevalent, with the death rate amongst miners being around 20% higher than the UK average.[99]

However, it was in the twentieth century that occupation-related respiratory disease in the coal mining industry reached epidemic proportions. The *extent* of this tragedy has tended to be overlooked. In part, this was the consequence of a fixation within government, and recently within the occupational health historiography, upon the asbestos problem, with the sustained growth in mesothelioma mortality from the late 1960s. However, as Melling and Bufton have shown, there was a sharp rise in the numbers of miners diagnosed with silicosis in the 1930s, and after Coal Workers' Pneumoconiosis was officially recognised (and made compensatable) in 1942, the numbers diagnosed with the disease rocketed.[100] After the war, in the late 1940s, deaths of miners with pneumoconiosis reached 700–800 a year. At peak, from the early 1950s to the late 1960s, the mortality rate from pneumoconiosis amongst British coal miners topped 1,600 a year. To put this in perspective, deaths from silicosis (of iron workers, masons, quarrymen and so on) at this time averaged around 420 a year, and deaths from asbestosis less than 100. Even as late as the 1990s, mortality from Coal Workers' Pneumoconiosis (CWP) was outstripping mortality from all other pneumoconioses (including silicosis and byssinosis) by a ratio of 5 to 1.[101] Very quickly, around the middle of the twentieth century, dust became the major occupation-related killer in mining communities. By the late 1940s, recorded deaths from pneumoconiosis had outstripped deaths in British coal mining from accidents, and by the mid-1950s pneumoconiosis deaths outnumbered mining accident deaths by a ratio of 4 to 1.[102] The total *recorded* death toll of coal miners in Britain who died from CWP was more than 40,000 between 1930 and 1990. This is undoubtedly an underestimate, as for a number of reasons the official figures under-represent the number of deaths of miners from occupation-related respiratory disease (for example, many earlier cases were misdiagnosed as tuberculosis and silicosis, whilst bronchitis and emphysema were not recognised as occupation-related until 1993 – see Chapter 5). From the 1950s, however, the scourge of pneumoconiosis was beginning to be brought under control (see Figure 2.1). Newly diagnosed cases of pneumoconiosis peaked from the mid-1940s to the mid-1950s, and declined sharply

---

99 Church, *The History of the British Coal Industry*, vol. 3, p. 592. See also Oliver, *The Dangerous Trades*, pp. 159–60.

100 See M. Bufton and J. Melling, 'Coming Up for Air: Experts, Employers and Workers in Campaigns to Compensate Silicosis Sufferers in Britain, 1918–39', *Social History of Medicine*, vol. 18, no. 1 (2005), pp. 82–3; J. Melling and M. Bufton, 'From Sandstone Dust to Black Lung: The Origins of Pneumoconiosis Regulation in the UK and its Impact on Miners' Compensation c. 1935–1945', unpublished paper delivered to Dust at Work Conference, Glasgow Caledonian University, 28 May 2004. See also Melling and Bufton, '"A Mere Matter of Rock"'.

101 Health and Safety Commission, *Health and Safety Statistics, 1995–6*, p. 76; *1998–9*, pp. 86–7.

102 Ministry of Power, *Statistical Digest, 1957*, table 31, p. 44; *Annual Report of the Chief Inspector of Factories for 1959*, table 4, p. 38.

thereafter. The death rate from pneumoconiosis continued at a relatively high level, however, well into the 1960s, as Figure 2.2 indicates.

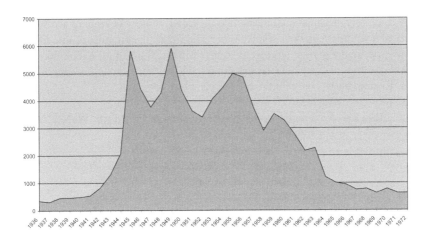

Source: Annual Reports of the Chief Inspector of Factories; Health and Safety Commission, Annual Reports.

Figure 2.1   Coal workers' pneumoconiosis: new diagnosed cases, UK, 1936–72

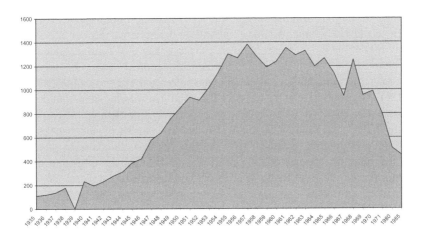

Source: Annual Reports of the Chief Inspector of Factories; Health and Safety Commission, Annual Reports.

Figure 2.2   Coal workers' pneumoconiosis deaths, England and Wales, 1936–86

Whilst pneumoconiosis was clearly a major cause of mortality within British mining communities in the twentieth century, as with accidents there was considerable variation in incidence across the coal fields. The disease was particularly prevalent in the early/mid-twentieth century within the South Wales coal field (see Table 2.6). Moreover, mainly because of the practice of Welsh miners beginning work at the coal face at a younger age than in most other coal fields, the prevalence rate in South Wales was particularly high amongst younger miners: 33% of all pneumoconiotics in the Aberdare Valley and 26% in the Rhondda Valley were under 40 years of age in the mid- to late 1950s, compared to a UK average of less than 15%.[103]

Table 2.6   New cases of pneumoconiosis in South Wales, 1939–55

	Total UK cases	South Wales	% of total UK cases
1939	465	418	89.9
1945	5,821	5,224	89.7
1951	3,154	1,222	38.7
1956	4,848	1,088	22.4

Source: Ministry of Fuel and Power, *Statistical Digests*.

By the 1950s, pneumoconiosis was recognised to be a problem throughout the UK coal fields, though cumulatively, as Table 2.7 indicates, South Wales continued to have a substantially larger disabled community than elsewhere.

Many more miners were disabled by the disease than died from it. Added to the 40,000 or so officially recorded deaths from pneumoconiosis in the UK, there were three or four times that number of miners who suffered the seriously incapacitating form of this disease (Progressive Massive Fibrosis). No wonder, then, that dust was such a recurring motif in Bert Coombes's evocative autobiography of working in the South Wales pits in the 1920s and 1930s and in Orwell's *Wigan Pier* (1937).[104] Orwell talked of the mine atmosphere at the face 'black with coal dust', that 'you cannot see very far, because the fog of coal dust throws back the beam of your lamp' and that the dust 'stuffs up your throat and nostrils and collects along your

---

103 *Hansard*, 30 July 1958, pp. 1,540–51, cited in Scottish Home and Health Dept Records, Department of Health for Scotland NAS/HH104/29. One of our oral interview respondents from South Wales recalled one colleague dying of pneumoconiosis in his early twenties. The first mass x-ray survey over the five years 1959–63 found 1,047 cases of pneumoconiosis amongst miners under the age of 35 (out of a total of 56,009 pneumoconiotics).

104 On Coombes, see Chris Williams, '"Is a Working Man any Greater Value than the Dust?" Lung Disease in the Writings of B. L. Coombes', unpublished paper delivered at the 'Dust at Work' Conference, Glasgow Caledonian University, 28–29 May 2004.

Table 2.7   Proportion of the mining labour force in each region with pneumoconiosis, 1959–63

Region	%
South Western (South Wales)	25.3
South Eastern	15.5
Durham	14.3
Yorkshire	12.5
North Western	11.9
West Midlands	10.7
Northumberland and Cumberland	8.7
East Midlands	5.8
Scotland	5.7
Average	12.1*

Note: * 56,009 out of 462,999.

Source: NCB, Results of Periodic Chest Surveys. Letter, C.G. Gooding (Divisional Medical Officer, NCB Scottish Division) to Chief Medical Officer, Department of Health for Scotland, 11 September 1964, NAS/HH 104/42.

eyelids'.[105] Similarly Zweig was shocked in his 1948 study *Men in the Pits* by the extent of disability in mining communities: 'Nowhere else', he commented, 'can you see the same relative numbers of disabled men as in a colliery village.'[106] From his conversations with miners in the late 1940s, Zweig concluded that from the men's point of view, 'enemy number one in the pits is dust'.[107] Dust even featured in a rare depiction of mining life in the boy's comic/story book *The Rover* in 1950.[108] A few years later, in one pioneering epidemiological study in the Rhondda valley in South Wales in the early 1950s (using the relatively new x-ray surveillance techniques), it was discovered that over a third of the coal mining workforce had some level of pneumoconiosis.[109] Moreover, even more were afflicted with varying degrees of impairment to respiratory function in the bronchial tubes and airways. A mining area GP in Scotland (Dr Bell) recalled of the immediate post-Second World War period:

---

105 Orwell, cited in Thomas (ed.), *The Oxford Book of Work*, p. 385.

106 Zweig, *Men in the Pits*, p. 6.

107 Ibid., p. 118.

108 *The Rover* (22 July 1950). In this case, though, it was giant rats who threatened the 'heroic' group of six miners furiously digging to rescue colleagues buried by a pit explosion. We are indebted to Hilary Young for this reference.

109 For a full discussion of the Rhondda Fach study, see Chapter 4.

The miners, the older miners, middle-aged and older miners accepted the fact that the longer they worked in the pits the more breathless they became and the cough developed, got worse ... It was just one of these things they developed was this chronic bronchitis.[110]

In 1955, Dr Ian Jones, Chief Medical Officer of the Fife Health Board, began looking at the health records of 427 coal miners working at the Nellie pit, Lochgelly, Fife. He followed the progress of these men for 22 years. By 1977, he found that only 1 in 4 of the miners was in good health; 2 out of 3 of them had some form of disability related to mining, and 1 in 3 had chest problems; 1 in 4 of them had visited their GP in the previous two weeks – the average for Scotland regarding this was a little over 1 in 10. Jones concluded: 'It is clear that these miners and ex-miners experienced a considerable amount of ill health, especially when one bears in mind the very high level of health demanded of recruits into this industry.'[111]

The exact number of miners disabled by bronchitis and emphysema caused or exacerbated by working in dusty conditions will never be known. After these diseases were belatedly prescribed for benefit purposes in 1993, an average of almost 2,000 new cases were being diagnosed every year to the turn of the century.[112] However, some sense of the historical legacy can be gauged from the fact that at the 2004 deadline for miners and their families to register for compensation under the 1998 bronchitis and emphysema litigation against British Coal, a staggering 570,000 claims had been made.[113] Whilst it would be erroneous to claim that all coal miners had their breathing impaired from working underground in the heyday of deep-mining in the first three-quarters of the twentieth century, none the less occupation-related respiratory disease was a common, chronic and persistent problem which affected hundreds of thousands of mineworkers and their families in the twentieth century, whilst blighting whole mining communities.

Mining towns and villages were characterised by older ex-miners, wheezing and coughing up black phlegm, unable to walk short distances without a rest, and seeing out their days excluded from the social activities healthier men took for granted. Their experience of living with respiratory impairment is examined in some depth in Chapter 9, where we incorporate miners' own narratives provided in oral interviews and other personal testimonies. One comment we would make here, though, is that within such communities there was a great deal of acceptance of injury and erosion of bodily capacity, especially amongst the older generation. Davie Guy described prevailing attitudes in the Durham coal field in the 1950s:

I think in particular the old miners, they never went to the doctors with chest complaints because they witnessed the fathers and the grandfathers who had also worked in the mines, who had also suffered chest problems and I think they almost felt it was almost

---

110 Dr George Bell GP, Bellshill, Motherwell Museum Oral History Transcript, Interview 7 October 1992. We are indebted to Neil Ballantyne for this reference.

111 Labour Research Department, *The Hazards of Coal Mining* (London, 1989), p. 7.

112 *Annual Abstract of Statistics* (London, 2001), table 9.7, p 134.

113 Mick Antoniw, Interview C28 (SOHC).

inevitable that at some point in time in their lives they would start having problems with their chest, and there wasn't any real effective treatment for it. And so, they were *so hardy* people that the only occasions that they went to the doctors was when there was a broken limb involved or an amputated finger or something of that nature. You wouldn't get them going to the doctor for influenza or things of that nature, they didn't. The more recent generation, the younger ones, were more prone to go to the doctors, but the older ones, for whatever reason, people in my Dad's category … I can remember my Dad puncturing a hole in his foot with a windy-pick. And he came home, he took his shoe off and I could *see the hole, he must have broken bones in his foot*, and he was *wanting to go to work the next day*. He said it would be all right. He was reluctant to have any medical, or even hospital treatment for it. He eventually had to go to hospital with it, but the *willingness* wasn't there.[114]

What is evident is that miners were a diverse and complex collection of individuals, from markedly different coal field cultures across the country. Recent research has done much to refine the stereotypical image of the archetypal proletarian and to establish miners as part of a very heterogeneous community, with greatly contrasting work cultures, customs and practices prevailing across different coal fields. The same might be said about the impact of work upon the body, because social, economic and environmental conditions varied considerably from coal field to coal field, and even from pit to pit. Dusty pits, for example, had different effects upon the body than wet pits, and narrow seams affected posture differently to high seams.

All this inevitably begs a cluster of questions: Why did the most significant of Britain's occupational health tragedies occur? Who were responsible? When and how effectively was dust controlled in the pits? How did miners and their collective organisations react to this health crisis? And how were miners and their communities affected by the epidemic of dust disease? Amongst the most important factors affecting health and safety standards in the mines were the attitudes and policies of the employers and the state (in the labour market and as regulators), medicine and medical knowledge, changes in production methods, including mechanisation and automation, the strategies of the mining trade unions, and the prevailing lifestyles and work culture of men themselves. Discussion of the role of these key forces in relation to occupation-related respiratory disease in coal mining will ensue in the chapters that follow, as well as evaluation of workplace culture and detailed analysis of the impact of such occupational disability and death within mining communities. For the latter, we have relied heavily upon personal testimony, reconstructing miners' experience from a series of oral interviews. The dangers and risks associated with mining work had a fundamental impact upon miners' attitudes and consciousness, contributing to what Supple has called 'a most sensitive interdependence' of miners in the workplace and to the militancy of their trade unions and the bitterness of capital–labour relations.[115] These issues are explored in more detail in Parts III and

---

114 David Guy, Interview C44 (SOHC).
115 Supple, *The History of the British Coal Industry*, vol. 4, p. 431.

IV of this book. We turn initially, however, to the evolution of medical knowledge on respiratory disease in coal mining in the following three chapters.

PART II
Advancing Medical Knowledge on Dust Disease

Chapter 3

Coal Workers' Pneumoconiosis: Discovery and Denial

This chapter traces the emergence of coal miners' lung disease in the UK up to the early 1940s, with some reference to other countries. Important research on the evolution of silicosis as an industrial disease has been conducted by Melling and Bufton, and the reader should refer to their work for a full account of such developments.[1] What we want to do in this chapter is sketch in the foundations upon which the recognition of coal workers' pneumoconiosis (CWP) rested. As we will see in this and the following two chapters, the road towards having CWP, and later emphysema and bronchitis, accepted as compensatable diseases was a tortuous one with many detours and reversals. The whole process of disease recognition in coal mining revolved around an interaction of capital, the state, the medical profession, organised labour, and the workers themselves. Therefore, to some degree our research and conclusions relate to commentators who suggest that economic and social factors and issues of compensation are as important as advances in medical knowledge when it comes to state recognition of industrial disease.[2]

---

1   M.W. Bufton and J. Melling, '"A Mere Matter of Rock": Organized Labour, Scientific Evidence and British Government Schemes for Compensation of Silicosis and Pneumoconiosis among Coal Miners, 1926–1940', *Medical History*, vol. 49, no. 2 (1 April 2005), pp. 155–78; M.W. Bufton and J. Melling, 'Coming Up for Air': Experts, Employers and Workers in Campaigns to Compensate Silicosis Sufferers in Britain, 1918–1939', *Social History of Medicine*, vol. 18, no. 1 (2005), pp. 63–86; also J. Melling and M. W. Bufton, 'From Sandstone Dust to Black Lung: The Origins of Pneumoconiosis Regulation in the UK and its Impact on Miners' Compensation c. 1935–1945', unpublished paper delivered to 'Dust at Work' Conference, Glasgow Caledonian University, 28 May 2004; see also S. Morrison, 'The Factory Inspectorate and the Silica Dust Problem in the UK Foundries, 1930–1970', *Scottish Labour History*, vol. 40 (2005), pp. 31–50, and also her forthcoming PhD Thesis, 'The Impact of Silicosis in Scotland' (Glasgow Caledonian University); C. Mills, 'The Kinaird Commission: Siliceous Dust, the Pitfalls of Cause and Effect Correlations and the Case of the Cornish Miners in the Mid-nineteenth Century', *Scottish Labour History*, vol. 44 (2005), pp. 13–31.

2   A.E. Dembe, *Occupation and Disease: How Social Factors Affect the Conception of Work-related Disorders* (New Haven, CT, 1996), pp. 3–21, and *passim*. See also R. Gillespie, 'Accounting for Lead Poisoning: The Medical Politics of Occupational Health', *Social History of Medicine*, vol. 15, no. 3 (1990), pp. 303–31; B. Harrison, *Not Only the 'Dangerous Trades': Women's Work and Health in Britain, 1880–1914* (London, 1996); P. Bartrip, *The Home Office and the Dangerous Trades* (Amsterdam, 2004).

Early Recognition of Miners' Lung

Mining in all its forms has since earliest times been noted for being a dangerous and unhealthy occupation. It is from mining in the fourth-century BC that we get the first reference to an occupational illness, when Hippocrates recorded what seems to have been the symptoms of lead poisoning amongst miners. Later, Galen remarked on visits to Cyprus copper sulphate mines where the miners worked naked because sulphurous fumes destroyed clothing. We know that in the second century AD, those who toiled in gold, silver, lead and mercury mines tried to shield themselves from dust by wearing primitive bladder-skin masks. And in the mid-sixteenth century, Agricola and Paracelsus described a form of lung disease peculiar to miners.[3] As far as Britain was concerned, long before industrialisation, mining had a reputation for its notoriously unhealthy work processes.[4] However, it would be much later – in the nineteenth century – that the British medical profession began to take the health risks associated with breathing mine air seriously. In 1831, the Yorkshire physician Thackrah noted that miners suffered from asthma,[5] and in the same year another Scottish doctor Gregory, writing in the *Lancet*, also referred to what he called 'miners' asthma'. Gregory drew his evidence from the example of a 59-year-old patient named John Hogg who had worked in a Dalkeith colliery for twelve years – and it is interesting that Hogg himself had come to the conclusion that his disability had been caused by his work.[6] Gregory went so far as to warn medics in coal mining areas to be on the look out for the disease, appealing to:

> … these practitioners who reside in the vicinity of the great coalmines, and who may have charge of the health of miners, to the existence of a disease, to which that numerous class of the community would appear to be particularly exposed.[7]

At this time, most doctors presumed that the illness which miners like Hogg were succumbing to was the result of contaminated air caused by blasting or by exposure to soot from oil lamps.[8] In 1833, though, Marshall noted the occurrence of what he referred to as 'Black Spit' (*melanoptysis*) in the lungs of three long-serving Lanarkshire coal miners, and he attributed this to the excessive dustiness of some of the region's dry seam mines. Marshall also found that the lungs of the dead miners were ridden with black nodules and cavities which convinced him that the prime

---

3   G. Rosen, *A History of Public Health* (Baltimore, MD, 1993), pp. 22–3.

4   R.I. McCallum, 'Pneumoconiosis and the Coalfields of Durham and Northumberland', *Transactions of the Institution of Mining Engineers*, vol. 113 (1953–54), p. 99.

5   See C. Mills, 'The Kinaird Commission: Siliceous Dust, the Pitfalls of Cause and Effect Correlations and the Case of the Cornish Miners in the Mid-nineteenth Century', *Scottish Labour History*, 44 (2005), pp. 16–17.

6   A. Derickson, *Black Lung, Anatomy of a Public Health Disaster* (Ithaca, NY, 1998), p. 5.

7   P.F. Holt. *Pneumoconiosis, Industrial Diseases of the Lung Caused by Dust* (London, 1957), p. 160.

8   D. Hunter, *Diseases of Occupations* (London, 1975), p. 994.

cause was the inhalation of fine coal dust.[9] Further revelations followed. In 1837, the physician Thomson described a number of fatal lung cases from the Scottish pits of which the main symptoms were breathlessness (*dyspnoea*) and cough with a sputum which eventually became black. After collecting autopsies from nine dead miners, he found the lungs were infiltrated with black matter. The same year, Stratton from the North East of England became the first to use the term *anthracocis* – named after anthracite coal – to describe a particular lung disease of colliers; and it was around this time that a father-and-son team of Edinburgh doctors drew a clear distinction between the nodules found on the lungs of stone masons (silicosis) and the much darker agglomerations apparent in dead coal hewers' lungs.[10]

Towards the middle of the nineteenth century it became evident that the problem was widespread, as more and more cases of lung diseases amongst coal miners appeared in the medical literature. At the same time, the growing body of knowledge in Britain regarding the dangers of coal dust stimulated similar concerns in the USA.[11] Moreover, whereas some of the earlier authorities had posited that bad air and the use of explosives were the main causes, medical opinion began to slowly swing behind the notion that, as Gregory and Marshall had suggested, it was the mine dust itself that was causing the problems. In his 1861 Public Health Report, Sir John Simon drew attention to the relative freedom from chest complaints of miners in the north of England compared to those in Wales, and he attributed this to the differing standards of ventilation between the regions. The same report contained a survey by Dr Greenhow – based on statistics collected by local doctors – which indicated there was a prevalence of chest 'infections' in two Welsh regions, Merthyr Tydfil and Abergavenny. Greenhow then examined 53 miners from these regions and concluded that most of these men were suffering from a form of chronic bronchitis.[12]

For a hundred years or so after its first appearance in the medical literature, coal workers' lung disease was referred to by a range of terms, including anthraco silicosis, pseudo silicosis and miners' asthma.[13] In 1861, a committee appointed by Palmerston's government looked into dust disease in mines. Five years later, the general term pneumoconiosis was first used to describe this specific kind of condition, derived from the Greek words *pneumon*, meaning lung, and *conis* meaning dust. This name was to include eventually all the lung diseases thought to be caused by the inhalation of dusts, and included silicosis, brought about by inhaling silica; asbestosis, related to asbestos; sinderosis, caused by iron; byssinosis, caused by textile fibres, and – much later – coal miners' pneumoconiosis. The main point is that

---

9   Ibid.

10 Ibid., p. 995.

11 See Derickson, *Black Lung*, Chapter 1.

12 Medical Research Council (MRC), *Chronic Pulmonary Disease in South Wales: Coal Miners, Medical Studies* (1942), p. 140; henceforth MRC *Medical Studies*. It is interesting that these regions were to the east of the modern anthracite fields.

13 Ministry of Fuel and Power, *Dust Prevention and Suppression, Instructional Pamphlet No. 1: Water Infusion, a Means of Dust Control. By the South Western Committee on Dust Prevention and Suppression* (1955), p. 1.

by the 1860s it was accepted that coal miners suffered from a distinctive respiratory disease caused by inhaling coal dust, which, amongst other symptoms, caused the production of black spit, and ultimately, black lesions in the miners' lungs.

From the 1880s, the number of reported cases of anthracosis or miners' asthma declined. In his textbook on occupational health written in 1892, Arlidge noted this change in direction, saying there was 'a widespread belief at the present day that serious lesions of the lungs associated with the calling of coal getters, belong to past history …'.[14] However, it was clear that he believed such lesions were simply being attributed to other causes:

> That the lesions are deemed unusual, is due to the circumstances that they are not looked for. Their sufferers enter hospital wards for cough, and get labelled as having bronchitis or asthma, and thus fail to excite pathological interest. By this indifference to pathological research, we are deprived of a full and clear insight into the morbid anatomy of the miners' lungs.[15]

Crucially, in 1892 Arlidge described what would be accepted forty-five years later as the main characteristics of coal workers' pneumoconiosis:

> The inspired dust … enters within the lung tissue, colours it both superficially and deeply in proportion to the amount and duration of its inhalation, and provokes subinflammatory lesions ending in fibrosis, and marked by the symptoms of chronic bronchitis and by dyspnoea.[16]

However, the notion that miners' pneumoconiosis was disappearing from the pits persisted, and twenty years after Arlidge's pronouncements, the leading occupational health specialist Sir Thomas Oliver could boldly state:

> So much have the conditions of labour in the mines improved, that, apart from explosions coalmining is now a healthy occupation … Coal miners' phthisis or anthracosis is in this country in decline.[17]

And in 1914 Shufflebotham, an expert in Workmen's Compensation from Staffordshire – drawing much of his evidence from a Departmental Committee on Industrial Diseases in 1906–7 – remarked: 'at the present time in Great Britain fibrosis of the lungs amongst miners could be said to be practically non existent'.[18] Medical opinion of the time linked this apparent decline of miners' lung to a number

---

14 J.T. Arlidge, *The Hygiene Diseases and Mortality of Occupations* (London, 1892), p. 265.

15 Ibid.

16 Ibid., p. 262.

17 MRC, *Medical Studies*, p. 141.

18 Ibid.

of factors, including fifty years of improving mine ventilation, coupled with shorter working periods underground.[19]

However, it was no doubt the case that – as Arlidge had suggested – many thousands of miners continued to die from pneumoconiosis during the nineteenth and early twentieth centuries, but their deaths were recorded as tuberculosis, chronic bronchitis or asthma. It is also significant that much of the evidence pointing to a reduction in cases of anthracosis in the UK was derived from English and Scottish coal fields. However, little information was being collected from Wales, where in the 1880s and 1890s coal was being cut in increasing quantities in dusty pits using blasting. This lack of information was to have serious and unexpected repercussions, for in 1934, twenty years after Shufflebotham's optimistic observations, a Welsh Medical Officer of Health sounded the alarm: 'silicosis has caused a heavy toll in the anthracite district ... The miner in your area today is terror stricken by the thought of developing silicosis.'[20] One of the reasons for the sudden upsurge in silicosis cases was that miners were being exposed to increasing amounts of coal dust as well as rock dust. We return to analyse silicosis as a complicating dynamic in the understanding of miners' lung later in this chapter. Before this, though, we turn to other complicating medical issues.

Complicating Factors: Tuberculosis (TB) and Bronchitis

It is important to contextualise miners' lung disease against the background of general health in the UK in this period, when by far the most serious public health issue was TB.[21] Due to the contested nature of medical knowledge we should avoid interpreting medical understanding of miners' lung as a smooth upward trajectory. In 1896, for example, Greenhow – following on from his earlier conclusions – doubted that miners' lung disease was directly caused by dust, and suggested that chronic bronchitis aggravated by dust caused a form of pneumonia. As we will see in Chapter 5, it was only in the 1990s that bronchitis and emphysema were eventually but reluctantly accepted as diseases of coal miners – that is, with coal dust as the causal agent – despite the fact that evidence for this had existed from very early on.

Regardless of the growing body of evidence relating to miners' health, the notion that miners succumbed to a particular type of lung disease caused by dust inhalation was rejected by most doctors in the late nineteenth and early twentieth centuries, and one of the reasons for this was the difficulty in differentiating between TB and dust-induced respiratory disease. However, the picture was made even more complicated by the fact that several leading experts argued that mine dust *protected* miners from TB. The notion that coal dust was good for miners' health can be traced back to the eighteenth century. In 1763, a doctor named Clapier reputedly successfully treated a TB patient by arranging for him to live for a while in a French coal mine. Although

---

19 Hunter, *The Diseases of Occupation*, p. 994.
20 MRC, *Medical Studies*, p. 141.
21 See T. Dormandy, *The White Death: A History of Tuberculosis* (London, 1999).

the apparent success of this somewhat radical course of treatment was attributed by Clapier to the patient's inhalation of sulphur while down the mine, other medics held that it was the carbon itself which had produced the beneficial effect – the idea being that ulcers in the lung had been neutralised when they became coated with coal dust.[22] By the 1860s, doctors across Europe – including Greenhow in the UK – were speaking about the beneficial effect of coal dust in relation to the relatively low levels of TB amongst miners.[23] This was a compelling argument which reappeared in the 1880s and 1890s – although one that was rejected by Arlidge.[24] In the 1880s, Dr Smart argued that the low prevalence of TB amongst miners was the result of carbon's antiseptic characteristics, and in an address to the Edinburgh Health Society in 1883 he made these views crystal clear:

> Coal dust – or to call it by its proper name, carbon – from its highly antiseptic properties acts as an excellent protective to the pulmonary organs.[25]

In 1882, Koch discovered that TB was caused by a germ. This meant that from now on the distinction between TB and dust-induced lung disease was much easier to define. The invention of x-rays by Roentgen in 1895 also made for more accurate studies of the course of lung disease. However, the idea that miners were being guarded against TB by the nature of their working environment persisted throughout the late nineteenth century and into the twentieth. By 1924, for example, Sir Thomas Oliver – echoing Smart in the 1880s – argued that the copious amount of black spit which miners produced was doing them more good than harm, and other experts would stake their reputations on the beneficial effects of coal dust well into the 1930s.[26] Cummins, for instance, repeating medical opinion regarding the absorbing properties of coal dust voiced a hundred years earlier, suggested that coal dust absorbed the tuberculin of TB, which also made the presence of TB difficult to recognise in miners. Consequently, he argued, many deaths from TB had been recorded as silicosis or bronchitis. Clinical evidence from studies in the USA, the Ruhr, the USSR and from South Wales failed to support this notion.[27] Once again, though, the prestige surrounding British research influenced medics on the other side

---

22 J.C. Gilson, 'Is Coal Dust Harmful to Man?', *PRU Collected Papers*, vol. 4 (1954–55), paper no. 95 (1955), p. 245.

23 Ibid.

24 Arlidge, *The Hygiene Diseases and Mortality of Occupations*; A. McIvor, 'Work and health, 1880–1914: A note on a neglected interaction', *Scottish Labour History Society Journal*, vol. 24 (1989), pp. 14–32.

25 A. Smart, 'Note on Anthracosis', *British Medical Journal*, vol. 2 (5 September 1885), p. 493; *The Scotsman* (26 November 1883), p. 3.

26 Quoted in Derickson, *Black Lung*, p. 44.

27 MRC, *Medical Studies*, p. 155.

of the Atlantic, where the argument that mine air was conducive to good health was also gathering strength.[28]

The medical uncertainty and controversy regarding the connection between TB and coal dust disease was to some extent replicated by similar confusion over pneumoconiosis and bronchitis. In 1915, Collis utilised x-ray technology to argue that bronchitis, and not anthracosis, was the 'chief of all the pneumoconioses'.[29] This was also a view adhered to by J.S. Haldane. Haldane had initially conducted important research on miners' phthisis – a common nineteenth-century term for tuberculosis – amongst Cornish rock drillers, and in 1904 alerted the Royal Commission on Health and Safety in Coal Mines that men drilling hard rock in coal mines throughout the UK faced the same dangers as the Cornish miners. Between 1916 and 1918, Haldane was Director of the Doncaster Coal Owners' Research Laboratory, and it was during this period that he began to examine the causes of the high death rate amongst older coal miners in England and Wales. His eventual conclusion was that the chief culprit was bronchitis, brought about by 'over-breathing' during periods of physical exertion, accentuated by poor ventilation – which caused a rise in carbon dioxide levels. As far as dust inhalation was concerned, though, he surmised:

> There is no real statistical evidence of harm resulting from the inhalation of coal dust or shale dust in the quantities ordinarily breathed by miners, and a strong presumption that the dust they breathe protects them from serious dangers.[30]

Haldane's views became widely known. In 1916, *The Scotsman* reported on one of his talks on dust disease under the headline 'Healthy Coal Dust: Miners' Immunity from Consumption':

> Dr. J. S. Haldane, in an address on 'The health of old colliers' at the annual meeting of the Institution of Mining Engineers yesterday, said it was well known that colliers suffered very little from phthisis ... Coal dust certainly did not kill germs, but it had come to be regarded by medical men as a preventive of phthisis ...

Interestingly, he went on to get it completely wrong about the dangers of smoking too:

> Town dwellers and smokers might also take comfort to themselves in the thought that, in introducing smoke particles into their lungs, they were educating their lung epithelium to deal with really harmful foreign bodies.[31]

In 1942, the Medical Research Council (MRC) concluded that there were three main faults in Haldane's theories. Firstly, in the period before x-rays, many of the

---

28 See Derickson, *Black Lung*, Chapter 3, 'The Atmosphere in the Mine is now Vindicated'.

29 MRC, *Medical Studies*, p. 141.

30 Ibid., p. 142.

31 *The Scotsman* (9 June, 1916), p. 6.

cases which were being reported as bronchitis were probably silicosis, or indeed coal workers' pneumoconiosis. Secondly, it was very likely that what Haldane referred to as 'over-breathing' – due to increased levels of carbon dioxide or physical activity – would have resulted in the miners inhaling more coal dust. And thirdly, the MRC researchers noted that Haldane had not studied the position in the South Wales anthracite area, where there was a higher incidence of respiratory disease, but where the physical activity levels would not have been any higher than in the lower-incidence regions in England.[32] However – as we hope to stress throughout this book – the rejection of old knowledge and the acceptance of the new is a slow process, and even in the early 1940s the MRC's conclusion regarding miners and TB was still on the fence:

> From the compensation figures, together with the autopsy and clinical studies ... the view emerges that rock workers in coal mines who suffer from pneumokoniosis [*sic*] are specially liable to develop clinical tuberculosis in addition; and that colliers with pneumokoniosis also have a tendency to develop this complicating infection, though often in a modified form so that it may not be easy to recognize clinically and may even be difficult to determine at autopsy. There is still no clear evidence that, apart from pneumokoniosis, coal miners have a special liability to tuberculosis; indeed they may even prove to have a reduced liability ...[33]

In the early 1930s, Haldane modified his position, but only very slightly, when he took account of new statistics relating to coal miners' health:

> The data for each successive period from 1881 to 1911 had shown that coal mining was an occupation associated with a lower death rate than the average for all occupations ... The data for 1921–1931 showed, however, that coal mining had lost its lead.

However, he still believed that the underlying explanation for the trend was nothing to do with increased dust levels in the mines:

> The probable explanation of this is that after the war, in consequence of the great temporary demand for coal and the Seven Hours Act, a large number of men of inferior physique and experience were taken into the industry from outside.[34]

Moreover, although holding on to the notion that the root cause of bronchitis in the pits was physical exertion, he did concede that miners' lungs which had already been damaged by bronchitis or emphysema could have had their dust elimination capacities impaired – although he remained convinced that exposure to coal dust

---

32 MRC, *Medical Studies*, p. 142.

33 Ibid., p. 157.

34 J.S. Haldane, 'Silicosis and Coal Mining', *The Colliery Guardian*, (16 January 1931), p. 226; from a paper read before the Institution of Mining Engineers, London, 15 January 1931, p. 226.

really did protect against lung disease, and utilised other workers as a yardstick to prove his point:

> The relative immunity produced by coal dust is indicated by the low phthisis rate for coal boat loaders, as compared to the rather high rates for ordinary stevedores and for other dock labourers.[35]

Interestingly, as we will see in a later section, it was to be evidence drawn from coal trimmers at the docks with which the MRC would strengthen its argument that coal miners were succumbing to a disease directly linked to coal dust.

Haldane's belief regarding the benign nature of coal dust was replicated in his views on silica dust. For, once again, he was convinced that the bulk of silicosis cases were actually bronchitis. However, in the early 1930s he had to take account of x-ray evidence being provided by research conducted by the Welsh Memorial Association. Melling and Bufton illustrate how important this organization was in highlighting the incidence of dust disease, with the first x-rays of miners being conducted by a TB expert. As early as 1926, Tattersall published a paper on silicosis drawing attention to the risks faced by miners working in hard rock. His paper, combined with a later publication in 1931, began to convince Haldane of the significance of the silica problem.[36] The research indicated that prolonged mine work – especially in the Welsh anthracite mines – produced a distinctive lung x-ray, which suggested silicosis. As far as Haldane was concerned, though, although accepting there was a danger from silica, the problem was very rare, and in the conclusion to a 1931 article he placed the emphasis firmly back on to bronchitis:

> Neither the Registrar-General's statistics nor any other evidence whatsoever show that any class of work in coal mining is subject to risk from silicosis except under very exceptional conditions that can be guarded against effectively. Nor is there any clear evidence that dust inhalation by coal miners is an ordinary cause of either bronchitis or pneumonia among them, *although it seems practically certain that excessive inhalation of coal dust or shale dust must cause bronchitis*, and ought therefore to be avoided.[37]

In 1933, he stated in an article entitled 'Silicosis in Coal-mining Employment': 'there were very few real cases of silicosis among coal-miners.'[38] By this time, Haldane was an Honorary Professor and Director of the Mining Research Laboratory at Birmingham University.[39] However, his prestige did not protect him from peer criticism. In 1934, for example, he became involved in a very public argument across the pages of the *Western Mail and South Wales News* with another occupational

---

35 Haldane, 'Silicosis and Coal Mining', p. 226.

36 Melling and Bufton, 'From Sandstone Dust to Black Lung'.

37 Haldane, 'Silicosis and Coal Mining', p. 315; emphasis added.

38 *Western Mail and South Wales News* (15 January 1935).

39 This unit was subsidised by SMRB and Imperial Chemical Industries; Safety in Mines Research Board (SMRB), *Second Annual Report* (1937), p. 110; also MSWCOA, Research Committee, *Eight Annual Report* (February 1943), p. 5.

health expert, Dr W.R. Jones, over Jones's work on the nature of silica dust damage. Jones argued that the chief mineral present in the lungs of damaged miners was not quartz or any form of free silica, but the needle-like fibres of sericite, a silicate of potassium and aluminium.[40] Haldane strongly disagreed, and in the exchange which followed, Jones accused Haldane of repeatedly contradicting himself, and of using 'his powerful influence' to oppose theories.[41] In criticising Jones's ideas, though, Haldane also took the opportunity to hammer home his own points of view regarding the centrality of bronchitis:

> I should like to add that any condition which tends to produce bronchitis or bronchial catarrh among men who are exposed to dust inhalation ought to be carefully avoided. The lungs can deal in the most wonderfully effective manner, so long as they are healthy, with all ordinary forms of dust, except concentrated free silica or active poisons; but they lose this capacity, more or less, if bronchitis is present.[42]

And a month later he reiterated this point in relation to the same anthracite coal regions where the MRC would very soon positively conclude that a disease called coal workers' pneumoconiosis existed:

> As regards the anthracite district in which they are so common ... They are, I believe, primarily cases of bronchitis, but aggravated by the secondary collection in the lungs of coal and other dust.[43]

It would appear, then, that coal was being now accepted as an 'aggravating' agent, and not a protective one.

In Haldane's last paper, published in 1939, soon after his death, his original thesis was again slightly modified. In this paper, he had to take account of x-ray evidence which was increasingly showing that Welsh colliers working at the coal face – and not just those working on hard rock – were succumbing to lung disease. Consequently, Haldane and his fellow researchers embraced the argument of Dr T.D. Jones, who was soon to acquire the nickname 'Spake Jones'. Most of the anthracite mines in Wales had no shafts, and access was by means of inclines. In most cases men entered and left the mine on trains, known as spakes, which usually ran in the main intake airway. Consequently, according to 'Spake' Jones, as the trains approached the surface, the men were exposed to the chilling effect of a considerable wind, and, when the spakes emerged from the warm mines in cold weather, to rapidly

---

40 *The Times* (3 May 1934), p. 15.
41 *Western Mail and South Wales News* (15 January 1935).
42 *Western Mail and South Wales News* (19 December 1934).
43 *Western Mail and South Wales News* (24 January, 1935).

falling temperatures.[44] It was this constant chilling, then, which was making the men especially liable to bronchitis.[45]

Even by the early 1930s, though, Haldane's arguments were already swimming against a tide of evidence that had been growing for some time. The availability of clinical and radiological studies, an increase in the number of miners' autopsies, and the accessibility of more accurate mortality statistics meant that the study of miners' lung diseases became much more precise.[46] Increasingly, it became more and more apparent that mine dust, and not TB or bronchitis, was the main culprit behind the escalation of miners' respiratory problems. However, as the next section will illustrate, for some time the hazards of coal dust were to be overshadowed by the focus on the silica danger.

Complicating Factors: Silica

The eventual recognition of the dangers of silica dust was a crucial stage in the history of miners' lung. However, the acceptance that rock dust in the mine air was hazardous to health would also act as a complicating factor which delayed the wider appreciation that dust given off when working with coal was dangerous too. Like many aspects of the work–health interaction, the history of silicosis is one in which much denial and delay preceded an eventual recognition of occupational causation.[47] The Second Report of the Royal Commission on Mines of 1906–11 referred to the dangers of inhaling dust when siliceous stone was being broken up, but concluded that it was only men who were using rock drills on hard rock who would be affected. By this time, the use of water on drills was obligatory in the Cornish tin mines, and the Royal Commission – taking on board Haldane's warning – recommended that this stipulation should be extended to such work in other areas.[48] This became a requirement under the 1911 Coal Mines Act. This Act replaced all regulations in mines which had been directed towards health and safety, and specified that inspections of working places and certain roadways had to be made during working shifts. More importantly from the point of view of miners' respiratory disease, the 1911 Act also attempted to specify standards of adequate ventilation.[49] However,

---

44 MRC, *Chronic Pulmonary Disease in South Wales Coal Miners, Environmental Studies* (1943), p. 68.

45 The MRC would later spend a considerable amount of time investigating the spake theory but concluded that as far as a cause of pulmonary disease was concerned sudden changes in atmospheric humidity was not a viable explanation; MRC, *Medical Studies*, pp. 77–8.

46 Ibid., p. 152.

47 Melling and Bufton, 'From Sandstone Dust to Black Lung'.

48 See C. Mills, 'A Hazardous Bargain: Occupational Risk in Cornish Mining 1875–1914', *Labour History Review*, vol. 70, no. 1 (April 2005), pp. 53–73.

49 Sir Andrew Bryan, *The Evolution of Health and Safety in Mines* (Letchworth, 1975), p. 74. Hunter, *The Diseases of Occupations*, p. 213.

although much of this would bring some benefit to men who dug coal, the emphasis was still very much on workers who drilled hard rock. This emphasis would disguise the much wider danger of respiratory mine dust for some time to come.

It was not until after the First World War that those suffering from the effects of silica dust inhalation were liable to any compensation, and one of the main difficulties here was differentiating between dust-induced disease and other respiratory diseases such as bronchitis, tuberculosis or pneumonia. The Workmen's Compensation (Silicosis) Act 1918 (introduced in 1919) allowed for compensation to be paid to men who could prove they had worked in rock which contained no less than 80% silica. Under this scheme, employers had to pay into a joint fund from which miners would subsequently be compensated. The 1918 Act also introduced periodic medical examinations, and from 1919, any men found to be suffering from silicosis, or silicosis with TB, were to be suspended from the industry. These regulations were amended in 1925, and in 1929, under the Various Industries (Silicosis) Scheme of 1928, compensation became payable to coal miners employed in drilling and blasting in siliceous rock, if they had been certified as disabled through silicosis – by a medical panel from 1931 – or from silicosis accompanied by tuberculosis. As Melling and Bufton have shown, the factors underlying the acceptance of the health-impairing effects of silica on mine workers were complex, with pressure from the miners' unions playing a crucial role in getting the restrictive 1928 silicosis legislation amended in 1935, when the provision that silicotics had to prove they had been working with rock containing free silica was dropped.[50]

As we will explore in some depth in Chapter 7, it was during this period that the South Wales Miners' Federation (SWMF) began pushing for more research into the coal dust problem in the anthracite districts of South Wales – where, by the 1930s, the vast majority of pneumoconiotics were to be found. Due in great part to trade union pressure, then, the silicosis scheme was extended to all underground colliery workers. A consequence of this legislation was that for the purpose of diagnosis and the issue of certificates, a large number of x-rays and coal miners' autopsies were collected from throughout the UK. It was from this growing mass of hard evidence that the peculiarities of the Welsh coal fields began to be discerned.[51] What became more and more evident was that the great majority of silicosis cases were from the anthracite districts of South Wales, and crucially, that many of these men had never worked on rock.

At this time, several eminent doctors were arguing persuasively that bronchitis was the principal respiratory condition suffered by coal miners, and that the main enemy in mining was silica dust, and not coal dust. Indeed, Collis suggested that in contrast to the beneficial protective effect of inhaling coal dust, exposure to dust containing

---

50 For a full account, see Melling and Bufton, '"A Mere Matter of Rock"'; also Melling and Bufton, 'From Sandstone Dust to Black Lung'.

51 MRC, *Medical Studies*, p. 152.

crystalline silica could cause TB.[52] The whole field of inquiry was becoming muddied and confused, so much so that in 1935 the mining engineer Cullen suggested that medical opinion should be ignored and that efforts should be targeted at eradicating all dust in the mine atmosphere, whether it contained silica or not.[53] By this time, the government was also coming under more and more pressure – much of this from the miners' trade unions – to look into the dust issue, and questions were being asked in the House of Commons by the Welsh MP James Griffiths. Investigative journalism, as we will see in Chapter 7, was also playing a significant role by exposing the conditions of pneumoconiotic miners in South Wales. The government's response to what was fast becoming a heated contest between conflicting medical opinions was to delegate the issue to the judgement of experts at the MRC's Industrial Pulmonary Disease Committee, and we shall be looking at this in some detail later on.

A similar set of circumstances was unfolding in the USA, where accumulating evidence that coal dust was harmful to miners was also being buried under the weight of attention being placed on silica. Much of this had initially been driven by British research.[54] However, in 1933 a large-scale study of Pennsylvania miners conducted by the US Public Health Service concluded that the increasingly common respiratory disease amongst the workforce was a modified form of silicosis.[55] The Pennsylvania survey team took medical and industrial histories, and conducted x-ray and clinical examinations of the miners. Investigations were also taken regarding the working environments, including temperature humidity and ventilation. Atmospheric dust concentrations were also ascertained, and the number of particle years per cubic foot of air for each employee was calculated to gauge the miners' total dust exposure over the course of their employment – expressed as the 'weighted average dust concentration'. The main conclusions of the Pennsylvania study were: that there *was* a serious incidence of disabling pulmonary disease attributable to dust amongst US anthracite miners; that this was common amongst colliers as well as those working on rock; that the degree of disability increased with the severity of the disease, and that periods of service and the concentrations of dust which the miners were exposed to were important factors. However, although the free silica content of the dust was a factor, the evidence for this was unclear.[56] This large-scale US study was later

---

52 Derickson, *Black Lung*, pp. 48–9. Collis's pronouncements had a big impact in the USA, where the spotlight was turned on the silica problem for some time to come.

53 NCB Scientific Department, *Pneumoconiosis Field Research, The Study of the Composition of Respirable Dust in the Pneumoconiosis Field Research* (1960), p. 2.

54 See D. Rosner, and G. Markowitz, *Deadly Dust: Silicosis and the Politics of Occupational Disease in Twentieth-century America* (Princeton, NJ, 1994); Derickson, *Black Lung*, p. 48.

55 MRC, *Medical Studies*, p. 148; for a full account of the Pennsylvania Miners' asthma study, see Derickson, *Black Lung*, pp. 94–7.

56 Ibid.

utilised as a model for the planning of the MRC's groundbreaking research in South Wales.[57]

Other countries also conducted important research into coal dust disease in the inter-war period. In the USSR between 1930 and 1935, a team from the Ukrainian Central Tuberculosis Institute and the Donetz Institute for Industrial Hygiene carried out an extensive field study of miners from an anthracite mine and two bituminous mines in the Donetz Basin. The home and working environments of the men as well as their medical conditions were assessed. As was the case with the US studies, the incidence of pneumoconiosis of anthracite miners was found to be higher than amongst those working in the bituminous mines – although the contrast was not as stark as that found by the American investigators. At this time, the Soviet authorities were taking steps to protect miners who were thought to be at risk from lung disease. New entrants to the industry were carefully vetted and medically examined; miners with evidence of dust damage were transferred to more suitable jobs; pensions were granted to pneumoconiotics at an earlier age than normal; selected miners received a month's annual holiday and an extra pint of milk a day, and at-risk miners were taught breathing exercises and offered treatment at spas and sanatoria.[58] In Australia, 477 non-anthracite miners in New South Wales were investigated in 1930, and 26 were found to have pulmonary fibrosis – a chronic lung condition characterised by shortness of breath. Similar studies with analogous findings were conducted in Germany in 1925; Sweden in 1926; France in the early 1930s; and Belgium in the mid-1930s. Most of these studies found that pulmonary fibrosis was most common amongst men with over ten years' service, and that this was the case with colliers as well as hard rock miners.[59]

Research was also conducted in Southern Rhodesia in 1938, but this was less conclusive. However, the experience of South African mining was utilised in other ways in the UK. In 1913–14, the Royal Commission on Metalliferous Mines and Quarries acknowledged the important research being carried out in South Africa, which at this time was ahead of the UK regarding knowledge of the silicosis hazard and measures to curtail it. By the early years of the twentieth century, the high incidence of silicosis and TB in South Africa had severely disrupted the gold mining industry, and x-rays were being used to detect the disease amongst miners. Moreover, South African Mines and Works legislation of this period gave the dust issue particular attention:

> No person shall in any part of the mine move any broken rock or ground, if such rock or ground is in a dusty condition, unless and until it and the floor, roof and sides of the

---

57 MRC, *Medical Studies*, p. 145; S.A. Roach, 'A Method of Relating the Incidence of Pneumoconiosis to Airborne Dust Exposure', *British Journal of Industrial Medicine*, vol. 10 (1953), p. 220.

58 MRC *Medical Studies*, p. 151.

59 Ibid.

working place, to a distance of at least 25 feet, have been effectively wetted and kept wet so as to prevent the escape of dust into the air during removal.[60]

The South African legislation also stipulated that dry mines had to have an adequate supply of water at every working place to prevent the formation of dust.[61] A good example of South African knowledge of the mine dust problem being utilised in the UK occurred in 1925, when the Health Advisory Committee of the Mines Department capitalised on the expertise of Dr H. Pirow, an Inspector of Mines of the South African Government, to investigate working conditions of rock drillers in Somerset and South Wales.[62] Pirow later extended his investigations into Scotland, Northumberland, South Yorkshire, Lancashire, and North and South Wales, and produced a detailed report of working conditions in these areas before he returned to South Africa.[63] In 1934, Cummins of the Cardiff Medical School illustrated there were clear similarities in the x-rays of South African gold miners and those miners working in South Wales.[64] And it is also interesting that one of the first dust particle counting machines, the Konimeter, was invented by the South African Sir Robert Kozé.[65] The British Mines Department was so impressed by this that it adopted an arbitrary standard based on the South Africa dust measuring initiatives. However, whereas South African legislation recommended that up to 300 p.p.c.c. (particles per cubic centimetre) was a safe working limit, the corresponding measurement in the UK was 450 p.p.c.c.[66]

Therefore, by the late 1930s the dangers of silica dust were widely understood in Britain and other countries, and advancing knowledge of the hazards and methods to combat them was being transferred between countries. The emphasis, though, was very firmly on silica. Therefore, although the majority of miners worked amongst coal dust, they were still not widely perceived to be at risk from lung damage.

The State, the Private Coal Companies and the Dust Problem in the 1930s and 1940s

As the growing medical awareness of miners' respiratory diseases unfolded, some of the earliest measures directed at the mine dust problem were implemented by coal companies in South Wales. By the early 1930s, employment in the South Wales coal

---

60 J.H. Davies, 'Methods of Preventing Miners' Silicosis and some other Lung Diseases in the Anthracite District', in South Wales Miners' Federation, Anthracite District, *The Prevention of Silicosis and Anthracosis* (n.d.), p. 6.

61 Davies, 'Methods of Preventing Miners' Silicosis' p. 6.

62 Safety in Mines Research Board, *Annual Report* (1926), pp. 38–9.

63 Ibid.

64 Melling and Bufton, 'From Sandstone Dust to Black Lung'.

65 *Royal Commission on Safety in Coal Mines Report* (1938), Cmd. 5890, p. 462.

66 Ibid.

industry was around half its 1920 figure.[67] However, coal mining was still the most important industry in South Wales, and was in the early stages of mechanisation. Several of the private coal companies here became proactive in addressing the silica dust problem, while at the same time perpetuating the notion that rock dust was the only danger to miners' respiratory health. The Monmouthshire and South Wales Coal Owners' Association (MSWCOA) set up its own Coal Dust Research Committee in 1937 and was conducting research at the same time as the MRC was becoming involved. This employers' research committee had a sound understanding of the complexities of dust-induced respiratory disease, fully realising that dust particles of less than 5 microns in size were the main cause of respiratory health problems. However, the Committee was convinced by the argument that silica dust and not coal dust was the main threat.[68] To some degree this is understandable given the medical uncertainly regarding the dangers of mine dust at this time, and the employers drew further reassurances from several speakers at the 1938 International Conference on Silicosis who also adhered to the silica argument.[69] Therefore, in contrast to the views of the Miners' Federation of Great Britain, the MSWCOA Coal Dust Research Committee was convinced that only men exposed to silica were in danger and in need of protection.[70]

The rising number of silicosis certifications in South Wales and the mounting costs of compensation were – according to several employers' accounts – pushing some coal companies towards bankruptcy.[71] Consequently, some mine owners began to devote serious attention towards developing and implementing dust suppression measures. The chairman of the Amalgamated Anthracite Company noted in 1937 that £800,000 in compensation had been paid out in South Wales for silicosis, and that this was 'reason enough to compel everyone to make an effort to rid the coal field of the worst menace that has ever confronted it'.[72] The following quote from the Chairman of the Monmouthshire and South Wales Coalowners' Association is further illustration of the alarm being felt by owners at this time:

> ... from the information supplied by experts, it is inevitable that there will be some extension of the regulations, and the owners must try and ensure these extensions are as small as possible. Silicosis affects South Wales more than any other district in the country, and medical examination might prove many men to be suffering from silicosis who were not previously aware of it. And resultant claims for compensation would be inevitable. It

---

67 M. Bloor, 'No Longer Dying for a Living: Collective Responses to Injury Risks in South Wales Mining Communities, 1900–47', *Sociology*, vol. 36, no. 1 (2002), p. 89.

68 Monmouthshire and South Wales Coal Owners' Association, Coal Dust Research Committee, *Ninth Annual Report* (July 1943), pp. 11–12.

69 Ibid., pp. 7–9.

70 Ibid., pp. 16–17.

71 Ibid.

72 *Western Mail and South Wales News* (18 April 1938).

is not thought to be in the interests of the trade to apply a medical examination to men at present in the employ of the owners.[73]

Notwithstanding the frequently hard-hearted nature of the employers' responses to the growing dust hazard, the knowledge base that was built up in South Wales regarding dust suppression – by the employers and by the South Wales Miners' Federation – was to prove vitally important to the NCB in the post-Second World War period in its attempts to tackle the dust problem. For although efforts were initially directed at protecting men drilling and handling rock which contained at least 50% free silica, important technological progress was made in the development of wet drilling, mist projectors and the spraying of faces with water before shot blasting.[74] Dust suppression efforts were also directed towards mechanical coal cutting. By 1942, the dust committee of the MSWCOA was beginning to realise that respirable dust generated by mechanical cutting was posing an even bigger threat to the future of the industry than coal dust's combustible potential:

It is true to say that the Coal Dust problem on machine cut faces in some of the South Wales collieries has reached such proportions that the days of coal cutters in these collieries were definitely numbered. Planning has taken place with the view of eliminating coal cutters in future faces.[75]

If mechanised coal cutting was to progress, then, dust suppression had to be utilised.

The oldest form of industrial dust control involved the use of water. Indeed, a patent was taken out in 1713 for a spraying process to address the dust problem in the pottery industry.[76] In 1901, a German book entitled *Ventilation in Mines* referred to a system which would later appear in the UK in the early 1940s as water infusion:

The Meissner system of wetting the coal face consists in drilling one to three holes to a depth of 40 inches in the coal during the shift preceding that in which the coal is to be worked. A half-inch iron pipe is then fitted into each hole by the aid of a wooden washer, and connected up with the supply pipe, the water pressure being then allowed to act on the coal for eight hours. In this manner the coal is so completely permeated with moisture that the formation of dust in winning coal is precluded. This method, however, does not act in the case of very hard or fissured coal, in which event, the working face and the won coal must be the more frequently and thoroughly sprinkled with the hose.[77]

---

73 Bloor, 'No longer dying for a living', p. 96.

74 NUM, South Wales Area Council, *Annual Conference Report, 1962–1963*, p. 11; also L.R. James, *The Control of Dust in Mines* (Cardiff, 1959), p. ix.

75 MSWCOA Research Committee, *Seventh Annual Report* (1942), p. 3.

76 L.R. James, *The Control of Dust in Mines* (Cardiff, 1959), p. 6.

77 Ministry of Fuel and Power, *Dust Prevention and Suppression, Instructional Pamphlet no. 1*, p. 4.

As we will discuss in Chapter 7, in the mid-1930s the South Wales Miners' Federation was suggesting to the mine owners methods to deal with the issue of mine dust, and in 1936 the owners came in for scathing criticism for inaction. However, by the early 1940s some employers were applying effective dust suppression techniques. In 1942, for example, a successful trial using water to suppress dust generated by coal cutters at Ferndale Colliery was looked upon as a lifeline by some of the South Wales coal owners. This 'Ferndale Method' which caused so much excitement involved directing water onto the coal cutting machine's jib, chain, and cutter picks:

> A large proportion of the water used is carried into the cut by the motion of the chain and picks, and this action ensures thorough mixing of the water with the cuttings at the point where the fines are produced, and where the turbulence and time aid in mixing the water and dust. In this way, the whole of the cuttings, coarse and fine, were effectively damped throughout the pile both inside and outside the cut.[78]

The employers were also pleased to learn that there were several important fringe benefits which accrued from using water on coal cutting machines. For example, the water acted as a lubricant which helped prevent the cutters jamming – or 'freezing', as the machinemen called it. It was also assumed that the use of water in coal cutting had the potential to reduce the danger of mine explosions caused by gas ignition.[79] Water suppression techniques spread throughout the South Wales coal fields, and to other mining areas soon after.[80]

The MSWCOA's Coal Dust Research Committee was also pioneering methods of sampling mine dust. The quantity and rate of fall of coarser dust particles was determined by catching the dust in flat metal trays placed on the ground. However, it was realised, even in this early period, that the main danger to the miners was from the finer dust that remained suspended in the air and was frequently carried some distance from its source. But the overriding problem was the fact that an accurate dust measuring device suited to mine conditions was not available.[81] As we will examine in some depth in Chapter 5, this technological problem would not be properly addressed for a long time to come.

Another technical problem related to the growing realisation of the dangers of mine dust was how to produce an effective dust respirator. As early as 1923, the Department of Scientific and Industrial Research was working on the development of such a device. [82] Early versions were inefficient and difficult to breathe through, but by 1934 a satisfactory respirator had been developed. According to the Mines Department's Health Advisory Committee, this respirator was suitable for workers

---

78 MSWCOA Research Committee, *Seventh Annual Report*, p. 3.

79 Ibid., pp. 12–13.

80 Ministry of Fuel and Power, *Dust Prevention and Suppression, Instructional Pamphlet no. 1*, p. 2.

81 MSWCOA, Research Committee, *Seventh Annual Report*, p. 5.

82 SMRB, *Annual Report, 1932–33*, p. 38.

in dusty processes in both mines and quarries. However, it was made clear by the Safety in Mines Research Board that the respirator was only to be used as a last resort when all other methods of dust suppression had failed:

> It can hardly be disputed that, in processes which give rise to much dust, the collection or extraction of dust as near as possible to the point at which it is produced is by far the best way of protecting the workers against the harmful effects or inconvenience of inhaling such dust. When, however, it is impossible to prevent the dust from entering the atmosphere which the workers breathe, the most practical method of protection appears to be the wearing of respirators.[83]

The new rubber mask fitted closely around the wearer's nose and lower part of the face, and had filter pads on each side which could be discarded when contaminated. According to the *Western Mail and South Wales News*, the mask was 'so comfortable to breathe through that all suggestion of fatigue is eliminated'.[84] The Royal Commission on Safety in Coal Mines Report of 1938 recommended that respirators were required in certain circumstances, and especially in mines where there was a history of silicosis.[85] However, as we will see in Chapter 5, the notion that masks were only to be used as a *last* line of defence was to become a cornerstone of dust control underground. One of the consequences of this was that it would be another fifty years before coal miners habitually put on dust masks before starting work at the coal face.

Clearly, then, although much of the effort was focused on the silica issue, state involvement and private initiative in the inter-war period, combined with trade union pressure and changing medical opinion, were vitally important in the preliminary attack on the coal dust problem. As the MRC began its investigations into pneumoconiosis in 1936, the Royal Commission on Safety in Coal Mines was under way (1935–38), at which the Miners' Federation of Great Britain was campaigning to extent the limited dust regulations of the 1911 Act. The Royal Commission expressed the wish that the MRC's investigation would throw much-needed light on the problem. However, no doubt in response to trade union demands, the Commission also recommended that something needed to be done in the interim:

> The rapid growth in the incidence of the disease, especially in South Wales, and the distress which it causes, are too serious to permit of indefinite delay while that knowledge is being sought, and we felt that such tentative measures of dust prevention as have proved reasonably effective ought to be enforced without delay wherever they appear to be necessary.[86]

When the MRC became involved with the mine dust hazard the media reported strong collaboration between the government, the owners and the miners and their

---

83 SMRB, *Annual Report, 1934*, p. 49.

84 *Western Mail and South Wales News* (22 July 1938).

85 *Royal Commission on Safety in Coal Mines Report* (1938), Cmd. 5890, p. 466.

86 Ibid., p. 460.

trade unions.[87] However, the fight against dust disease in the UK in the years before nationalisation was a factional one, and especially so in South Wales, where the company doctors were treated with mistrust by the miners. Moreover, although some employers paid lip service to the need to address the dust problem – by initiating dust suppression measures and by setting up investigative committees – much of this was driven by the necessity of ensuring that mechanisation was allowed to proceed unhindered. The government for its part was forced into responding to the dust problem by the escalating costs of compensation, the increasing political heat of the topic, and most importantly, by the determination of the miners' trade unions to challenge accepted medical opinion.

The Rediscovery of Coal Dust Disease: Medical Research Council (MRC) Research

The increasing attention directed towards miners' respiratory health in the inter-war period needs to be seen against the background of a growing awareness of the importance of workplace health in general. In 1913, the MRC was established, and a decision was taken at its first meeting that the investigation of certain industrial diseases should be part of its remit.[88] With the outbreak of the First World War, the MRC was drawn in to the urgent problem of how to increase war production, and one of the most pioneering state initiatives into the work–health interaction was the setting up of the Health of Munitions Workers' Committee (HMWC) in 1914. Although the HMWC was disbanded at the end of the war, the MRC decided that the high priority placed on workplace health and efficiency during the war should continue, and from this the Industrial Fatigue Research Board came into being in 1918, which changed its name to the Industrial Health Research Board (IHRB) in 1928.[89] The main difference between this organisation and the HMWC was that, whereas the HMWC had looked only at one sector (munitions workers), the IHRB began investigating the work–health interaction across a broad range of work activity.

In 1930, following a request from the Home Office, the MRC set up an Industrial Pulmonary Diseases Committee (IPDC):

> ... for further research into morbid conditions due to the inhalation of dust associated with occupation. The practical importance of the subject may be gauged by the fact that one of these conditions, silicosis, had been certified as the cause of over 300 deaths annually in

---

87 'Silicosis Inquiry Co-operation', *Western Mail and South Wales News* (18 April 1938).

88 P.D. D'Arcy Hart and E.M. Aslett, 'Chronic Pulmonary Disease in South Wales Coal Mines: An Eye Witness Account of the MRC Surveys (1937–1942)', *Society for the Social History of Medicine*, vol. 11, no. 3 (1998), pp. 459–68.

89 A. McIvor, 'Manual Work, Technology, and Industrial Health, 1918–39', *Medical History*, vol. 31 (1987), pp. 160–89.

England and Wales during the last three years, and has cost in compensation alone more than £100,000 in a single year.[90]

The IPDC was to play a vital role in the rediscovery of black lung in the UK. In the spring of 1935, Haldane informed the IPDC of the differences of opinion amongst medical experts regarding the silica problem in mine dust. At the same time, the Chief Medical Officer of the Silicosis Medical Board (SMB), Dr C.L. Sutherland, was keeping the Committee fully informed of the ever-increasing number of claims for compensation pouring in from South Wales. The ratio of rejected compensation claims to the total number had risen from 22% in 1933 to 50% in 1935.[91] It was against this background, then, that the IPDC decided to investigate. Subsequently, a meeting was arranged in Cardiff of medical specialists, disabled workers and workers' representatives, and this was followed by a meeting with Sutherland and other officials of the SMB.[92] The SMB produced radiographic evidence of a different type of respiratory disease to classic silicosis. The SMB called this new phenomenon 'disease x', and the IPDC noted in its minutes in 1936:

> There is amongst South Wales coal-miners a type of pulmonary disease which is disabling but which does not come within the radiographic definition of silicosis. This disease is due to employment and is prevalent.[93]

The IPDC was convinced of the need for a full investigation, and relayed this immediately to the MRC and then to the Home Office.[94] The IPDC had recently completed an analysis of dust inhalation amongst aluminium workers in Kinlochleven in the Scottish Highlands, and it was decided that any large-scale clinical and radiological study of coal miners would be based on this successful project. Dr Philip D'Arcy Hart – seconded from the MRC – was put in charge of the study, and he was assisted by Dr Edward Aslett of the Welsh National Memorial Association. The team also included mining engineers and pathologists.[95] After some departmental wrangling over who would pay for the two-year project, the IPDC was given the go-ahead to begin its investigations in 1937.

Before the research got under way, the IPDC suggested to the Home Office that compensation law be changed immediately to allow disabled workers and their

---

90 P. D'Arcy Hart, 'Chronic Pulmonary Disease in South Wales Coal Mines: An Eye Witness Account of the MRC Surveys', *The Society for the Social History of Medicine* (1998), p. 460.

91 Industrial Pulmonary Disease Committee (IPDC), Minutes, 28 May 1936, PRO, FD1/2884.

92 Letter from the Home Office to MRC, 23 May 1936; MRC to HO, 18 June 1936; Minutes of a Special Meeting of IPDC, Cardiff, 17 June 1936, PRO, FD1/2884.

93 IPDC Minutes, 16 July 1936, PRO, FD1/2884.

94 IPDC Minutes 23 October 1936; IPDC Memorandum, 20 November 1936, PRO, FD1/2884.

95 Hart and Aslett, 'Chronic Pulmonary Disease', pp. 459–61; see D'Arcy Hart's eyewitness account of the MRC project in this article, pp. 461–8.

families to claim relief. However, the Home Office rejected this on the grounds that it would set a dangerous precedent, because no other occupational disease had ever been scheduled without evidence of its causation.[96] It was also becoming apparent by this time that there were too many technicalities preventing compensation being paid even to those men who were positively diagnosed with silicosis. For example, on rejecting a miner's claim at Aberdare in 1934, a judge expressed his sympathy for the obviously disabled claimant. This particular miner had been working on the 'process' – meaning on silica rock – a month before he was certified, and also for a period in 1928. However, because he had not been drilling or blasting within the three years immediately prior to March 1933, his claim for compensation had to be disallowed.[97] Clearly, then, the IPDC investigation was timely.

In advance of commencing field work, the IPDC collected statistics on the rates of silicosis in the South Wales coal mines from HM Inspectors of Mines, and contacted the MFGB, whose assistance was thought to be essential for the success of the study. In December 1937, the main thrust of the research got under way with radiological and clinical examinations of 560 miners at Ammanford colliery – an anthracite mine. Over a six-month period, each man was clinically examined and x-rayed, and this information was then collated with detailed occupational histories. Three reports (numbers 243, 244 and 250) were subsequently published by the MRC as part of its Special Reports Series. The first, in 1942, related to the Ammanford study, and it was in this report that Drs Hart and Aslett described how CWP first showed up under x-ray examination as a faint reticular pattern on the lung – labelled reticulation – then progressed, as the disease became more severe, through various stages, including nodulation, coalescent nodulation, and finally multiple fluffy shadows.[98]

The second report published in 1943 encompassed a wider study of 15 mines throughout South Wales. During this phase of the research, Drs Bedford and Warner – members of the Scientific Department of the Industrial Health Research Board – correlated dust levels at some of these collieries with each mine's rate of CWP. In a 'practical suggestions' section of their paper, Bedford and Warner also suggested maximum dust concentration levels at which dust suppression personnel should aim. These were 650 particles per cubic centimetre (p.p.c.c.) for working in anthracite coal dust, 850 p.p.c.c for other types of coal dust, and 450 p.p.c.c. when men were working in stone. Bedford and Warner made it clear that these levels were not being suggested as definitive standards: 'We are in some doubt as to what concentrations should reasonably be taken as the basis of provisional standards for immediate practical application.'[99] Not only that, the Committee on Industrial Pulmonary

---

96 IPDC Memorandum, 20 November 1936, PRO, FD1/2884.

97 *News Chronicle* (21 March 1934).

98 Hunter, *The Diseases of Occupations*, p. 999; By 1950, the term 'reticulation' was later abandoned because x-rays showed a fine mottling of the lungs, and not a reticular pattern as had been assumed; C.M. Fletcher and J. Gough, 'Coal miners' Pneumoconiosis', *British Medical Bulletin*, vol. 7, no. 1 (1950), p. 42.

99 T. Bedford and C.G. Warner, 'Physical studies of the dust hazard and of the thermal environment in certain coalmines', Medical Research Council, *Chronic Pulmonary Disease*

Disease emphasised in the introduction to the report that these levels were indeed arbitrary:

> In their report, Dr Bedford and Dr Warner suggested certain standards of permissible dustiness in the air breathed by the miner. While the standards may serve as a target at which to aim at present, the Committee feel that it would be a mistake to lay down any rigid standards until the results of further investigations ... are available and additional information has been obtained about the extent to which concentration of air-borne dust can be reduced by methods that are practicable to the coalface.[100]

However, as we shall see later, although Bedford and Warner's rudimentary standards were not intended as a gauge to prevent miners contracting pneumoconiosis, necessity would dictate that this is exactly what would happen.

The MRC's third report also contained the results of the IPDC's study of coal trimmers in the South Wales docks. This was to be crucial, because although the work which the trimmers performed never brought them into contact with rock dust, a significant number of them were succumbing to 'disease x'. As we illustrate in Chapter 7, much of the credit for directing the MRC to examine these workers lay with the trade union compensation secretary, Harry Finch. Along with the South Wales Miners' Federation, the investigation of coal trimmers had the full support of the Amalgamated Anthracite Collieries and the Transport and General Workers' Union. The IPDC's initial study of the coal trimmers turned out to be inconclusive.[101] However, later, when Gough published the results of his post-mortem investigations of 12 Cardiff coal trimmers, the evidence began to look watertight, as 8 of the men had fibrosis, and 5 had definitely died of pneumoconiosis.[102] The MRC conducted a more extensive study of 470 coal trimmers from four South Wales ports in 1942. This study proved conclusively that although the men had not been exposed to silica rock, they were suffering from a dust-related lung disease. Therefore, the causal agent must have been the coal dust.[103]

The MRC team became convinced that there was a strong correlation between the incidence of pneumoconiosis and the concentration of coal dust particles below 5 microns in size. Research also pointed to the fact that some forms of dust were more dangerous than others. Hart and Aslett had suggested in their report on the Ammanford mine that anthracite dust was the most hazardous. The initial reasoning behind this 'rank of coal' hypothesis was that because the highest prevalence of the disease was

---

in South Wales, *Special Report Series* no. 244 (1943), p. 64.

100 Ibid., pp. vii–viii.

101 S.W. Fisher of Mines Department to Sir David Munro, IHRB, 3 January 1934. PRO, FD 1/2875.

102 MRC, *Medical Studies*, p. 160; see also C.M. Fletcher and J. Gough, 'Coal miners' Pneumoconiosis', *British Medical Bulletin*, vol. 7 (1950), p. 43.

103 *The Colliery Guardian* (October 1945), pp. 463–5; interestingly, a similar argument had been used in the USA using railway engine firemen as a control group; Derickson, *Black Lung*, p. 51.

in the anthracite areas – where the Ammanford pit was located – anthracite coal dust had to be the most dangerous. To some degree this theory was backed up by evidence from similar anthracite regions in America and Russia. However, Charles Fletcher – the first Director of the British Pneumoconiosis Research Unit established in 1946 – later reflected on this and noted that anthracite mines were not as well ventilated as non-anthracite pits, because there was less danger of coal dust explosion. Therefore, more cases of dust disease were reported from anthracite areas, not because of the type of coal dust, but because there was simply more dust in the mine air.[104] As we will see in Chapter 4, epidemiological research would reveal that the rank of coal hypothesis was indeed flawed.

The MRC's third report of 1945 also suggested that quartz was the major agent in the production of pneumoconiosis in South Wales. Increasingly, as coal dust became accepted as being dangerous to miners' respiratory health, the dangers of silica or quartz – interchangeable terms – were lost sight of by researchers. However, the centrality of quartz to miners' lung disease would later be corroborated by studies conducted by the Institute of Occupational Medicine (IOM) in the 1980s, and by further research at the beginning of the twenty-first century.[105]

The end result of the IPDC investigations in the early 1940s was that the MRC was able to recommend that compensation procedures should be changed:

> We recommended that the word silicosis should be dropped and instead the scheme should be called 'pneumoconiosis of coal workers', so it would include coal miners at the face, rock workers and the coal trimmers at the docks …[106]

Consequently, under the 1943 Coal Mining Industry (Pneumoconiosis) Compensation Scheme all miners who developed 'fibrosis of the lungs due to silica dust, asbestos dust, or other dust' were to be covered by the legislation if they had worked:

> … in any operation underground in any coal mine, and on the surface of any coal mine in any of the processes of tipping, screening, breaking, loading, handling or moving of coal or other minerals extracted from the mine.[107]

However, one of the consequences of the 1943 Pneumoconiosis Compensation Scheme was that certified miners were forced to leave the coal industry; and by 1945 the Silicosis Medical Board was suspending men from the South Wales Area at a rate of over a hundred per week.[108] Moreover, the government's intention to

---

104 C.M. Fletcher, 'Epidemiological Studies of Coal Miners' Pneumoconiosis in Great Britain', *Archives of Industrial Health*, vol. 2 (January 1955), p. 30.

105 NCB, Scientific Department, *Pneumoconiosis Field Research, The Study of the Composition of Respirable Dust in the Pneumoconiosis Field Research* (1960), p. 3.

106 D'Arcy Hart and Aslett, 'Chronic Pulmonary Disease', p. 464.

107 D.D. Evans, 'A Survey of the Incidence and Progression of Pneumoconiosis Related to the Environmental Conditions', pp. 4–5.

108 A. Stewart, 'Pneumoconiosis of Coal Miners: The Disease After Cessation of Exposure to Dust', cited in *Colliery Guardian*, vol. 177 (1948), p. 374.

introduce suitable rehabilitation schemes and retraining was thwarted by a lack of understanding as to the most suitable type of work to provide. Subsequently, between November 1945 and December 1946 the Ministry of Fuel and Power conducted a survey of men certified by the Silicosis Medical Board between 1931 and 1944.[109] Following the Report of the Advisory Committee on the Treatment and Rehabilitation of Miners in the Wales Region Suffering from Pneumoconiosis, the MRC became convinced that more research needed to be undertaken on the problem of miners' health. This conviction led to the setting up of the MRC's own Pneumoconiosis Research Unit in South Wales in 1946 to carry out investigations into aspects of pneumoconiosis.[110] The same year, to address the growing economic and social consequences of contracting pneumoconiosis, the Ministry of Fuel and Power formed the National Joint Pneumoconiosis Committee (NJPC), made up of representatives from the NCB, the trade unions, the Miners' Welfare Commission, as well as from the Ministry of Fuel and Power itself.[111] One of the first things the NJPC did was to carve out a scheme which passed through parliament in 1948 as the *Employment of Pneumoconiosis Cases* (Cd. 354). With the passage of this legislation, Bedford and Warner's suggested dust exposure limits were to be given unexpected significance.

The 1948 *Employment of Pneumoconiosis Cases* legislation allowed for the employment of 'seriously incapacitated' men in 'approved dust conditions' on the surface, and for the employment/re-employment of men in the earlier stages of pneumoconiosis in 'approved dust conditions' underground. This solution, it was thought, would be a benefit to the miners who had been thrown out of work, as well as to the manpower-starved coal mining industry in general. The NJPC also recommended that periodic medical examination of miners should be adopted as a way of curtailing the pneumoconiosis problem, with the assumption that the nascent NHS would bear the cost of this – which it would eventually do ten years later.[112]

However, for the moment two crucial points need to be noted. Firstly, before any dust-damaged miners were able to return to the pits, it was essential to ensure they would not be exposed to the same levels of dust that had caused them to contract pneumoconiosis in the first place – or to levels which would cause their pneumoconiosis to progress. But at this time no one really knew what constituted a safe dose of coal dust, and the only 'standard' which had been suggested by researchers was that included in Bedford and Warner's 1943 report. However, something had to be done in response to Cd 354, and done quickly. Therefore, Bedford and Warner's suggested upper limits of dust exposure were seized upon as standards to determine

---

109 Ibid., p. 375.

110 Ministry of Fuel and Power, *Dust Prevention and Suppression, Instructional Pamphlet no. 1*, p. 3.

111 Four sub-committees were formed as part of the NJPC, dealing with Dust Suppression, Medical Examinations, Medical Treatment and After Care, and Industrial Rehabilitation, Re-training and Re-employment; NCB, *Annual Report* (1947).

112 W. Ashworth, *History of the British Coal Industry, Volume 5. 1946–1982* (Oxford, 1986), p. 566.

'approved dust conditions'. Warner was especially unhappy about this, and in 1949, by which time he was Divisional Dust Suppression Scientist for the South West Area of the NCB, he expressed his concern at the decision:

> I think it is a fair question to ask the Ministry on what evidence … they have seen fit to suggest 650 p.p.c.c. for anthracite mines. Why not suggest 250 or any other low number for a condition which everyone concerned with the dust problem would be glad to see … the prescribing of standards of dustiness must be approached in a most guarded manner.[113]

As we shall see in Chapter 6, though, the approach taken was far from guarded, and Bedford and Warner's scale became the NCB's first line of defence against excessive mine dust for over twenty years.

Conclusion

Although coal dust-induced lung disease in the UK was identified in ancient times, and by the end of the nineteenth century was acknowledged to be an industrial disease of British coal miners, this upward curve of recognition dipped in the early twentieth century. Improvements in mine air quality from the late Victorian period went some way in reducing the number of miners succumbing to black lung, but the apparent decline of the disease was probably as much to do with its prevalence being camouflaged, in that lung disease coal mining deaths were recorded as other conditions extant in the non-mining population, such as asthma, bronchitis and TB. Advancements in medical knowledge of lung diseases in the Edwardian period, combined with further expansion of mining and an increased use of pneumatic drills in mines, underpinned a new awareness of the hazards of mine dust. By this time, though, the issue of compensation had become a significant factor, and it was primarily because of this that the 're-appearance' of coal workers' lung disease – linked as it was to the growing awareness of the dangers of silica dust – occurred amidst much conflict and denial.

The growing importance of coal mining to the British economy, combined with increased mechanisation of mining in the inter-war period and the reviving collective strength of the miners' trade unions from the early 1930s, were important factors in the 'rediscovery' of black lung. Concurrent with this were further advances in medical knowledge of lung disease. Throughout this period and well into the twentieth century – certainly until the discovery of drugs such as streptomycin – tuberculosis took precedence as the number one public health issue, and this overshadowed miners' lung disease. The insistence by some medical professionals that coal miners were succumbing to bronchitis – non-compensatable because, like TB, it was prevalent throughout the population – also retarded understanding and recognition of the dust hazard which miners were having to endure every day. Therefore, a serious

---

113 Cited in Judgment of Mr Justice Turner, 'The British Coal Respiratory Disease Litigation' (1998), p. 30.

consequence of the increased attention devoted by medical scientists to miners' lung disease was that the prolonged tussle over how best to medicalise dust-induced disease took time and cost lives. The mining engineer Cullen's plea in 1935 that attention be focused on eradicating mine dust regardless of the intricacies of its composition was apposite.[114] As we will see in the next chapter, this state of affairs was to continue for some time.

South Wales was the heartland of the mine dust problem, so much so that in 1944 the government was compelled – partly through pressure from the Miners' Federation of Great Britain, and partly due to a labour shortage in the pits – to make dust suppression compulsory in South Wales where airborne dust was considered dangerous to miners' health. It is significant that two HM Mines Inspectors were detailed specifically to deal with the dust problem in this area.[115] Here, the mine employers, the trade unions, the workers and the state came into conflict around the growing problem, with the first attempts at dust suppression being implemented as a defensive reaction by the owners to the swelling number of compensation claims and the threat to the future of mechanisation. In South Wales, the sheer scale of the problem became such that state intervention in the form of the MRC's IPDC was thought essential. The resultant investigations by the MRC substantiated what many in South Wales had known for some time: the inhalation of coal dust, and not just rock dust, was highly dangerous to health.

Therefore, by the end of the Second World War and the eve of nationalisation, CWP had been recognised, some preventive measures had been introduced in South Wales, and a significant network of interlocking initiatives had been created to undertake further research and monitor the health of the coal mining workforce. High-quality medical research underpinned the change in compensation procedures in 1943, with men at last being able to claim compensation for respiratory damage caused by coal dust as well as silica dust. However, as we shall see in the next chapter, only comprehensive long-term epidemiological research would eventually determine what constituted a safe limit of mine dust exposure. Therefore, the nascent NCB's adoption of Bedford and Warner's speculations as a measure to determine approved dust conditions for the re-employment of pneumoconiotics, and as a protective shield for miners in general, was – as Warner himself noted – ill advised. As we shall see in the following chapters, it is from this act of expediency that much of the NCB's difficulties regarding the coal dust problem were to derive.

In the next chapter, we focus again on the continuing medicalisation of miners' lung in the second half of the twentieth century.

---

114 NCB Scientific Department, *Pneumoconiosis Field Research, The Study of the Composition of Respirable Dust in the Pneumoconiosis Field Research* (1960), p. 2.

115 *The Miner* (October 1944), p. 11.

Chapter 4

Social Medicine and Pioneering Epidemiology

The previous chapter illustrated how, by the early 1940s, Coal Workers' Pneumoconiosis (CWP) had been identified, and how efforts to check the virulence of this serious lung condition were beginning to be put into place. Much of this activity, though, was focused on South Wales, and indeed the CWP problem was looked upon as a Welsh problem for some time to come. In this chapter we take the analysis further by exploring how, from the 1940s, the issue of CWP began to be perceived as having more national importance than had previously been assumed. We also highlight how efforts to find out about and curb CWP fitted into the growing social medicine movement of this period, and how for some medical professionals, such research became almost a crusade. We also illustrate how coal miners' respiratory health was to benefit from growing expertise in epidemiology from the 1950s onwards, while conversely, the discipline of epidemiology gained substantial prestige from path-breaking research on coal miners.

Contextualising Occupational Health in Mining in the 1940s

It is understandable that when the social medicine movement began to gather momentum, the archetypal proletarian miners would derive some benefit. The high unemployment of the inter-war years was one of the reasons that the roots of social medicine began to flourish. This new approach captivated several of the medical professionals who would eventually play an important role in the fight against miners' lung disease. Archie Cochrane – of whom much more later – fought with the International Brigade in the Spanish Civil War, and recounted how, when he was a student at Cambridge, he had 'felt the sap of radicalism rise up in him', saying: 'I took to socialism because of the terrible unemployment in the thirties. It was also beginning to be pretty popular at Cambridge at the time.'[1] In a similar way, Julian Tudor Hart, who, like Cochrane, was to become heavily involved with epidemiology in the post-Second World War period, also held strong political convictions when he was a medical student:

---

1   'The Health Thinkers', *Health and Social Service Journal* (24 November 1978), p. 1,337.

My politics was more important than medicine, and it still is. Politics, in the sense of changing the world, is an overall context within which medicine operates, so in that sense it is more important. I had wanted a way to be a useful person, politically changing the world while actually doing something useful with my hands.[2]

And to some extent Philip D'Arcy Hart's reasons for joining the MRC were driven by the same basic desire:

Why did I join the MRC? Well it's rather confessional, but I wanted to get out of consultant medicine, because I found that I wanted to do research with a small 'r', and I found that I couldn't do it, because I had to earn my living. And therefore I was looking for ways of getting out. Out of the blue, Sir Thomas Lewis on the [Medical Research] Council heard about this demand from the Home Office or the Government to do something about pneumoconiosis, and they were looking for somebody to do it. And he knew me ...[3]

Richard Schilling has similar memories of early socialist tendencies:

My mother asked her Tory Member of Parliament what she could do with her youngest son, who had become a Socialist. At that time I was a doctor in Birmingham, witnessing the devastating effects of long-term unemployment during the economic slump of the 1930s. The MP told her that some Socialists were quite nice people and young ones tended to get over it.[4]

Concomitant with the rise of the social medicine movement in the UK, organisations emerged to promote the idea of an international public health research network, and occupational health was frequently an integral part of their agenda. The US-backed Rockefeller Foundation was one such organization, as was the League of Nations Health Organization, and the International Labour Office (ILO).[5] The ILO was established in 1919 with representation from politicians, employers and workers. The organisation's initial concern was to protect women and children at work, and to secure adequate maternity leave and an eight-hour working day. The ILO also ran conventions in which industrial health problems were discussed – such as lead and phosphorus – after which the ILO made recommendations. However, it was entirely up to the governments of individual countries whether they took any notice of what the ILO was saying – Britain, for example, refused to implement the eight-hour day or ratify a convention relating to maternity leave. The ILO set up its own industrial hygiene section in 1920, but found co-ordinating research and gathering

---

2   Interview with Julian Tudor Hart, Wellcome Institute for the History of Medicine, *Witness Seminar. The MRC Epidemiology Unit (South Wales)*, vol. 13 (November 2002), p. 37; henceforth Wellcome Witness Seminar (2002).

3   Dr Philip D'Arcy Hart, Wellcome Witness Seminar (2002), p. 3.

4   R. Schilling, *A Challenging Life: Sixty Years in Occupational Health* (London, 1988), p. 11.

5   P. Weindling, 'Social Medicine at the League of Nations Health Organization and the International Labour Office', in P. Weindling (ed.), *International Health Organization and Movements, 1918–1939* (1995), p. 135.

statistics throughout Europe problematic. In general, then, although the ILO looked good on paper, nothing much was done by the organisation to improve workers' health in Britain in the inter-war period. This was also the case with the League of Nations Health Organization, which by the 1920s was engaged mostly in scientific and technical research, and hardly gave any attention to industrial welfare.[6]

During the Second World War, the British government placed a higher priority on workers' health than had been the case in the inter-war years, and this was reflected in the passage of legislation which compelled employers to appoint factory doctors and nurses, and to ensure that companies initiated safe and healthy working environments for their staff.[7] Another important manifestation of the keen interest in workers' health during the war was the appearance in 1944 of the *British Journal of Industrial Medicine*. This was the brainchild of the Association of Industrial Medical Officers, whose members had managed to get the British Medical Association to support the project. One of the first editors of the journal was Donald Hunter, an occupational health expert who was to go on to publish a comprehensive influential textbook on industrial diseases in 1955: *The Diseases of Occupation*. The publication of the *British Journal of Industrial Medicine* gave British occupational health increased status, and many medical experts were convinced that the post-war years would see the new emphasis on industrial health and welfare continue to grow. This optimistic tone was further bolstered by the publication of the Beveridge Report in 1942, with its proposals for health, social security, and the maintenance of full employment. The war, then, had intensified a drive towards a more socially inspired post-war era, and the landslide victory of the Labour Party in 1945 was a clear indicator of the prevailing mood of the time.

Social medicine became even more prominent in the new post-war political climate, and for a while in the UK, society was placed at the heart of medical investigation – something which the ILO was trying to do on an international basis. John Ryle had been Professor of Medicine at Cambridge, and his 'social pathology' approach posited that certain population groups were prone to particular diseases because of the conditions in which they lived.[8] Ryle became the first director of the Institute of Social Medicine at Oxford. The Institute had been set up during the Second World War to investigate how social, genetic, environmental and domestic factors impacted on human diseases and morbidity. Ryle was to play a major role in motivating a generation of British epidemiologists in post-war Britain when environmental factors affecting health, including the working environment, were

---

6   Ibid., p. 143.

7   R. Johnston and A. McIvor, 'The War and the Body at Work: Occupational Health and Safety in Scottish Industry, 1939–1945', *Journal of Historical Studies*, vol. 24, no. 2 (2005), pp. 113–36.

8   Society for Social Medicine Website, http://www.socsocmed.org.uk/history.htm; see also D. Porter, 'John Ryle and the Making of Social Medicine in Britain in the 1940s', *History of Science*, vol. 30 (88, Part 2) (June 1992), pp. 137–64.

moved closer to centre stage. One medical professional summed up the underpinning principles of the movement in this way:

> Society largely determines health; ill-health is not a personal misfortune due often to personal inadequacy, but social misfortune due more commonly to social mismanagement and social failure.[9]

The Socialist Medical Association (SMA), established in 1930, was another manifestation of the leftward trend in medicine.[10] The SMA in the early 1950s was deeply interested in the coal dust issue, and its Edinburgh and South East Scotland branch wrote to the Secretary of State for Scotland in 1954 demanding that the government do more to address the dust problem in the mines.[11] Julian Tudor Hart reflected on the political and ideological dimensions of the social research that was beginning to emerge in post-war Britain, to which he would soon be fully committed:

> In America the Cold War was already going on. Very early on the Cold War stopped the liberal social programme in America, which never since has managed to get round to providing a health service for the whole of the American people … Already collectivism was equated with communism, and they were looking for individual solutions for everything. We weren't like that. It is of course true that if you focus on pneumoconiosis as a topic then you are going to go to an industrial working class area with a militant political tradition.[12]

Four university chairs in social medicine were established throughout the UK, and in 1946 Richard Schilling – then secretary of the MRC's Industrial Health Research Board – suggested that the MRC should set up its own Social Medicine Unit. This came in to being in 1948, superseding the IHRB. To some degree, then, social medicine emerged from occupational medicine – a trend paralleled in the USA, as the work of Sellers has shown – and it is interesting that Schilling was the man responsible for the appointment of Charles Fletcher as Director of the Pneumoconiosis Research Unit which would play an important role in developing an understanding of miners' lung disease.[13]

---

9   S. Murphy, 'The early days of the MRC Social Medicine Research Unit', *Social History of Medicine*, vol. 12, no. 3 (1999), p. 390.

10   For the politics of the SMA, see J. Stewart, *'The Battle for Health': A Political History of the Socialist Medical Association* (Aldershot, 1999).

11   Letter from SMA to Secretary of State for Scotland, 18 November 1954, Department of Health for Scotland, HH 104/1 (HOS/15/15).

12   Testimony of Julian Tudor Hart, Wellcome Witness Seminar (2002), p. 37.

13   Murphy, 'The early days of the MRC Social Medicine Research Unit', p. 392; Sir Christopher Booth, Wellcome Witness Seminar (2002), p. 26; Schilling, *A Challenging Life*, pp. 48–9. Chris Sellers argues convincingly that environmental medicine emerged out of occupational medicine in the USA; see C. Sellers, *Hazards of the Job:From Industrial Science to Environmental Health Science* (Chapel Hill, NC, 1997).

The science of epidemiology was to prove central to the understanding of miners' lung in the UK, and much of this was linked to the new post-1940 social medical approach. Epidemiology has been defined simply as 'the study of how diseases occur in different groups of people and why', and has a long history which can be traced back to ancient times.[14] However, despite the importance of early studies, it was really from the 1940s onwards that epidemiology was accepted as a science in its own right, and one of the initial driving forces was the need to gain an understanding of the health hazards of smoking.[15] The work of Bradford Hill at the London School of Hygiene and Tropical Medicine was influential in the post-war development of epidemiology, and several of his students, including Richard Doll, Jerry Morris, Richard Schilling and Archie Cochrane, were to gain prestigious reputations in this field.[16]

Simultaneous with the coming of socially inspired medicine, the NHS arrived on the scene. The introduction of the NHS in 1948 meant that Britain now provided free medical care to its entire population – and it would be another twenty years before another country, Sweden, did the same. However, whereas many medics and trade unionists had hoped that an *occupational* health service would be set up as part of this new health care system, this was not to be.[17] Several of the big nationalised enterprises set up their own health services, including the National Coal Board (NCB). The NCB's medical service – looked at in some detail later in this chapter – was a comprehensive undertaking.[18] There was also a medical service set up in the docks by the National Dock Labour Board – which, although really an accident service, had seven full-time medical officers. The nationalised railway network also had its own health service employing full-time and part-time medical officers.[19]

Therefore, it is within the context of a fresh approach towards workers' health and safety in the years following the Second World War that we need to contextualise the miners' coal dust problem and the efforts to tackle it. By the 1950s, medical scientists were finding out more and more about dangerous work hazards. The increased use of organic insecticides focused attention on the risks these posed to workers, and similar attention was devoted to radiation in the 1950s. In 1953, the MRC set up its own Toxicology Unit, and in the early 1960s the increased use of plastics in industry

---

14 R. Coggon et al. (eds), *Epidemiology for the Uninitiated*, 3rd edn (London, 1997), p. 1; for a short but detailed online account of the evolution of epidemiology, see R. Saracci, *The History of Epidemiology*, http://www.oup.co.uk/pdf/0-19-263066-0.pdf.

15 Ibid.; see also V. Berridge and K. Loughlin, 'Smoking and the New Health Education in Britain, 1950s–1970s', *American Journal of Public Health*, vol. 95, no. 6 (June 2005), pp. 958–64.

16 Schilling, *A Challenging Life*, p. 53.

17 See R. Johnston and A. McIvor, 'Whatever Happened to the Occupational Health Service?', in C. Nottingham (ed.), *The NHS in Scotland* (Aldershot, 2001), pp. 79–106.

18 A. Meiklejohn, 'Sixty years of industrial medicine in Great Britain', *British Journal of Industrial Medicine*, vol. 13, no. 3 (July 1956), p. 158.

19 *Report of a Committee of Inquiry on Industrial Health Services* (1951), Cmd 8170, p. 9; henceforth the Dale Committee.

meant attention was focused on dermatitis caused by handling chemical compounds. There was also research being done on heart disease and TB rates amongst workers, and in 1953 the British Occupational Hygiene Society was founded.[20] Other notable developments were the founding of a Department of Occupational Health at the London School of Hygiene under the control of Richard Schilling. This establishment (which closed in 1990) would quickly gain a reputation as being the leading department of occupational medicine in the world.[21] On top of this, the Nuffield Foundation plugged some of the gaps in occupational health coverage by giving large sums of money to universities to set up departments of industrial health. As part of this incentive, Manchester and Durham founded professorships of occupational health, while Glasgow set up a lectureship. Interestingly, Dundee University – which also received a grant – emerged as the most important Scottish institution, with a vibrant and world-renowned department of industrial health set up in the 1960s led by Alex Mair, from which would emerge the pioneering Dundee and District Occupational Health Service.[22] Therefore, professional interest in the field of occupational health was steadily growing, and the appearance by the 1950s of the *Journal for Industrial Nurses* and *Industrial Welfare* further illustrates this.

The Pneumoconiosis Research Unit (PRU)

In 1945, due to the serious nature of occupational disability emerging in Britain's premier heavy industry, the MRC set up a Pneumoconiosis Research Unit (PRU) at Llandough Hospital, Penarth, in South Wales, in which the various aspects of the dust problem would be investigated. When Charles Fletcher was appointed as its Director, some of his contemporaries reflected on what seemed at the time to be a mismatch appointment for a position requiring day-to-day contact with coal miners:

> I mean, an Old Etonian, Trinity College, rowed in the boat race in 1933, won against Oxford … You'd think that that was really a man with quite extraordinarily wrong qualifications to go to talk to coal miners in South Wales. Nothing could be further from the truth, because there was nobody who really managed to get people eating out of his hand in South Wales better than Charles Fletcher. He was incredibly successful in his relationship with all the people there and he deserves very great credit for that.[23]

Fletcher later reflected on his reasons for accepting the position at the PRU: 'I saw that too many doctors were trying to treat diseases and not enough were trying to prevent them. Here was a chance to do something to prevent a really serious

---

20 Meiklejohn, 'Sixty years of industrial medicine in Great Britain', p. 160.

21 A. Dalton, *Safety, Health and Environmental Hazards at the Workplace* (London, 1998), p. 19.

22 Johnston and McIvor, 'Whatever Happened to the Occupational Health Service?', pp. 89–90.

23 Sir Christopher Booth, Wellcome Witness Seminar (2002), p. 9.

disease.'[24] The unit became one of the largest of the MRC establishments, and was to remain in existence until 1985. One of its most important characteristics was the sheer breadth of research backgrounds which were drawn upon to address the coal dust problem. These included physicians, physiologists, pathologists, physicists, bioengineers and statisticians. John Gilson – who had been at Cambridge with Fletcher – was made Deputy Director. Gilson had been researching respiratory problems of aircrew during the war, and would succeed Fletcher when he left to take up the post of Reader, then Professor of Epidemiology, at the Postgraduate Medical School in London in 1952.[25] Next in the hierarchy came Archie Cochrane. Cochrane was 40 years old when he joined the PRU. Educated at Cambridge, he had served as a House Physician at West London Hospital before becoming a Research Assistant at the Medical Unit of University College Hospital in London. During the war, he was captured, and worked as a doctor in several prisoner of war camps, work for which he was awarded an MBE. After the war, a Rockefeller Fellowship enabled him to take a Diploma in Public Health at the London School of Hygiene and Tropical Medicine. Before joining the PRU, he also gained important experience at the Henry Phipps Institute in Philadelphia – again on a Rockefeller fellowship – where he researched the study of pulmonary TB using x-rays, and studied observer error in reading the x-ray films.[26] Cochrane was to become a giant of epidemiology, a founding father of evidence-based medicine, and an early advocate of the use of randomised control trials.[27]

Fletcher told an American audience in 1955 that he and his co-workers had two prime objectives when it came to investigating mine dust disease: firstly, they wanted to determine whether the great differences in certification rates across the country were attributable to varying dust concentrations, or were in fact caused by the differing nature of coal dusts; secondly, the Unit wanted to determine safe dust levels which men could be exposed to without them succumbing to pneumoconiosis.[28] Like most of his co-researchers at the PRU, Fletcher was deeply touched by the sheer extent of the problem in South Wales, and his empathy with the miners clearly stiffened his convictions:

> Throughout the coalfield men in their thirties and forties with young families, sat around, too breathless for the labouring jobs which were all they could be offered … I found it

---

24 C.M. Fletcher 'Fighting the Modern Black Death', *The Listener* (28 September 1950), p. 407.

25 W.E. Miall, Wellcome Witness Seminar (2002), p. 33.

26 See A.L. Cochrane's online biography: http://www.cardiff.ac.uk/schoolsanddivisions/insrv/libraryservices/research/cochrane/biography.html.

27 Cochrane's papers have been catalogued and are available at the Cochrane Archive at Llandough Hospital.

28 C.M. Fletcher, 'Epidemiological Studies of Coal Miners' Pneumoconiosis in Great Britain', *Archives of Industrial Health*, vol. 11 (January 1955), p. 29.

tragic, to see the wasted lives – the wasted lives of these cultured friendly men, for what has struck me most about the Welsh miners is their culture and friendliness.[29]

By the early 1950s, research into the coal dust problem in the UK was being conducted by several agencies, and was being well financed. The MRC was spending around £77,000 a year on pneumoconiosis work, and the PRU at Cardiff had a staff of 70. At the same time, the Ministry of Fuel and Power's Safety in Mines Research Establishment was dedicating £75,000 a year to pneumoconiosis, primarily as wages for its 48 staff working in Sheffield.[30] The SMRE first came into being as the Safety in Mines Research Board in 1947, but changed its name to the Safety in Mines Research Establishment (SMRE) in 1950. In the same year, the Safety in Mines Research Advisory Board (SMRAB) was set up to advise the Minister for Fuel and Power on matters relating to the organisation and progress of the Ministry's research work on safety in mines.

Some indication of how seriously the dust disease problem was being taken at this time was the number of agencies becoming involved. Soon after the PRU had been established, Fletcher expressed some concern that too many interest groups were trying to tackle the same problems. In 1943, there was some departmental rivalry between the MRC's Industrial Pulmonary Disease Committee and an Industrial Advisory Committee (IAC) which Bevin had set up. Of most concern to the MRC was that a sub-committee had been initiated by the IAC to investigate the nature of industrial dust, and according to a letter from the MRC to Sir Henry Dale in 1943, was 'so arranged as to eliminate those who have been working for us [the MRC] who have naturally developed great experience in such matters during the past four years'. The MRC representative went on to state:

> It is just rather disturbing to find the action of one government department or departments is all towards going their own way, when to an ordinary person it would have seemed desirable to have maintained the closest relations.[31]

Certainly, by 1948 the field was becoming even more obscured, and Fletcher drew attention to the pitfalls of potential overlap to Sir Edward Mellaby of the MRC. In a letter that year he referred to:

> ... the crop of committees which are now springing up in relation to the pneumoconiosis problem. There is the National Joint Pneumokoniosis Committee [sic] with its four Sub-Committees, there are the Regional Dust Prevention Committees, and the Regional Joint Consultative Committees on Pneumokoniosis of the Coal Board and the National Union of Mineworkers and there is the Joint Pneumokoniosis Research Committee. Lastly there is the Dust Panel of the Ministry of Labour and, of course, the Industrial Pulmonary Disease Committee ... I also believe that the Coal Board are proposing in the future that

---

29 Fletcher, 'Fighting the Modern Black Death', p. 407.

30 *Hansard*, 19 March 1956, PQ 247/56.

31 Letter from MRC to Sir David Dale, The Royal Institution, 7 June, 1943. National Archives of Scotland, FD 1/2880.

their Medical Officers might undertake radiological surveys of pits. It is very important that we know of and be consulted in any such ventures.[32]

Fletcher was asked by the government to draw up a statement on how the problem of overlap should be addressed. He recommended that an Advisory Group be formed within the MRC – which included members from the PRU, the Coal Board's Scientific Staff, and other interested agencies – to co-ordinate medical and environmental aspects of research into pneumoconiosis.[33] The setting up of this group made for a much more clearly defined research strategy.

By the early 1950s, it was accepted that pneumoconiosis was really two entities: simple and complicated. Simple pneumoconiosis was characterised by multiple coal foci scattered throughout the lungs, surrounded by small areas of emphysema. The second form of the disease was what the pathologist Dr Jethro Gough of the Welsh National School of Medicine referred to as 'infective' pneumoconiosis. Gough's method of slicing lung tissues into sections was very effective in revealing the devastation caused to the lung by the lesions of the disease. This complicated form of the disease was also known as progressive massive fibrosis (PMF), and was the most feared. Initially, PMF was thought to have been the result of TB being superimposed on the coal dust-laden lung – indeed, Gough found that 40% of 1,000 post-mortems conducted on miners with PMF showed evidence of TB.[34] This presumed link between TB and PMF would be the subject of intense epidemiological study.

Fletcher realised that one of the first requirements for an effective x-ray study of pneumoconiosis was to have a consistent radiological grading system in place. Only with such a system could observer error be minimised, the prevalence of the disease gauged, and its progression over time measured. To this end, along with Cochrane and Davis, he classified radiographs into four categories, from 0 (which was normal) through stages 1, 2, and 3 CWP, to correspond with the increasing number of opacities revealed as the disease progressed, and this classification was later adopted by the ILO at its Third International Conference of Experts on Pneumoconiosis in 1950. All men with x-rays classified as Category 1, 2 or 3 were recorded as having simple pneumoconiosis. However, Category 1 was not recognised for purposes of diagnoses under the 1946 National Insurance (Industrial Injuries) Act, and indeed, by the early 1950s the PRU was unsure whether the very slight evidence of dust exposure known as Category 1 – at one time referred to as reticulation – should be counted as a disease at all.[35] However, men reaching the stage corresponding to Category 2 faced a risk of developing PMF superimposed upon simple pneumoconiosis. Complicated pneumoconiosis (or PMF) was definitely disabling, and could kill, and it was this

---

32 Letter from C.M. Fletcher, PRU, to Sir Edward Mellanby, dated 14 April 1948, NA/PDI/214.

33 Ibid.

34 J.C. Gilson, 'Pathology, Radiology, and Epidemiology of Coal Workers' Pneumoconiosis in Wales', *Archives of Industrial Health*, vol. 15 (June 1957), p. 469.

35 A.L., Cochrane, 'Pulmonary Tuberculosis in the Rhondda Fach', *British Medical Journal*, vol. 2 (18 October 1952), p. 8.

which needed to be eradicated from mining communities. The problem was, though – as the researchers well knew – that because of the nature of the industry, a certain level of dust disease would have to be accepted:

> For all practical purposes as long as there is dust there will be some pneumoconiosis, and it is first necessary to consider just how much or how little pneumoconiosis can be tolerated in the colliery. This will depend not only on the number of men involved, but also the extent to which their health is affected by pneumoconiosis.[36]

The PRU also devised standard questions to determine grades of breathlessness in miners. This scale – referred to as Fletcher's Scale after the publication of his 1959 *BMJ* article – reads like a sad catechism of a miner's gradual loss of lung function, either through emphysema or coal workers' pneumoconiosis:

> Grade 1: Is the patient's breath as good as that of the other men of his own age and build at work, on walking, and on climbing stairs?
> Grade 2: Is the patient able to walk with normal men of own age and build on the level but unable to keep up on hills or stairs?
> Grade 3: Is the patient unable to keep up with normal men on the level, but able to walk about a mile or more at his own speed?
> Grade 4: Is the patient unable to walk more than about 100 yards on the level without a rest?
> Grade 5: Is the patient breathless on talking or undressing, or unable to leave his house because of breathlessness? [37]

Miners who lived in hilly regions – such as in South Wales – normally became aware of dyspnoea first thing in the morning rather than when at work; while miners with Grade 3 dyspnoea frequently complained of leg cramps. Those with Grade 5, though, usually had severe emphysema or had x-ray evidence of PMF.[38] As we will see in forthcoming chapters, many of the men we interviewed for the present study clearly remember gauging their health against their ability to keep up with their fellow workers.

Pioneering Epidemiology: The Rhondda Fach Study

The PRU was to very quickly emerge as a world leader in occupational epidemiological studies, and one of its most important early surveys was conducted in the Welsh valley called the Rhondda Fach ('the little Rhondda') – in the early 1950s. It was Cochrane's idea to set up a large-scale epidemiological experiment to test the

---

36 A.S. Roach, 'A Method of Relating the Incidence of Pneumoconiosis to Airborne Dust Exposure', *British Journal of Industrial Medicine*, vol. 10 (1953), pp. 220–24.

37 C.M. Fletcher, 'The Clinical Diagnosis of Pulmonary Emphysema – an Experimental Study', *Medical Research Council, Pneumoconiosis Research Unit, Papers 1952–1953*, paper no. 49.

38 *Postgraduate Medical Journal*, vol. 75, nos 275–9 (May 1999), p. 3.

hypothesis (mentioned earlier) that PMF was a TB lesion modified by the presence of coal dust. However, this hypothesis could not be tested using animal experiments, primarily because animals did not react to the inhalation of coal dust in the same way as humans. There had been several attempts to use animals in this way. For example, in 1939, guinea pigs were kept underground in some Welsh anthracite collieries so that their lung contents could later be examined in the SMRE laboratory; at the same time, animals were kept for nine months in a bituminous colliery in North Staffordshire so their lungs could be compared with those exposed to anthracite.[39]

However, the plan to use 'human guinea pigs' in a controlled experiment was much more adventurous, and was expected to provide definitive answers. The idea was to measure changes in the rate of appearance of PMF – the 'attack rate' – in a region where simple pneumoconiosis and PMF were prevalent, but after the area had been made as free from TB infection as possible. For this, Cochrane needed to study a fairly manageable enclosed region, and it is interesting that he reflected on his wartime experience as a prison camp doctor responsible for thousands of patients who were suffering from hunger and TB:

> I got attracted to epidemiology by studying everybody in a community beautifully defined by wires. I was lecturing in Germany recently and I thanked them for leading me into this productive field as a prisoner of war.[40]

The Rhondda Fach is a narrow, winding valley which in the early 1940s had a population of just under 30,000, lying between Aberdare Valley and the Rhondda Fawr ('the big Rhondda'). The prevalence of pneumoconiosis in the Rhondda Fach, measured by certifications under the Workmen's Compensation Act/National Insurance (Industrial Injuries) Act, was higher than the average for the whole of Wales, and had soared with the introduction of the pneumoconiosis compensation scheme in July 1943.[41] Within the valley, eight small towns were grouped around five collieries in which most of the men were employed. Up to this point, mass x-rays of communities had rarely included more than 30% of a targeted population. However, it was crucial for Cochrane and his team to get as close to 100% coverage as possible. To try and ensure this, before the survey took place lectures were delivered throughout the valley, and a propaganda campaign was carefully orchestrated utilising wireless, television, lectures, posters and home visits.

The first phase of the research took six months. To reduce the likelihood of mistakes occurring in the reading of x-rays – an important part of Cochrane's earlier medical training in the USA – all radiographs were read by two observers working separately. Any individuals suspected of having TB had their sputum tested, and those whose sputum revealed the presence of TB were sent for treatment to one of two 27-bed wards which had been made available by the Welsh Regional Hospital

---

39 Safety in Mines Research Board, *Eighteenth Annual Report* (1939).

40 'The Health Thinkers', *Health and Social Service Journal* (24 November 1978), p. 1,337.

41 Cochrane, 'Pulmonary Tuberculosis in the Rhondda Fach', p. 2.

Board (WRHB). A team from the WRHB also contributed to the survey by testing all the schoolchildren in the valley for TB, in order to obtain an estimate of the prevalence rate of the disease. The x-raying process began in September 1950 in six centres in the valley, with two teams working in each town. The PRU teams based themselves at the pit heads, while researchers from the WRHB were located in local halls and chapels.

Cochrane's team comprised two doctors, one male nurse, three ex-miners – one for transport and two for census and coding – and one secretary.[42] Initially, Cochrane's PRU colleagues bet amongst themselves that he would get no more than 50% of the area's population signed up for the study.[43] However, thanks to the help of the former miners and the success of the propaganda campaign, an impressive 89% coverage was soon achieved. Moreover, when the appearance rate began to flag, members of the team made home visits, and as Cochrane later recounted, a certain amount of cajoling was sometimes required to get the most reluctant to take part: 'Repeat visits were often successful, some obstinate persons agreeing at the sixth attempt.'[44]

By the end of the first phase of the project, 91.7% of males and 86% of females in the Rhondda Fach had been x-rayed, with most lapses recorded amongst the non-miners and the elderly. The new radiological classifications initiated by Fletcher were utilised, and the survey found that around 30% of miners and ex-miners in the Rhondda Fach showed some signs of pneumoconiosis, while 15% had PMF. At the same time, the testing of schoolchildren in the valley showed that the prevalence rate of TB was not atypical compared to the rest of the UK. In all, 122 people were hospitalised, with only two infected cases refusing to go, and those who returned to the valley still infected were given advice on sputum control and monitored by members of the team. Consequently, the researchers were highly confident that they had brought about a marked reduction in TB infectivity in the region, while, at the same time demonstrating that it was possible to x-ray 90% of the adult population of a community.[45]

A second survey was conducted in 1953. This time the BBC broadcast a 50-minute radio programme which helped publicise the study, and the Welsh edition of the *Radio Times* also reported on the scheme. Under the headline 'X-raying a Welsh Community', readers were given an up-beat background to the PRU research:

> Dr. A. L. Cochrane proposed a bold scheme. 'Why not', he asked, 'join forces with the Mass Radiography Service? Why not attempt to discover, in a selected mining area, how much TB of the lungs there was, and then try to wipe it out?'[46]

---

42   J.C. Gilson and A.L. Cochrane, *Advisory Committee on Medical Research, Report of Pneumoconiosis Group, Appendix A: Summary of Evidence*, p. 3, National Archives of Scotland, HH104/46.

43   'The Health Thinkers', *Health and Social Service Journal* (24 November 1978), p. 1,339.

44   Cochrane, 'Pulmonary Tuberculosis in the Rhondda Fach', p. 2.

45   Ibid., p. 8.

46   *Radio Times* (7 November 1953), p. 12.

However, although the Rhondda Fach studies were monumental regarding their success in placing the population of a large area under the microscope, the question of why some men developed PMF and others did not remained unanswered.[47] In an article in the *British Journal of Industrial Medicine*, Cochrane acknowledged this defeat: 'An attempt to investigate the importance of exogenous tuberculous infection by comparing the attack rate [of PMF] in two mining valleys, in one of which great efforts had been made to eradicate tuberculosis, failed. The reasons for the failure are discussed.'[48] From the 1950s, TB was on the decline throughout the UK, with the MRC playing no small part in this by testing the effectiveness of streptomycin in 1948.[49] Because of this decline, Gough's hypothesis that simple pneumoconiosis progressed to PMF because of TB could not now be fully tested. There was, though, gathering evidence that this was not the case. For one thing, the drop in TB rates did not result in a similar decline in the rate of PMF. Also, trials in the USA using therapy against TB to prevent PMF failed to influence the development of the latter disease.[50] Julian Tudor Hart reflected in 1999 on the quest to link PMF and TB:

> It is an interesting thing historically, but we know beyond question that tuberculosis has nothing to do with it. But it was an extremely attractive hypothesis. A hypothesis that seems so self-evidently true that you can hardly believe that you need evidence to prove it.[51]

From the early 1950s, the reputation of the PRU crossed the Atlantic. In the USA, although many researchers clung to the notion that silica dust was the main problem, several were convinced by the new British research and arranged for the PRU team to give lectures on their work in the USA.[52] An offshoot to the PRU appeared in 1960 with the opening of the MRC's Epidemiology Unit in South Wales, with Cochrane as its Director (this unit closed in 1999). As well as being crucially important for research into respiratory disease, PRU data also helped to prove the existence of Caplan's syndrome. This condition was first described by the medical scientist Caplan in 1953, and involved rheumatoid arthritis showing up as nodular fibrosis of the lung, similar to, but at the same time distinguishable from, the massive fibrosis

---

47 P.E. Enterline and M. Jacobsen, 'Epidemiology', in J. Rogan (ed.), *Medicine in the Mining Industry*, p. 370; *Postgraduate Medical Journal*, vol. 75, nos 257–9 (May 1999), p. 2.

48 A. Cochrane, 'The attack rate of progressive massive fibrosis', *British Journal of Industrial Medicine*, vol. 19 (1962), pp. 52–64.

49 MRC, 'Streptomycin treatment of pulmonary tuberculosis: and MRC investigation', *BMJ*, vol. 2 (1948), pp. 769–82.

50 B.G. Staley, 'Coal workers' Pneumoconiosis', *Colliery Guardian* (November 1973), p. 405.

51 Julian Tudor Hart, Wellcome Witness Seminar (2002), p. 12.

52 A. Derickson, *Black Lung: Anatomy of a Public Health Disaster* (Ithaca, NY, 1998), p. 128. For the influence of British research in the USA at this time, see Chapter 6 of Derickson's book.

which appeared with complicated pneumoconiosis.[53] Other studies conducted in the Rhondda were important too. Cochrane's colleague and fellow prisoner of war Bill Miall developed a research programme to investigate hypertension in which he examined 1,228 people in the Rhondda and 1,640 in the Vale of Glamorgan. Miall reflected on how the important epidemiological work carried out in the Rhondda Fach fed into a broad range of projects:

> From the early 1950s we recognized the potential of the Rhondda Fach as a field for epidemiology research into other conditions ... Having the Rhondda Fach population defined by private census and on Hollerith cards – the nearest approach to computerization in those days – we were in a position to obtain representative samples of the general population and become involved with research into other conditions.[54]

Included in this work was key research in the early 1960s into glaucoma, when over 4,000 people in the Rhondda were examined to gauge the presence of the disease. Similar research was conducted on anaemia, when Elwood and his colleagues examined 900 women in the Rhondda Fawr in the late 1960s.[55] When the PRU was set up, it was given a broad remit, and although its early work focused on coal dust disease, a broad range of projects was subsequently undertaken by its researchers. By the late 1960s, the PRU was becoming increasingly involved with the asbestos problem. The South African pathologist Chris Wagner discovered the relationship between asbestos and mesothelioma, an incurable cancer of the lining of the lung. This work was initially carried out by Wagner in South Africa, but was continued by him under the auspices of the PRU at Llandough Hospital.[56] Peter Elmes, who was appointed Director of the PRU in 1976, was also heavily involved in asbestos research, and continued as an independent consultant in asbestos-related diseases until he was 75.[57]

A glance through the index of the PRU's papers reveals the changing nature of its research agenda. Over the 1948–51 period, all but six of the papers published by the unit relate to miners' dust disease; between 1962 and 1963, though, whilst still predominantly concerned with miners' lung, the PRU was now publishing on pulmonary blood pressure in patients with chronic lung disease, the hereditary factors in arterial blood pressure, mesothelioma, and factors influencing arterial blood pressure in the population of Jamaica. By the early 1970s, moreover, the activities of the researchers at the PRU were even more diverse, and were encompassing, as well as the aforementioned asbestos issue – now a prime area of study – breathing difficulties of Lancashire cotton mill workers, the influence of exercise on young

---

53 W.E. Miall et al., 'An epidemiological study of rheumatoid arthritis associated with characteristic chest x-ray appearances in coal-workers', *BMJ*, vol. 4,848 (5 December 1953), pp. 1,231.

54 W.E. Miall, Wellcome Witness Seminar (2002), p. 37.

55 *Postgraduate Medical Journal*, vol. 75, nos 257–9 (May 1999), p. 3.

56 S. Kilpatrick, Wellcome Witness Seminar (2002), p. 28.

57 Queen's University Belfast, *Alumni Magazine* (Autumn 2004), p. 3.

adults, the effects of aerosols produced for dentistry, and lung disease in New Guinea Highlanders.[58]

The PRU closed its doors in 1985, two years before the NCB became the British Coal Corporation. For forty years it had been the most important think tank on industrial dust disease in the UK, and the high quality of its work had made an immense contribution to medical science and to the understanding of the coal dust problem throughout the world. By the 1980s, though, the research environment had changed, and a letter to *The Times* from a medical scientist based at the University of Newcastle illustrated this point:

> The MRC have just closed the pneumoconiosis unit, destroying in the process hundreds of thousands of chest radiographs and associated records. The material on tin workers, coal trimmers and slate workers – not yet fully analysed – is irreplaceable. This university department, affected by sparse accommodation in our new medical school and a reduced grant, have likewise melted down irreplaceable radiographs for the contained silver. Apart from the institute [of Occupational Medicine] in Edinburgh, the pneumoconiosis medical panels of the DHSS are the principal remaining repository of research material and it is to be hoped that here pressures to unload will be resisted successfully ...[59]

The NCB's Health and Safety Infrastructure

As we shall see in Chapter 6, the NCB's main priority in the early years was to win coal. However, despite this prioritisation – and notwithstanding the heavy pressures which the Board was under from day one – the NCB took its responsibility for workers' well-being seriously, and this included a very early commitment to controlling pneumoconiosis.[60] This was manifest in a broader determination to make working in the industry a less onerous experience than it had been before

---

58 J.E. Cotes et al., 'Effect of breathing oxygen upon cardiac output, heart rate, ventilation, systemic and pulmonary blood pressure in patients with chronic lung disease', *Clinical Science*, vol. 25 (1963), pp. 305–21; W.E. Miall and P.D. Oldham, 'The hereditary factor in arterial blood-pressure', *BMJ*, vol. 1 (1963), pp. 75–80; W.E. Miall et al., 'Factors influencing arterial pressure in the general population in Jamaica', *BMJ*, vol. 2 (1962), pp. 497–506; W.J. Smither et al., 'Diffuse pleural mesotheliomas and exposure to asbestos dust', *Lancet*, vol. 2 (1962), p. 1,228; J.C. Wagner et al., 'Mesothelioma in rats after inoculation with asbestos and other materials', *British Journal of Cancer*, vol. 28 (1973), pp. 173–85; G. Berry et al., 'A study of the acute and chronic changes in ventilatory capacity of workers in Lancashire cotton mills', *British Journal of Industrial Medicine*, vol. 30 (1973), pp. 25–36; J. E. Berry et al., 'Cardiac frequency during sub-maximal exercise in young adults: Relation to lean body mass, total body potassium and amount of leg muscle', *Quarterly Journal of Experimental Physiology*, vol. 58 (1973), pp. 239–50.

59 Letter to editor from Dr J.E. Cotes, Department of Occupational Health and Medicine, The Medical School, University of Newcastle on Tyne, *The Times* (6 October 1985), p. 15.

60 NCB *Annual Report, 1947*: 'The Board will not be satisfied until the disease is completely under control.'

nationalisation, and much of this was fuelled by early idealistic expectations in which the NCB saw itself as setting standards for private industry:

> Any organization must deal honestly with its workpeople if it is to prosper, but a nationalized industry, existing only to serve public ends, must set an example in the way it treats its employees, enlarges their opportunities and encourages their efforts.[61]

Certainly, there was a genuine desire to fulfil and go beyond statutory minimum standards regarding health and safety. Indeed, of all its duties, the NCB claimed, 'none was more important' than health and welfare.[62] Most of the miners we interviewed recognised this watershed and conceded that occupational health improved substantially after nationalisation.

The evolution of the Mines Medical Service is a good example of this determination. The basic layout was inherited from a scheme launched by the Minister of Fuel and Power during the Second World War to provide medical facilities for miners over and above the then statutory obligation – in which any mine employing more than 100 persons had to provide a first aid room in the charge of a doctor, nurse or qualified first aid man. Prior to nationalisation, some of the larger colliery companies retained the services of doctors to deal with accidents and to advise the companies on insurance claims. However, very few of them employed a full-time medical officer dedicated to ensuring the long-term health of the workers.

One factor which drove the government into initiating a more comprehensive service for miners was that accident rates in mining were notoriously high.[63] In 1944, then, the Chief Mines Medical Officer of the Ministry of Fuel and Power drew up a scheme, under the direction of the Miners' Welfare Commission, for the creation of a Mines Medical Service. This involved the erection of medical treatment centres at the larger mines which were to be accessible from the 'clean side' of the pithead paths – with the understanding that every new pithead bath would incorporate a treatment centre while established pithead baths would be modified to include one. This scheme developed very slowly, and by 1947 there were only five new prototype centres and five adaptations of first aid rooms in place, with a further 24 centres under construction. However, despite the fact that only 45 nurses were employed across the coal fields, these new nurse-staffed centres proved to be very popular, with miners voluntarily attending in much greater numbers than had been the case with the old first aid rooms.[64]

---

61 Ibid., p. 14.

62 Ibid., p. 50.

63 'The Provision of a Mine's Medical Service', Memorandum by Lord Citrine, 1947. NA/Coal 43/2, NCB.

64 NCB General Purpose Committee, Mines Medical Service, Memorandum by Sir Geoffrey Vickers, 1948. NA/Coal 43/2.

Many saw nationalisation as an opportunity for the special problems of miners' health to be tackled comprehensively.[65] In 1948, the Chief Medical Officer of the NCB (Dr Capel) set out what he saw as the Board's moral responsibility towards the workforce:

> The miner spends about a third of his life at his place of work, exposed to conditions and hazards often of a very specialized nature. The purpose of a Medical Service for the coalmining industry should be to advise the Management of these factors insofar as they affect health, to see that the man is physically fit for the work he has to do, and to organize emergency treatment for accidents and illnesses arising at work ...[66]

Subsequently, a Chief Medical Officer was appointed at the NCB's national headquarters, and this was followed by the appointment of Medical Officers in each of the Divisional Boards.[67] From the outset, the application of the broad principles underlying the Mines Medical Service were to be left up to the individual Divisional Boards, who would act upon the advice of their Medical Officers. As a rough guide to the Divisions, though, it was recommended that a full-time doctor should be appointed to serve units of approximately 5,000 men, that these medics should not have had any previous association with compensation in the coal industry, and that their work should involve limited handling of any matters involving compensation.[68] By this time the Board fully realised that this would be a costly venture. The erection of the proposed new 217 medical centres across the UK was likely to cost £1,400,000, and running costs were expected to be in the region of £200,000 a year over the first four years. This was a considerable outlay on health and safety, especially coming on top of an existing expenditure of £380,000 a year to which the Board was already committed for doctors' fees, medical examinations and the payment of full-time first aid attendants.[69] Therefore, given the dire economic situation which the NCB stepped into in 1947, a pledge to focus on health and safety and ensure that coal workers were covered by a medical service was highly commendable.

By September 1948, six Divisional Medical Officers had been appointed. Below these were to be colliery doctors employed either on a full-time or part-time basis. At this stage, though, the Board was very reluctant to interfere in any way with the creation of the National Health Service, and informed the Divisions that, given the shortage of GPs, the engagement of an 'excessive number' of full-time doctors was

---

65 See, for example, Ministry of Fuel and Power, 'A Proposal for a Miner's Medical Service', A. Tudor Hart, 1946. NA/Coal 43/2.

66 Ministry of Fuel and Power, NCB General Purpose Committee, Mines Medical Service, paper by Dr Capel, 1948. NA/Coal 43/2.

67 NCB *Annual Report, 1947*, p. 3.

68 Ministry of Fuel and Power, NCB General Purpose Committee, Mines Medical Service, paper by Dr Capel, 1948. Coal 43/2, p. 3.

69 NCB *Annual Report, 1950*, p. 4.

to be avoided.[70] From the end of 1948, the Divisions quickly began to build up their health services. However, everything was put on hold in 1949, when the government set up a Committee under the Chairmanship of Judge E.T. Dale to consider the relationship between the NHS and the various health services being provided by industry. Consequently, the Prime Minister asked all branches of industry to postpone any further developments of industrial health services until the Dale Committee had made its recommendations.[71] The Board, then, was forced to implement an interim policy in which it completed those centres already under construction and staffed them with State Registered Nurses. However, no new centres were built, and no full-time doctors were taken on.

The Dale Committee – to which the NCB gave evidence – sat through 1950, and eventually fully endorsed the Board's policy regarding medical services, giving the go-ahead for the recruitment of full-time doctors if required. The committee also heard evidence from the NCB that its medical service was already one of the most comprehensive in the UK. The Chief Medical Officer was assisted by 65 Coal Board doctors and 300 nurses, and 20,000 workers across the mining regions of the UK were trained in first aid.[72] Consequently, by the end of December 1951, 119 medical centres were in operation at pit level.[73] There was, though, a considerable disparity regarding the number of employees per doctor, ranging from one doctor for 6,188 men in the South Eastern Division to one for 34,074 men in the North Eastern Division.[74] By 1953, the 200 medical centre target was reached, and by this time there were also 473 smaller 'medical units' operating at smaller collieries.[75]

The Medical Officers in each Division were responsible for running the treatment services. Below these, the NCB doctors were normally deployed on a Divisional or Area basis, while the nurses were on hand at the collieries. As well as carrying out routine visits to mines and quarries, the Mines Medical Officers carried out special investigations into a wide range of subjects, including pneumoconiosis, Weil's disease, dermatitis and nystagmus, as well as operating the 'Morphia Scheme' in which specially selected men were allowed to administer morphine to alleviate shock

---

70 NCB, Manpower and Welfare Department, 'Mines Medical Service', September, 1948. NA/Coal 43/2.

71 We have engaged with the subject of industrial health services elsewhere. Johnston and McIvor, 'Whatever happened to the Occupational Health Service?', pp. 79–106.

72 *Report of a Committee of Enquiry on Industrial Health Services* (1951), Cmd 8170, pp. 8–9; henceforth the Dale Committee.

73 NCB, 'Medical Centres Programme, 1948–1951', 15 January 1953, table 1, NA/POWE10/259.

74 Ministry of Fuel and Power, Letter from M.J. Bentley, Medical Branch of the NCB, to Dr T.D. Spencer, Divisional Medical Officer, North Eastern Division, dated 15 January 1953, NA/POWE10/259.

75 W. Ashworth. *The History of the British Coal Industry, Volume 5. 1946–1982: The Nationalized Industry* (Oxford, 1986), p. 559.

and pain underground.[76] This was vitally important given the difficulties involved of getting injured men to the surface, but could only be authorised, by the Home Office, in pits where first aid facilities were of a sufficiently high standard. Clear evidence, then, of the rapid improvements in colliery first aid treatment is the fact that during 1947 alone, 99 collieries employing 87,000 men received this authorisation – bringing the total to 467 collieries employing half a million men.[77] Throughout the period from the early 1950s to the 1970s, the service expanded to become the largest industrial health service in Britain, employing around forty medical officers and over two hundred nurses.[78] Treatment in the centres and units, though, was intended only to be of an emergency nature, and the staff at each colliery had to always ensure that good links were in place with local hospitals, social services and GPs.[79]

As well as administering initial first aid treatment, the main role of the Mines Medical Service was to medically examine new entrants to the industry and to monitor miners' health. Prior to nationalisation, all new entrants to the industry had to be medically examined, and this examination included a chest x-ray for all Welsh miners – because Wales was seen at the time as the prime danger area for pneumoconiosis. These statutory examinations, as well as the role of x-raying all Welsh entrants – normally conducted by the Ministry of Labour and National Service doctors – were taken over by the NCB in 1952. Over and above this, though, the NCB went beyond its statutory duty by adopting a policy of medically examining all adult miners.[80] Also, during 1955 the NCB made arrangements with the Ministry for Pensions and National Insurance for the Board's doctors to receive, in professional confidence, full medical information about each man with pneumoconiosis who had been examined by a Pneumoconiosis Panel, providing the man consented to this disclosure.[81]

The periodic x-raying of all miners became one of the NCB's statutory duties in 1959.[82] There were three principal objectives to the mass x-ray scheme: firstly, it would provide a medical check on the effectiveness of dust control in the industry; secondly, it would afford all mineworkers the safeguard of a regular chest x-ray examination, and thirdly, it was thought that routine x-raying would help eradicate TB from the pits. The NCB fully realised that the implementation of this new scheme would reverse the downward trend in the number of pneumoconiosis cases, due to the simple fact that more cases would be discovered. However, it was very confident at this time that the battle was already being won:

76 Sir Andrew Bryan, *The Evolution of Health and Safety in Mines* (Letchworth, 1975), p. 116.

77 NCB *Annual Report, 1946*, p. 6.

78 Bryan, *The Evolution of Health and Safety* , pp. 116–17.

79 Ashworth, *History of the British Coal Industry*, p. 559.

80 D. Hunter, *Diseases of Occupations* (London, 1975), p. 1,008.

81 Ashworth, *History of the British Coal Industry*, p. 560.

82 NCB *Annual Report, 1952*, p. 18; Hunter, *Diseases*, p. 1,009.

Such a rise will result from greater x-ray facilities and the disclosure of cases at present
undiagnosed. It will not reflect a deterioration in dust conditions which have been, and still
are, improving as a result of the considerable measures taken in the industry to prevent
and suppress airborne dust.[83]

By late summer of 1959, then, the mass x-ray scheme, mooted by the NJPC ten
years earlier, was finally operational, and by the end of that year 80,000 miners
at 116 collieries across the UK had been x-rayed.[84] From this time on, the NCB
offered all mine workers an x-ray to check for the presence of pneumoconiosis. This
process was to be repeated every five years, with the frequency increasing in 1974
to every four years. Although there was no obligation on the men to come forward
for examination, from the outset attendance rates were over 85%, and in 1980 the
rate was 90%.[85]

As well as the Mines Medical Service, the NCB had other departments dedicated
to health and safety in the industry. Each Area and Division had Safety Engineers
under the direct control of the Chief Safety Engineer based in London, while the
larger collieries had their own Safety Officers. There were also two Standing
Committees which oversaw health and safety: the Safety Conference, and the Rescue
Advisory Committee, which was chaired by the Chief Safety Engineer. The Safety
Conference was made up of Divisional Safety Engineers and enlisted specialists to
ensure uniform action on health and safety matters throughout the UK.

The degree of consultation built into the infrastructure of the NCB was also
impressive. By the late 1950s there was the National Consultative Council, Divisional
and Area Councils, as well as around a thousand Colliery Consultative Committees.
More specific to the dust problem, at the national level there was the National Joint
Pneumoconiosis Committee, the Safety and Health Committee of the Coal Industry
National Consultative Council, and the Safety in Mines Research (Advisory) Board,
specifically designed to advise ministers on the progress of any research relating to
mine safety. All of these national committees had representation from the NCB, the
trade unions, managers and HM Inspectors.[86] This extensive consultative machinery
was further enhanced in 1952 with the setting up of four Advisory Panels to deal
specifically with medical and human problems associated with pneumoconiosis.
These were the Epidemiology Panel, the Psychology Panel, the Physiology Panel
and the Industrial Medical Panel. All of these panels were informed by experts in
their respective fields.[87]

---

83 NCB *Annual Report, 1958*, p. 8.

84 Ministry of Fuel and Power, National Coal Board Periodic Chest X-ray Scheme:
Results for 1959. NJPC No 113.

85 Ashworth, *History of the British Coal Industry*, p. 568.

86 Sir G. Nott-Bower and R.H Walkerdine, *The NCB: The First Ten Years* (London,
1958), pp. 45–6.

87 See, for example, the high-calibre list of members of the Industrial Medical Panel,
which included Gilson of the PRU, Rogan of the NCB, and the Chief Medical Officer of ICI;
Colliery Guardian (20 March 1952), p. 359.

By the 1950s, research work on coal dust was divided between the NCB, the Ministry of Fuel and Power – through its Safety in Mines Research and Testing Branch – and the PRU. There had been a long history of state interest in mine safety dating back to the mid-nineteenth century, and more importantly, from the passage of the 1911 Coal Mines Act which introduced the post of Chief Inspector of Mines. When the NCB came into being, it inherited 70 small laboratories which had been used for coal mining research in the era of private ownership. The Board's aim, though, was to locate laboratories and staff in each area, and by 1951 a further 31 were built, while 38 of the original 70 laboratories were extended and modernised.[88]

Important work was also carried out by the NCB's Scientific Department and by its Divisional Scientific Service. One of the main tasks of the Scientific Department was to analyse dust samples from underground roadways to ascertain their explosive potential. However, the Scientific Department became increasingly committed to the respiratory dust problem too, and by the end of 1951 over a hundred scientific staff were engaged in full-time sampling and the measuring of dust concentrations – we'll come back to issues of dust monitoring and control in Chapter 6. By 1952, the NCB's Scientific Service was costing £1,200,000 a year and was staffed by around 160 scientists and 1,200 technical officers. Half of this outlay went on analysis of coal output and the testing of coal preparation plants, while a tenth was allocated to dust sampling to address the pneumoconiosis problem.[89] By the mid-1950s, then, the NCB was annually bankrolling 15 separate research projects from this £121,000, the major one being the Pneumoconiosis Field Research (PFR) scheme which began in 1952, looked at in some depth in the next section. A further arm of research was added in 1969 in the form of the Institute of Occupational Medicine (IOM), based in Edinburgh. The IOM had four branches engaged in research: one for long-term research into pneumoconiosis and respiratory disability; one dedicated to environmental factors including dust exposure; one for physiological aspects of mining, such as working in hot conditions, and a statistics department which worked closely with the other departments in the planning and execution of research projects and the management and analysis of data.[90]

Clearly, then, the NCB, by dint of the high degree of expertise on which it was able to draw, was well equipped to deal with miners' health, safety, living conditions, and general well-being. However, as far as CWP was concerned, by far the most comprehensive manifestation of its commitment to miners' respiratory health was the Pneumoconiosis Field Research, and it is to this that we now turn.

The Pneumoconiosis Field Research (PFR): The 25-pit Scheme

In the early 1950s, the PRU researchers were strongly advocating that a long-term approach to the dust disease problem was required. According to Cochrane:

88 NCB *Annual Report, 1951*, pp. 5–6.
89 NCB *Annual Report, 1952*, p. 9.
90 Bryan, *The Evolution of Health and Safety*, p. 118.

Since the factors which may make coal dust dangerous are not yet known, the precise level of dust concentration in different pits which may be regarded as safe are uncertain, and indeed they cannot be established until a generation of coal miners has been exposed to them for their working life and has been shown to remain healthy.[91]

From 1947, the PRU had carried out extensive dust sampling of a range of mining conditions, with 8,000 dust samples taken by 1951.[92] These were related to x-ray evidence, and a detailed industrial history was taken of every man x-rayed, with special attention paid to periods of exposure at the coal face.[93] Owen Wade joined the PRU as a junior researcher in 1948, and could clearly remember Cochrane's determination to leave no stone unturned in these early studies:

> It was Archie Cochrane's conviction that the total population of any colliery be identified and when we went to visit a mine … we should interview and x-ray every man who was there. An enormous amount of work went into preparation beforehand. All of us in the unit were made to visit the colliery and meet the miners. A series of lectures was arranged. Any ability I have as a lecturer was, I am sure, because I had to go and speak in pubs, or clubs as they call them, because the pubs shut on Sunday … it didn't matter which day of the week, the procedure was always the same. The presiding chairman would introduce you, and you went up and explained to them what pneumoconiosis was, how it affected them, and why it was necessary for us to see every man in the colliery – 80 per cent wasn't good enough, 90 per cent wasn't good enough, 95 per cent wasn't good enough. We wanted to see every man.[94]

To compare dust inhalation between collieries more effectively, the PRU researchers concentrated on what they referred to as 'ten-year pure face workers', meaning men whose only significant dust exposure had been at the coal face at the same colliery for ten years immediately preceding the survey.[95] However, Fletcher had to admit there were still serious flaws in the research:

> The weakest point in the evidence is that the figures for dust dosage are based upon what can only be rough estimates of the dust concentrations prevailing in the 10 years before our dust measurements, during which time we know there have been considerable changes.[96]

---

91 A.L. Cochrane et al., 'The Role of Periodic Examination in the Prevention of Coal workers' Pneumoconiosis', *British Journal of Industrial Medicine*, vol. 8 (1951), p. 53.

92 P.D. Oldham, 'The Nature of the Variability of Dust Concentrations at the Coal Face', *British Journal of Industrial Medicine*, vol. 10 (1953), p. 227; NCB, *Annual Reports, 1951*, p. 61.

93 C.M. Fletcher, 'Epidemiological Studies of Coal Miners' Pneumoconiosis in Great Britain', *Archives of Industrial Health*, vol. 11 (January 1955), p. 31.

94 O. Wade, Wellcome Witness Seminar (2002), p. 16.

95 Fletcher, 'Epidemiological Studies', p. 32.

96 Ibid., p. 34.

Therefore, the PRU was not able to conclude from these surveys whether varying types of coal dust had different effects on miners. Moreover, although these studies – the longest of which lasted three weeks – produced evidence of the prevalence of dust disease in selected mines, they failed to answer important questions because of the uncertainties surrounding dust conditions which the men had been exposed to in the past. What was required, then, was a 'forward looking study relating the dust exposure of selected men to x-ray changes over a number of years'.[97] Three factors underpinned the rationale for such a scheme. Firstly, it would provide immediate protection for coal workers in what was seen as an interval before safe dust levels were defined and mine dust could be effectively suppressed. This would be possible because the PRU team was now fully aware that the progressive nature of the disease meant crucial radiological changes became apparent before serious injury could be done to the lungs. At such an early stage the worker would show signs of having simple pneumoconiosis and could be removed from dusty conditions. Therefore, the PRU team was confident that by advising men whose x-rays revealed ominous changes to work in reduced dust conditions, PMF could be avoided.[98] Unfortunately, nothing much could be done for the 'victims of the past' who already had PMF, as they would not derive any benefit from periodic x-rays, or indeed from changing to less dusty jobs.[99] The second rationale for implementing a comprehensive long-term study was that a UK-wide x-ray scheme would reveal to engineers in which mines, seams or districts the disease – despite the imposition of dust suppression measures – was still apparent. This would facilitate the targeting of resources to the most appropriate areas. And thirdly, if routine x-raying of miners was combined with the routine collection of dust samples at the places where the miners worked, it would be possible to determine the level of dustiness which had *not* brought about a rise in pneumoconiosis. Therefore, a long-term survey would eventually determine what was an unequivocal safe standard of dustiness.

Not all occupational health experts agreed that x-ray schemes were worthwhile. Sir Andrew Meiklejohn, Lecturer in Industrial Health at Glasgow University and the NUM's honorary medical adviser, was certainly very critical of the idea. For one thing, he argued that the men and their trade unions would simply want to know if they had contracted pneumoconiosis, not whether they had reached a critical level of severity. Meiklejohn was also worried that the propensity for error in reading the x-rays was too high, that there was a danger of producing just as many cases of neurosis as the number of cases of pneumoconiosis that would be prevented, and that such a scheme might also reveal so much pneumoconiosis in the UK that large

97 J.C. Gilson and A.L. Cochrane, *Advisory Committee on Medical Research, Report of Pneumoconiosis Group, Appendix A: Summary of Evidence*, p. 3, NAS/HH104/46.

98 This assumption, though, was based on early studies of PMF, and much later research would show that even men with simple pneumoconiosis could progress to PMF; M.D. Attfield and E.D. Kuempel, 'Pneumoconiosis, coal mine dust and the PFR', *Annals of Occupational Hygiene*, vol. 47, no. 7 (2003), pp. 525–9, p. 528.

99 Cochrane et al., 'The Role of Periodic Examination', p. 58.

numbers of the mining workforce would have to leave the industry.[100] His main concern was that the rise in the morbidity rates in South Wales and at some other coal fields was simply a result of the more thorough investigation which had been given to the disease in these areas. He also pointed out that a high incidence of pneumoconiosis appeared to be related to a high accident rate, which suggested that the psychological effects of the disease might have the effect of rendering men less alert, or more dubiously, that the fear of contracting pneumoconiosis was giving rise to a subconscious desire to be injured and escape from an unhealthy working environment.[101] However, the PRU team disagreed. Their views reflected a changing opinion that Hart and Aslett's conclusion – drawn from their South Wales study in the early 1940s – that the rank of coal was the main factor was wrong, and that much more attention had to be paid to the total quantity of dust inhaled, irrespective of its composition.[102]

By 1952, due to official figures of certifications of the disease, the NCB was well aware of the extent of pneumoconiosis across the UK, and the notion that the disease was confined to the Welsh coal fields was now a thing of the past. However, the difficulty lay in teasing out the degree to which the rising number of certifications reflected working conditions:

> The increase in certifications outside South Wales in 1949–52 does not necessarily mean that more men are getting the disease at the present time … in some places more men ask to be medically examined as they become aware of the possibility that they might have got pneumoconiosis. The Board are trying to find out the facts …[103]

Clearly, the NCB's accumulating x-ray evidence was not an indicator of the correlation of new cases of CWP with current working conditions, because of the preponderance of old cases – the result of past working conditions – which were being picked up.

In May 1951, a special committee was set up by the NJPC to examine proposals for field research in coal mines. Five meetings later, in January 1952, this sub-committee had:

> … no hesitation in recommending that a special survey should be undertaken at a representative sample of mines throughout the coalfields. The method would be over a period of years to relate the dust conditions in the selected mines to the prevalence and rate of attack and progression of pneumoconiosis among the workers in them. The quality as well as the quantity of dust would be taken into consideration.[104]

---

100 Ibid., pp. 59, 60.

101 *Colliery Guardian* (6 September 1951), p. 275.

102 NCB, Scientific Department, Pneumoconiosis Field Research, *The Study of the Composition of Respirable Dust in the Pneumoconiosis Field Research* (1960), p. 4.

103 NCB, *Annual Report*, 1952.

104 *NJPC Report of the Field Research Sub-Committee* (1952), NJPC Report no. 39.

The NCB accepted these recommendations without question, and invited Cochrane to be the survey's Scientific Adviser. Cochrane quickly began the organisation and training of two teams of researchers required for the project, and both teams were trained 'on the job' in the second Rhondda Fach survey which began in April 1953.[105]

The NCB, then, intended to 'find out the facts' by conducting a long-running field study. What emerged was the Pneumoconiosis Field Research (PFR), a grand-scale experiment in epidemiology designed to last at least ten years – for it was fully understood that for much of the early phase of the programme, the problem of old cases of CWP being recorded would be significant. The scheme was initially referred to as the '20-pit Scheme', although five more pits were subsequently added to the list. The NCB's Scientific Director described the study in 1955 as 'one of the biggest pieces of cooperative research that has ever been undertaken'.[106] Certainly, the co-operative elements of the programme were impressive. The study was undertaken in close collaboration with the MRC's Pneumoconiosis Research Unit, with a steering committee drawn from the NCB, the NUM, the Ministry of Fuel and Power, and the MRC, with the Ministry of Pensions and National Insurance sending an observer.[107] The NUM played a significant role too, though, exemplified in its insistence that the Shotts mine in Lanarkshire be added to the initial list of pits because it was notoriously dusty, as we discuss in Chapter 7.

The PFR's objectives were to establish definitive safe levels of dustiness in which men could work without damaging their health, and ascertain an accurate indication of the true prevalence of pneumoconiosis. Twenty-five pits were subsequently selected from the NCB Divisions stretching from Scotland down to Kent. Five were in Scotland, three in Northumberland and Cumberland, two in Durham, three in Yorkshire, one in Lancashire, one in North Wales, on in the East Midlands, two in the West Midlands, six in South Wales, and one in Kent. Four main factors thought relevant to the causation of pneumoconiosis underpinned the selection process: the range of coal in the seams; the dust concentrations experienced at the coal faces on the coal getting shifts; the average ash content of the coal seam; and the sandstone content of the roof and floor.[108] However, one of the limitations of the plan was that no account was taken of the nature and amount of the so-called 'dirt bands' between the coal seams. Therefore, because the size of dirt bands varied greatly between the seams in each colliery – and even within the same seam – only a very rough indication of the quartz content of the roof and floor strata of the working places in the selected pits would be possible.[109]

---

105 *Report of the Work of the PRU Pneumoconiosis Field Research 20 Pit Scheme* (November 1952), NJPC Report no. 46.

106 *The Miner* (January/February 1955), p. 18.

107 Donald Hicks, 'The 20-Pit Scheme', *The Miner* (January/February 1955), p. 18.

108 B.G. Staley, 'Coal workers' Pneumoconiosis', *Colliery Guardian* (November 1973), p. 410.

109 NCB, Scientific Department, *The Study of the Composition of Respirable Dust in the Pneumoconiosis Field Research*, p. 5.

The intention was to x-ray all the men in the selected mines every two years and keep detailed records of the dust and environmental conditions in every part of the mine. To accomplish this mammoth task, two Leyland Comet lorries were commissioned, towing 22 foot-long, 7 foot 6 inch-wide trailers equipped with state-of-the-art mobile x-ray apparatus. One unit was based in Edinburgh, closely associated with Edinburgh University Department of Diseases of the Chest, and the other was centred on Cardiff in close liaison with the PRU. Each of the units was staffed by a Medical Officer assisted by radiographers and clerical personnel. The trailers were divided into two compartments: an x-ray compartment, and a darkroom which had its own automatic film processing unit.[110] In all 60 people were involved with the on-site monitoring and the checking of working places, while a team of scientists and their assistants at the NCB's Hobart House analysed the data as it came in from around the country. Samples of the roof and floor strata at the working faces were collected on all production seams at the selected collieries, and these were then chemically examined. The whole scheme was directed by Dr J.M. Rogan, the Board's Chief Medical Officer, with, as noted earlier, Cochrane acting as Scientific Adviser. Every three months the Research Programme was reviewed by a steering committee made up of representatives from the NUM, the MRC, the Ministry of Fuel and Power, and the NCB itself, with the Ministry of National Insurance also sending an observer.[111]

In 1955, due to the increasing number of x-rays being conducted by the NCB, there was a rise in the number of certified cases of pneumoconiosis. The NCB accepted that this rise would continue until the gap between the number of men certified and the number who were certifiable had narrowed. However, once again the dominant tone was optimistic: '… the true prevalence of the disease is almost certainly decreasing as more and more progress is made with the Board's measures to suppress dust underground'.[112] We shall be looking closely at the NCB's dust suppression measures in Chapter 6. For the moment, though, the important point is that only the PFR's painstaking survey of dust exposure and x-ray evidence would be able to reveal how the incidence of the disease across the coal fields related to dust levels.

In 1957, a decision was taken to expand the scope of the PFR from concentrating only on CWP, to investigating occupational chest diseases in general. Rogan explained the reasons for this change:

> According to the existing plan the research should terminate with a statement of dust levels, which, if established over a man's working life, would prevent the great majority of mine workers from developing certain radiological appearances. Clearly, it was now desirable to extend the research so as to obtain information, if possible, about chest symptoms and about disability. Then, finally, it should be possible to examine the relationship between

110 *Colliery Engineering* (December 1953), p. 525.
111 *The Miner* (January/February 1955), p. 18.
112 NCB, *Annual Report 1955*, p. 15.

the symptoms, disability, and radiological abnormality and to establish the relationship between all three and the dust environment.[113]

To this end, when the second phase of the study commenced in 1957, two new elements were introduced. Firstly, all the men x-rayed were given respiratory function tests in order that the relationship between dust exposure, x-ray appearance *and* the extent of pulmonary disability could be correlated.[114] The second innovation was that every man was given a short questionnaire of chest symptoms. In this way information on cough, sputum, breathlessness, wheeze and the effects of weather on the chest and chest illnesses could be better understood.[115]

We need to keep in mind that while the PFR was in progress, miners throughout the UK were supposed to have been working in so-called 'approved dust conditions'. However, as we saw in Chapter 3, these were being determined by an inappropriate standard. The PRU researchers fully realised this was an unsatisfactory situation, and in 1951 Cochrane, Fletcher et al. described the NCB's provisional levels – 850/650/450 p.p.c.c. – for approved dust conditions as being 'based on scanty evidence'.[116] However, the state of affairs was made even more serious by the fact that many miners were working under conditions which did not even meet these highly questionable standards – and we explore this in some depth in Chapter 6. Therefore, the sooner the PFR produced definitive evidence of what constituted a safe dust level, the better for the health of the workers. But, due to the long-term nature of the research, this would not be forthcoming until 1970.

From 1961, the second round of the PFR medical surveys was slowed down to give the researchers time to overcome difficulties they were encountering with the radiological diagnoses, and to analyse the respiratory symptoms questionnaires in more depth. Eventually, though, the second surveys revealed little progression of pneumoconiosis since the first survey had taken place. However, the research also began to illustrate quite clearly that miners were suffering from higher rates of bronchitis.[117] In 1962, the NCB decided that the field research should continue for some years, but stated that it would review the situation around 1968. This caused consternation in the NUM, as the union wanted the surveys to carry on until a definite result had been obtained. Consequently, the Board was asked by the union to dispel any doubts regarding the future of the PFR. In reply, the NCB pointed out that the PFR was only supposed to last ten years, which had now elapsed, so it was only

---

113 J.M. Rogan, 'Pneumoconiosis: chest disease in coal miners, with special reference to the Pneumoconiosis Field Research', *The Mining Engineer* (November 1960), pp. 108–9.

114 NCB *Annual Report, 1957*.

115 Rogan, 'Pneumoconiosis: Chest disease in coal miners'.

116 A.L. Cochrane et al., 'The Role of Periodic Examinations in the Prevention of Coal workers' Pneumoconiosis', *British Journal of Industrial Medicine*, vol. 8 (1951), pp. 53–61, p. 53.

117 National Joint Pneumoconiosis Committee, *27th Report of the Field Research Steering Committee*, NJPC 116, 1961. NA/PIN 20/325.

reasonable that the NCB should want to review the research from time to time. The Board would not commit to an indefinite period of research.[118]

The main fruit of the PFR appeared in 1970 when an Interim Standards Study (ISS) was undertaken. From the masses of data collected, the researchers were at last able to produce estimates of the probability of miners developing simple CWP if exposed to mine dust for 35 years. A seminal paper was published by Jacobsen, Rae, Walton and Rogan, and this was subsequently used as a basis for recommending that more stringent dust levels be introduced in coal mining.[119] The PFR had furnished clear evidence that the control of CWP lay with reducing levels of respirable dust in the mines, that gravimetrically based measurement was much more effective than particle counting, and that the concentration of dust and the length of time exposed to dust were the two most important variables – although the evidence regarding the significance of quartz in coal miners' pneumoconiosis was still equivocal.[120] The PFR's use of gravimetric sampling had also demonstrated that the once-popular 'coal rank effect' was in fact the result of earlier studies' use of particle count sampling.[121] Very quickly, in 1971, the NCB voluntarily adopted new dust regulations based on a gravimetric scale. These stipulated that dust levels had to fall below 8–7 milligrams per cubic metre (mg/m^3). The general enforcement of this new standard marked a belated improvement over that adapted in 1948 from Bedford and Warner's unintentional dust datum. Further, in 1975 the state imposed a statutory duty on the industry to adhere to these standards with the introduction of the Coal Mines (Respirable Dust) Regulations of that year. However, as we will see, further research was to eventually demonstrate that even more stringent measures needed to be taken, and this resulted in another major review of dust standards in 2004.

Despite the NUM's misgivings regarding the NCB's lack of dedication to the PFR, the research was continued for another twenty years. The detailed monitoring of miners' exposure to respirable dust was carried on continuously up to 1968 at all the initially selected mines. After this, it was trimmed back to ten collieries which remained under closer supervision until the 1980s. The ISS analysis was based on working miners performing the dustiest jobs. However, realising that this could have resulted in a bias due to the selection of healthy workers, later studies of the PFR examined workers in other jobs as well as retired miners.[122] The final thrust of the

---

118 NJPC, Minutes of 21st Meeting held at the Ministry of Power on 18th October 1962. NA/LAB 14/799.

119 M. Jacobsen et al., 'New Dust Standards for British Coal Mines', *Nature*, vol. 227 (1970), pp. 445–7; see P.E. Enterline, in Rogan (ed.), *Medicine in the Mining Industry*, p. 369.

120 NCB, Scientific Department, *The Study of the Composition of Respirable Dust in the Pneumoconiosis Field Research*, p. 21.

121 See M. Jacobsen et al., 'The relation between pneumoconiosis and dust exposure in British coal mines', in W.H. Walton (ed.), *Inhaled Particles*, vol. III (Surrey, 1971), pp. 903–19.

122 M.D. Attfield and E.D. Kuempel, 'Pneumoconiosis, coal mine dust and the PFR', *Annals of Occupational Hygiene*, vol. 47, no. 7 (2003), pp. 525–9, p. 529.

PFR occurred in the mid-1980s, when miners at three mines in the PFR – one in South Wales, one in Yorkshire, and one in the North East of England – took part in another medical survey in which 1,671 men were examined.[123] And data from the PFR was also to eventually help prove that miners were especially susceptible to other diseases linked to dust inhalation, especially bronchitis and emphysema.

The 25-pit Scheme was a monumental example of high-quality epidemiological research, and a considerable body of knowledge was amassed by a large number of researchers over the thirty-odd years of its life – indeed, as early as 1957, sampling and x-raying in the 25 pits had provided continuous exposure histories of 35,000 men.[124] Writing in 1998, one expert on dust disease summed up the work of the PFR in this way:

> The National Coal Board embarked on a massively costly programme of research into dust control in mines alongside its medical research and, in full cooperation with the mining unions, progressively implemented the research results into its practical management of the pneumoconiosis problem. As an example of enlightened management in dealing with work related ill health this endeavour is unparalleled. The pneumoconiosis statistics tell the story, the disease having largely been eliminated.[125]

By the early 1970s it was clear that the prevalence of pneumoconiosis was falling in the UK. Clearly, then, there had been some success in improving dust suppression in the mines during the first twenty-odd years of nationalisation. However, although the overall trend was down, as we see in Figure 4.1, it was only after the imposition of the tighter 1970s dust regulations – which the NCB had a statutory duty to comply with in 1975 – that the decline became pronounced. Therefore, the more stringent

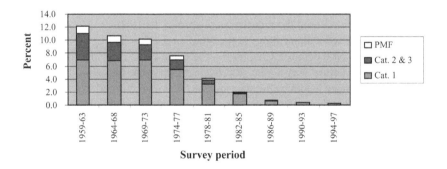

Figure 4.1   Prevalence of pneumoconiosis in British miners, 1959–97

123 D. Coggon and A.N. Taylor, 'Coal mining and chronic obstructive pulmonary disease: A review of the evidence', *Thorax*, vol. 53 (1998), pp. 398–407, p. 400.

124 Rogan, 'Pneumoconiosis: chest disease in coal miners', p. 108.

125 A. Seaton, 'The new prescription: Industrial injuries benefits for smokers?', *Thorax*, vol. 53 (1998), p. 1.

1970s dust datum went some way towards ensuring that dust suppression efforts were taken much more seriously by management and miners alike.[126]

Conclusion

In Chapter 3, we saw how various factors underpinned the recognition of coal dust disease. These included growing medical awareness and knowledge of occupational dust disease, the growth of the coal mining industry, increased mechanisation and the rise in dust levels, and the growing strength of the miners' trade unions. A similar fusion of economic and social factors lay behind the attention devoted by researchers to pneumoconiosis from the 1940s onwards. Certainly, one of the most important socio-economic factors was the urgent need for the NCB to re-employ pneumoconiotic miners who had been removed from the coal industry on account of their lung condition. As we saw in the last chapter, it was this which would result in the 'approved/non-approved' faces principle, and a long adherence to an arbitrary standard of maximum dustiness which was not rigorous enough.

Much of this medical effort to research the coal dust disease problem was related to the new worker-oriented approach to medicine taken by many medical professionals in the post-war period, carried along by the impetus of the rise of social medicine. As the archetypal proletarians, it was perhaps understandable that miners would be an obvious group for a new breed of ideologically infused medical scientists to study. The setting up of the PRU and its epidemiological method of inquiry into miners' health can be seen as part of the social medicine movement – and certainly, several leading medical experts of the time identified with the plight of miners. Moreover, despite a decline in social medicine in the late 1950s – which coincided with the atrophy of the mining industry – the inter-relationship between medicine and miners was sustained, right up until the industry's collapse in the 1980s.

Although there were major flaws in the NCB's coal dust strategy – and we will examine these in some detail in Chapter 6 – there can be no denying that its health and safety infrastructure was a vast improvement on what had gone before. The commitment to miners' health by the state and the NCB over this period was related to an understanding that those who worked in the most dangerous of industries required special consideration, coupled with an awareness of the strength of the NUM, which remained potent until the 1980s. There was also a sense that the government's flagship public corporation had to set an example for the rest of industry to follow. The NCB's 25-pit Scheme was a natural corollary of the path-breaking epidemiology undertaken by the PRU, and conclusions from the PFR in 1970 provided the long-awaited rationale for stricter dust regulations in the UK. However, the NCB knew from the outset that it would take at least ten years for the project to provide such results, and could possibly have done much more to protect its workers from dust

126 A.S. Afacan and D.A. Scarisbrick, 'Respiratory Health Surveillance in the UK Coal Mining Industry', *Transactions of the Institute of Mining and Metallurgy* (February 2001), p. 5.

exposure in the interim. Chapter 6 will examine ways in which the NCB struggled to address the coal dust problem within the workplace while at the same time trying to ensure that production was sustained in a shrinking coal market. Before addressing the NCB's strategy, however, we turn our attention in Chapter 5 to the other main respiratory diseases of coal miners – bronchitis and emphysema.

Chapter 5

The Last Gasp:
Bronchitis and Emphysema

In the concluding chapter of this part, we take the analysis of advancing medical knowledge on miners' respiratory disease up to 2006. By the 1990s, the British underground coal mining industry had virtually disappeared, with production centred on privately owned open-cast mines where machinery was much more important than labour power. However, as was the case with most of Britain's decaying and decayed heavy industries, although the supporting infrastructure and landscape traces had largely vanished, those who had spent their lives working in such industries were still bearing psychological and physiological scarring in the form of unemployment or redeployment, work-related ill health, or a combination of all these. We have illustrated in the previous two chapters that the fight against coal miners' respiratory disease was taken up by British medical science, and became for some medical professionals almost a crusade. We further illuminate the complexities surrounding the recognition of occupational dust disease in this chapter. For, as we will see, although leading medical scientists such as J.S. Haldane had since the beginning of the twentieth century adhered to the notion that bronchitis was the source of all miners' respiratory problems, it would only be towards the end of the twentieth century that this condition, along with emphysema, was accepted as being industrially linked.

The final acts in the long drama of miners' lung disease were played out against the background of a crumbling coal industry in which a major change in its relationship with government had taken place. When coal mining was nationalised in 1947, demand for coal was high and 750,000 people were employed. However, with the sharp decline of the household coal market in the 1960s, virtually all British coal was consumed by the production of electricity. Moreover, after the election of a Conservative government in 1979, there was strong political pressure to reduce Britain's dependence on coal as much as possible. The discovery of North Sea gas, combined with other factors including increased coal imports, saw consumption of domestic coal continue to fall, and between 1980 and 1994 total coal production fell from 130 million to 50 million tonnes. This caused employment in mining to drop from around 230,000 to about 8,400 – see Table 2.1. The increasing number of pit closures led to a series of miners' strikes, culminating in a year-long dispute in 1984–85. Throughout this pivotal struggle, Margaret Thatcher's Conservative government remained determined not to give in, and the strike left bitter divisions within mining communities. In 1987 the NCB changed its name to the British Coal

Corporation, and in 1992 the industry received another blow when the government announced it was closing down a further 30 pits – although at this point the Trade Secretary Michael Heseltine agreed to a reprieve for some of these. It was shortly after this that British coal mining was privatised, with Richard Budge's RJB Mining paying £800 million to take over what was left of the industry.

It was against this background that the British medical and legal professions deliberated over the question of whether coal miners were especially prone to contracting – and therefore deserving of compensation for – respiratory diseases other than coal workers' pneumoconiosis. As this chapter will illustrate, one of the main reasons why the struggle to have bronchitis and emphysema listed as occupational diseases of coal miners was so protracted was that these diseases were widespread throughout the non-mining population. However, the long tradition of high-quality research into miners' lung disease was sustained even when the British coal industry was in its death throes. This research would eventually lead to the recognition of these 'new' miners' dust-induced diseases, and would underpin the decision of the High Court in 1998 to compensate former employees of the NCB/British Coal Corporation for the damage caused to their respiratory systems by being exposed to dangerous levels of mine dust. However, this legal breakthrough was the culmination of a long, hard struggle, and the notion that bronchitis and emphysema were linked to working down the pits had been widely accepted by miners and their trade unions for a very long time before the 1990s. Once again, the contested nature of occupational disease is clearly illustrated.

The steady reduction in the incidence of pneumoconiosis across the UK from the 1950s onwards was related to improved methods of dust control and increasing surveillance of the mining workforce. However, this success was tempered by the growing realisation that miners were succumbing to other debilitating respiratory conditions which became grouped under the heading of Chronic Obstructive Airways Diseases (COAD). Unlike coal workers' pneumoconiosis, though, bronchitis, emphysema and asthma were prevalent throughout the general population, and indeed, were becoming more and more common. Consequently, a barrier which would prevent the recognition of these as conditions industrially caused was growing bigger. At its 1960 Congress, a TUC delegate from the Medical Practitioners' Union put the issue in perspective:

> The problem is essentially a difficult one because it is so extraordinarily difficult to differentiate between what is caused by an industrial hazard and what is caused by a non-industrial hazard … If you live in a smog-ridden town and are subject to bronchitis, how is it possible to say whether the bronchitis comes from smog in the town or the conditions in the factory in which you work? … The Industrial Injuries Advisory Committee has little latitude in this matter. It can accept only direct evidence of a connection.[1]

Moreover, such diseases were also closely connected with rising smoking rates. The seminal *Smoking and Health* report was approved by the Royal College of Physicians

---

1   TUC, *Congress Report* (1960), p. 372.

in 1959 and published in 1962. From this time on, the anti-smoking message began to be pushed strongly in the UK.[2] It also became more and more accepted that smoking was the principal cause of bronchitis. By the late 1950s, 25,000 people died each year from bronchitis, and the disease was causing 10% of all absences from work – resulting in 25 million working days being lost every year.[3] This was practically a British disease, as the big differences in national mortality rates illustrated. The rate in England and Wales stood at 80 deaths per 100,000, Scotland at 50 deaths per 100,000, Ireland at 42 per 100,000, while the rates in France, Norway and the USA stood at only 5, 4 and 2 deaths per 100,000 respectively. Occupation, though, was understood to have a significant impact, and some important research indicated that miners recorded much higher absence rates because of bronchitis than any other occupational group. As Table 5.1 illustrates, while the national average was 3.3%, the rate for miners was nearly three times as high.[4]

Table 5.1   Spells of sickness absence, men aged 17–67 (Ministry of Pensions and National Insurance, 1959)

	Population (000s)	*Total number of spells (000s)*	*No. of spells due to bronchitis (000s)*	*Spells due to bronchitis per 100 workers*	*% of all spells due to bronchitis*
All	14,400	4,843	476	3.3	9.8
Agriculture, horticulture and forestry	1,052	238	15	1.4	6.3
Coal mining	630	535	51	8.1	9.5
Foundry work	141	65	9	6.4	13.8

Source: I.T.T. Higgins, 'Bronchitis', paper given at the Annual Provincial Meeting of the MRC, 8 September 1960, PRU, Paper no. 243, p. 124.

Up until the 1950s, little research had been devoted to bronchitis in industry.[5] The MRC had set up its own Committee on the Aetiology of Chronic Bronchitis in

---

2   V. Berridge and K. Loughlin, 'Smoking and the New Health Education in Britain, 1950s–1970s', *American Journal of Public Health*, vol. 95, no. 6 (June 2005), pp. 958–64.

3   I.T.T. Higgins, 'Bronchitis', paper given at the Annual Provincial Meeting of the MRC, 8 September 1960, PRU, Paper no. 243, p. 124.

4   For further details, see also I.T.T. Higgins, 'An Approach to the Problem of Bronchitis in Industry: Studies in Agricultural, Mining and Foundry Communities', in E.J. King and C.M. Fletcher, *Industrial Pulmonary Diseases* (London, 1960), p. 124.

5   Ibid., p. 195.

the early 1950s. This was made up of leading experts on lung disease, and included several who were connected with research into coal workers' pneumoconiosis, such as Gilson, Gough and Fletcher.[6]

In contrast to pneumoconiosis, the MRC defined chronic bronchitis as a functional rather than disease-based condition.'[7] The disease was caused by inflammation of the tubes going into the lungs from the windpipe. Thick mucus was produced and coughed up daily, and the symptoms tended to be worse in the morning – although to be classed as 'chronic', the condition needed to have lasted for at least two years. As far as coal dust was concerned, it was the aggravation caused to the bronchial tubes by inhaling dust which did the damage, and not scarring of the lungs by smaller particles of dust as was the case with pneumoconiosis. It had long been acknowledged that coal miners were especially prone to contracting bronchitis whenever they were subjected to high levels of coal dust. However, many medical scientists clung to the belief that bronchitis was the only major respiratory disease to which coal miners succumbed for a long time. Collis used x-ray evidence to illustrate this point in 1915, and Haldane staked his reputation on the notion that the higher-than-average death rate amongst elderly coal miners in England and Wales was chiefly due to them having bronchitis.[8] In 1924, a study in Germany found the prevalence of bronchitis in coal miners was double that for staff who worked in the mine offices.[9] By 1931, Haldane was still unambiguous on the issue: '… it seems practically certain that excessive inhalation of coal dust or shale dust must cause bronchitis, and ought therefore to be avoided'.[10] In the early 1950s, another German study, this time of hospital patients, found that the frequency of bronchitis was 29.1% amongst miners, compared to 15.5% for non-miner patients. And in 1956, American researchers discovered that miners in the USA had more chronic bronchitis, emphysema and bronchial spasm than other workers of the same age.[11]

Emphysema was caused by very small particles of dust or smoke being inhaled over long periods of time. This disease is characterised by permanent abnormal enlargement of the lung's alveoli – the minute airspaces deep within the lung – with eventual destruction of the alveoli walls. The gradual atrophy of the alveoli

6   Medical Research Council, 'Definitions and Classification of Chronic Bronchitis for Clinical and Epidemiological Purposes, a Report to the Medical Research Council by their Committee on the Aetiology of Chronic Bronchitis', *The Lancet*, vol. 1 (10 April 1965), pp. 775–9. Again, this is another example of the interesting parallel with what C. Sellers argues happened in the USA from the 1890s with the transition of occupational hygienists into public and environmental health: C. Sellers, *Hazards of the Job: From Industrial Science to Environmental Health Science* (Chapel Hill, NC, 1997).

7   Higgins, 'An Approach to the Problem of Bronchitis in Industry', p. 121.

8   Medical Research Council (MRC), *Chronic Pulmonary Disease in South Wales. Coal Miners, Medical Studies* (1942), pp. 141–2; henceforth MRC Medical Studies.

9   Higgins, 'An Approach to the Problem of Bronchitis in Industry', p. 197.

10   J.S. Haldane, 'Silicosis and Coal Mining', *Colliery Guardian* (16 January 1931), p. 315.

11   Higgins, 'An Approach to the Problem of Bronchitis in Industry', p. 197.

causes the lungs to work harder in order to get more oxygen into the blood supply, which results in breathlessness as the body becomes starved of oxygen. In more advanced stages, the sufferer takes on a characteristic barrel-chested appearance. Early diagnosis of emphysema was problematic. In the late 1950s, researchers at the PRU noted how the diagnosis of emphysema – both clinically and radiologically – was uncertain except in the most advanced stages, and even by the 1990s the pathology of emphysema remained unclear.[12] What was known, though, was that there were two types (*panacinar* and *centriacinar*), although during the British Coal High Court litigation, intense debate revolved around the existence of a third type, referred to as *focal dust emphysema*. Asthma was also implicated as a distinctive coal mining disease. As we saw in Chapter 2, what was referred to as 'miners' asthma' had been recorded by doctors since the 1830s, and indeed was the term used to describe miners' lung disease before the word pneumoconiosis entered the medical vocabulary in the 1860s. In the modern accepted version of the disease, though, asthma is characterised by a variety of symptoms. At times air flow is seriously limited, but at other times sufferers are able to breathe normally. Once again, though, this was a disease which was prevalent, and became increasingly more prevalent, in the general population throughout the twentieth century.

As was the case with the quest to eradicate pneumoconiosis throughout Britain's coal fields, the PRU – and later the IOM – was to play an important role in enhancing knowledge of chronic bronchitis and emphysema. Research undertaken by Fletcher in 1952 had demonstrated the variability in the ability of doctors to detect and quantify the physical signs of bronchitis. This suggested that physical examination by medics was too blunt an instrument for tracing the epidemiology of the disease.[13] Consequently, when the PRU set out to gauge the prevalence of this disease amongst British miners, it was decided to rely upon reported symptoms only. Between 1954 and 1960, PRU researchers studied bronchitis rates in five different regions, two rural and three industrial, one of which was the Rhondda Fach. Every respondent's breathing capacity was measured, and a standardised questionnaire recorded respiratory symptoms and smoking habits. The study revealed that whereas the prevalence rate for bronchitis of men living in rural areas was only 6% – and 10% for non-miners living in urban areas – amongst the miners in the sample, the rate was 24%.[14] Research by the PRU also suggested that in general, the average breathing capacity of miners seemed to be significantly lower than that of non-miners. However, the evidence was acknowledged to be too equivocal to draw general conclusions.[15] Cochrane's Rhondda Fach studies, as we noted in Chapter 4, also made a significant

---

12 T. J.C. Gilson, 'Bronchitis and emphysema in coal workers' pneumoconiosis', PRU, Paper no. 160 (1957), p. 495; Judgment of Mr Justice Turner, 'The British Coal Respiratory Disease Litigation' (1998), p. 117; henceforth Turner.

13 Gilson, 'Bronchitis and emphysema in coal workers' pneumoconiosis', p. 491.

14 Higgins, 'Bronchitis', p. 122.

15 A. Coggon et al., 'Coal mining and chronic obstructive pulmonary disease: A review of the evidence', *Thorax*, vol. 53 (1998), pp. 398–407, p. 398.

contribution to the understanding of bronchitis and emphysema, because it was clear that it wasn't just miners with PMF in the Welsh valleys who had reduced breathing capacities. In 1958, Cochrane speculated on the reasons for this, and his first hunch was very close to the mark: 'There may be a type of industrial emphysema which affects miners with and without pneumoconiosis and causes the low average ventilatory capacity and the increased mortality in miners with Category 0 or simple pneumoconiosis'.[16]

Smoking was identified as a problematic factor very early on. A PRU survey in the late 1950s found a higher prevalence of respiratory symptoms in smokers than amongst non-smokers, or even ex-smokers – with the incidence of persistent cough and sputum production rising with the amount smoked.[17] The health risks of smoking were becoming more and more understood from the 1950s onwards, thanks in great part to the work of Doll and his co-researchers. In 1994, Doll summed up the main conclusions of his years of research into smoking in one chilling sentence: 'It now seems that about half of all regular cigarette smokers will eventually be killed by their habit.'[18] At one point, around 80% of working coal miners in the UK smoked.[19] Consequently, according to Doll's predictions, even if they had never worked in coal mining – where the effect of inhaling coal dust added yet another risk factor – half of these men would probably have been killed by their smoking habit. Moreover, by the 1960s it was understood that smoking was the main cause of bronchitis and emphysema. Therefore, the argument that coal mine dust was a significant causal agent in bringing about these diseases – and that miners should be compensated, including those who smoked – was going to a difficult one to win. In 1960, though, notwithstanding the increasing awareness of the dangers of smoking, researchers at the PRU were keeping an open mind, and were still uncertain regarding just how much damage could be attributed to smoking compared to the harmful effects of exposure to dust:

> In all groups the non-smokers had higher average M.B.C. [Maximum Breathing Capacity] than the smokers, but within the smoking groups there was no consistent trend with increasing tobacco consumption. Generalizing, smoking was associated with a reduction of M.B.C. of about 10 litres/minute. But smoking cannot explain the miners' disability since their habits were not significantly different from the non-miners.[20]

A breakthrough occurred in the mid-1970s with the publication of important research into chronic bronchitis and emphysema by Fletcher et al. This research found that it was only a minority of smokers – those who had a special susceptibility to tobacco

---

16 A. Cochrane, 'Epidemiology of Coal Workers' Pneumoconiosis', in E.J. King and C.M. Fletcher (eds), *Industrial Pulmonary Diseases* (London, 1960), pp. 224–5.

17 Higgins, 'Bronchitis', p. 122.

18 Turner, p. 200; see R. Doll et al., 'Mortality in relation to smoking: 50 years' observations on male British doctors', *BMJ*, vol. 328 (26 June 2004), 1,519–33.

19 Turner, p. 283.

20 Higgins, 'An Approach to the Problem of Bronchitis in Industry', p. 205.

smoke – who were liable to get bronchitis or emphysema through their smoking habit.[21] Such research was to prove crucial in the 1998 High Court case regarding the supposed failure of British Coal to protects its workers from respiratory disease. The implication of Fletcher et al.'s research was that high rates of Chronic Obstructive Pulmonary Disease (COPD) could be caused by the inhalation of coal dust, as well as by the inhalation of tobacco smoke. During the court proceedings, then, the plaintiffs successfully argued that because there was a 'common causal pathway' regarding respiratory damage caused by smoke and respiratory damage caused by mine dust, neither factor could be ruled out as the cause.[22] Most medical scientists accepted this was the case. However, some, although not disputing the case made by the plaintiffs in the High Court Decision, have suggested that the role which smoking played in rates of miners' COPD needs further investigation.[23] We return to the influence of smoking later on.

The Industrial Injuries Advisory Council (IIAC) Investigates

As a consequence of the growing unease surrounding the incidence of miners' respiratory diseases other than CWP, the IIAC began an investigation in 1985. The IIAC was set up in November 1947, and its duty was to advise on the making of any regulations under the 1948 National Insurance (Industrial Injuries) Act. Therefore, it fell upon the IIAC to decide whether bronchitis and emphysema should be considered as occupational diseases. Although there had been important changes to coal miners' compensation since 1945, by the 1980s there was only limited recognition that emphysema and bronchitis were caused by the mining environment, even although – as we have seen – numerous studies suggested that miners were particularly liable to contracting these diseases. Indeed, under legislation passed in 1967, bronchitis and emphysema were only accepted to confer *additional* disability to the damage which had already been caused by simple or complicated pneumoconiosis. The prevailing medical orthodoxy was that pneumoconiosis weakened the respiratory organs and led to the onset of bronchitis and emphysema.

Under the 1946 National Insurance (Industrial Injuries) Act, benefit could only be paid for occupational diseases if they were without doubt 'due to the nature' of the person's employment – a phrase derived from the era of Workmen's Compensation.[24]

---

21 C. Fletcher et al., *The Natural History of Chronic Bronchitis and Emphysema* (NewYork), p. 120; Turner, p. 203.

22 See R. Rudd, 'Coal miners' respiratory disease litigation', *Thorax*, vol. 53 (1998), pp. 337–40.

23 See M. Jacobsen, 'Reply to WRK Moran and NL Lapp', *American Review of Respiratory Disease*, vol. 138 (1998), pp. 1,643–6; also N.R. Anthonizen, 'The British Hypothesis Revisited', *European Respiratory Journal*, vol. 23 (2004), pp. 657–8.

24 *Report of the Departmental Committee Appointed to Review the Disease Provision of the National Insurance (Industrial Injuries) Act* (1955), Cmd 9548, p. 6; henceforth Beney Committee.

However, the door had been left slightly ajar regarding the inclusion of certain diseases common in the population by the Beney Committee, set up to review industrial diseases in 1953 – and we look at the Beney Committee in relation to the trade unions in Chapter 7.[25] The Beney Committee was made up of representatives of employers, trade unionists and government. The eventual majority decision of this committee was that there should be no extension to existing provision. However, its three trade union members could not subscribe to this view, and it was because of this that a majority and a minority report were produced. At the end of the day, though, definite proof of occupational causation – the *raison d'être* of the Industrial Injuries Scheme – was what was required, and the majority report made this quite clear:

> ... decisions relating to individual causation are fundamental to the Industrial Injuries scheme, the whole purpose of which is to provide benefit for injuries and diseases caused in a certain way, namely by the actual conditions of a workers' employment.[26]

The trade unionists on the Beney Committee, though, argued that it was possible to widen the scope of the act while maintaining its necessary rigour. Their suggestion was that that consideration should be given only to cases where *the balance of probability* was on the side of the claimant. This common-sense approach would eventually, in the 1980s, become the basis of IIAC policy regarding the prescription of occupational disease.[27] Moreover, although split over the issue of the prescription of new diseases, the Beney Committee members were unanimous in their recommendation that much more research should be carried out into the nature of industrial respiratory diseases:

(a)   A vigorous and sustained research effort was essential if prescription was to work effectively.

(b)   The greatest need was for more field research, especially research making full use of statistics to give a quick indication of areas where attention should be considered.

(c)   Research was needed specifically for the purpose of prescription over and above other forms of research.

(d)   [There is a] need for a small highly qualified specialist research staff.[28]

In 1966, the government bowed to increasing pressure and brought in a limited measure of improvement. Under the National Insurance (Industrial Injuries) (Amendment) Act 1967, men diagnosed as having over 50% disablement through pneumoconiosis were allowed to have their accompanying bronchitis and emphysema treated as part of the disease, although only 3,000 men fell into this category.[29] Once again, the main stumbling block towards full acceptance that bronchitis and emphysema

---

25   Ibid., p. 6.
26   Ibid., p. 13.
27   Ibid., p. 27.
28   TUC, *Congress Report* (1961), p. 145; Beney Committee, pp. 20–22.
29   TUC, *Congress Report* (1967), p. 183.

were occupationally caused was the prevalence of the diseases throughout the wider population.

This situation prevailed for some time, and by the 1980s the position was that under Section 108 (2) of the Social Security Contribution and Benefits Act of 1982, a disease or injury could be prescribed if the Secretary of State was satisfied that two main requirements were in place: the disease had clearly to be a risk deriving from occupation alone and not a risk common to all persons, and secondly, the attribution of cases to the nature of employment needed to be established *with reasonable certainty*.[30] The IIAC, then, posed three main questions in 1985 regarding bronchitis and emphysema:

1. Does occupational exposure to dust produce an adverse effect on the lung in addition to pneumoconiosis?
2. If there is an adverse effect on the lung, does it lead to disablement?
3. If there is disablement, can it be attributed to occupational causes with reasonable certainty?

The findings of the IIAC were published three years later. These reflected the current state of medical opinion regarding the complicating factor of smoking. Although agreeing that exposure to coal dust could cause a certain amount of airflow obstruction, the IIAC was forced to concede that:

> On the current evidence, we cannot say that occupational causation can be presumed with reasonable certainty in individual cases. This is because it is impossible to distinguish between airflow limitation due to smoking, which is the commonest cause of bronchitis and emphysema, and the probably smaller effects of occupational dust exposure. Among smoking miners it is far more likely that any airflow limitation is due to smoking than to dust exposure. There is insufficient evidence on non-smoking populations for accurate assessments to be made of the effects of dust exposure alone.[31]

The report went on to relate how expert witnesses had argued that the only way that this disease could be prescribed was if claimants were able to show evidence of having Category 1 pneumoconiosis. This procedure was put into practice in 1992, and clearly marked an improvement on the previous requirement of 50% disablement through pneumoconiosis. However, the Council was nevertheless perturbed at the failure of medical research to come to a decision regarding the relative impact of cigarette smoke compared to that of coal dust, and – as the Beney Committee had done many years earlier – ended its report with an appeal for more research:

> There is a need for more studies of non-smoking dust-exposed workers. We urge researchers in this field to collaborate if necessary to obtain study populations large enough to yield

---

30 Turner, p. 271.
31 Ibid., p. 272.

statistically valid results. We intend to review bronchitis and emphysema again when such evidence on non-smoking miners becomes available.[32]

However, a great deal of research was already being conducted.

Even though the British coal industry atrophied in the 1970s and 1980s, research into coal dust-related illnesses continued relentlessly into the era of privatisation. For example, in a study commissioned by the HSE in the mid-1980s, the IOM was asked to look into the relationship between exposure to coal mine dust and disabling lung damage other than pneumoconiosis. For this the IOM researchers were able to draw upon the reams of epidemiological evidence that had been produced by the PFR's years of painstaking x-raying, interviewing and dust sampling. Subsequently, an analysis of 7,000 coal miners who had worked at nine of the initial PFR collieries in the late 1970s was undertaken.[33] The researchers found a significant association between low FEV1 (Forced Expiratory Volume in 1 second) and miners' exposure to mine dust.

Through the 1980s and 1990s, more and more studies along these lines pointed to the fact that miners were suffering much more from breathing difficulties than any other group of workers, and were also enduring higher rates of chronic bronchitis and emphysema than the rest of the population. Another study in the 1980s compared the respiratory capacities of miners and telecommunication workers, and found that 31% of miners had symptoms of chronic bronchitis, compared to only 5% of telecommunication workers. Also, the miners' FEV1 averaged less than 80% of that predicted for their age and height. The main conclusions of this particular study were mirrored by research published in Belgium in 1987 which compared non-smoking coal miners with non-smoking steel workers. Again the findings were unambiguous, with miners recording significantly lower FEV1s than the non-miners.[34] Many other reports were published utilising the data from the PFR studies, and several were of particular importance regarding the final recognition that emphysema and bronchitis should be classed as diseases of coal miners.[35]

However, one of the most important pieces of research, and one which was to go a long way towards convincing the IIAC to change compensation procedure, was published by Marine et al. in 1988 – and it is interesting to note that Jacobsen, one of

32 Ibid.

33 Safety and Health in Mines Research Advisory Board, *Annual Review* (1999), p. 5.

34 Coggon and Taylor, 'Chronic mining and chronic obstructive pulmonary disease', p. 398.

35 For example, see J.M Rogan et al., 'Role of dust in the working environment in the development of chronic bronchitis in British coal miners', *British Journal of Industrial Medicine*, vol. 30 (1973), pp. 217–26; R.G. Love and B.G. Miller, 'Longitudinal study of lung function in coal-miners', *Thorax*, vol. 37 (1982), pp. 193–7; C.A. Soutar and J.F. Hurley, 'Relation between dust exposure and lung function in miners and ex-miners', *British Journal of Industrial Medicine*, vol. 43 (1986), pp. 307–20; J.F. Hurley and C.A. Soutar, 'Can exposure to coalmine dust cause a severe impairment of lung function?', *British Journal of Industrial Medicine*, vol. 43 (1986), pp. 250–56.

the authors of the paper which led to the new 1975 respirable dust regulations, was a co-author of this paper. The main rationale of this study was to weigh up the damage caused by smoking compared to damage caused by exposure to respirable dust. Once again, PFR data was re-examined, this time relating to 3,380 smoking and non-smoking coal miners. Each miner's FEV1 was compared with the level predicted for his age and height, and the results were incorporated into regression equations for four conditions: FEV1 less than 80%; chronic bronchitis; chronic bronchitis with FEV1 less than 80%; and FEV1 less than 65%. Increases in prevalence in each of these four categories with increases in exposure to dust were found to be statistically significant for smokers as well as for non-smokers. Therefore, the main conclusions were that both smoking *and* dust exposure could cause clinically important respiratory dysfunction, and that the risk of contracting chronic bronchitis and emphysema was double for miners exposed to high levels of dust, *whether they smoked or not.*[36]

Although the Marine et al. paper was something of a breakthrough, cross-sectional studies on their own were still not convincing enough to produce the statistical significance required for a conclusive answer to questions surrounding COPD and coal workers.[37] Several important studies of mortality statistics – some conducted in the mid-1970s – were also drawn upon to increase an understanding of the significance of COPD in coal mining. For example, Cochrane and his co-researchers used data from the Rhondda Fach studies to illustrate that over a thirty-year period there was a marked excess of deaths from bronchitis among miners in the study cohort compared to the national population.[38] In 1976, as part of his PhD research, Jacobsen concluded:

> With the exception of lung cancer deaths, the highest mortality occurred among men who had symptoms of persistent cough and phlegm, and who complained of breathlessness. This was so for both smokers and non-smokers ... A previously published association between cumulative dust exposure and loss of FEV1 is confirmed both among smokers and non-smokers. The effect is estimated as approximately 150 ml reduction in FEV1 for the maximum working life exposure consistent with current British dust standards.[39]

Several years later, Miller and Jacobsen studied mortality in over 26,000 miners in 20 collieries in England and Wales who had taken part in the first PFR survey over

---

36 W.M. Marine et al., 'Clinically important respiratory effects of dust exposure and smoking in British coal miners', *American Review of Respiratory Disorders*, vol. 137, no. 1 (January 1988), pp. 106–12. During the High Court proceedings, British Coal's opening position was that the research which formed the basis of the Marine paper was flawed. However, because of the sheer weight of medical evidence marshalled against them, British Coal's lawyers were forced into what the judge referred to as a 'sea change' and fully accepted that the data upon which the Marine paper was based was indeed rigorous; see Turner, pp. 132 and 143.

37 Coggon and Newman Taylor, 'Coal mining and chronic obstructive pulmonary disease', p. 406.

38 Ibid., p. 402.

39 Turner, p. 163.

the 1953–58 period. They found that although total mortality was lower than that in the general population, there was a clear increase in deaths from bronchitis and emphysema with increasing exposure to dust. They concluded, therefore:

> Miners exposed to excessive amounts of respirable coal mine dust are at increased risk of premature death, either from PMF or from chronic bronchitis or emphysema.[40]

Finally, post-mortem studies helped to complete the picture. Cockcroft et al. carried out post-mortem examinations of coal workers and non-coal workers in the early 1980s and found excessive rates of emphysema in the former group compared to the latter.[41] Also, two years later Ruckley et al. reported on their study of men who had taken part in the PFR. Four hundred and fifty coal miners were examined, the majority of whom had dust exposure records which could be correlated with their breathing capacities. Again a clear relationship was demonstrated between dust exposure and the presence of emphysema in those with PMF.[42]

The IIAC Reconsiders

The growing volume of evidence eventually convinced the IIAC that the limits of compensation legislation had to be extended. In the light of the new studies, the IIAC re-examined emphysema and bronchitis in 1993. According to the Council, the new research had:

> … provided answers to the questions we addressed in our previous report. They have demonstrated that cumulative coal dust exposure is associated with a clinically important reduction in FEV1 in both smokers and non-smokers, that coal dust has an important effect independent of tobacco smoking and that the risk of disabling loss of lung function is increased by more than two-fold in both smokers and non-smokers.[43]

On the basis of this research, the IIAC made new recommendations:

> That chronic bronchitis and emphysema be prescribed in relation to current and past coal miners who have worked underground. Prescription should be based on:
>
> 1. An objective measure of impairment likely to be associated with clinically important disablement. Accordingly, we recommend a reduction in FEV1 from the mean value for age and height of one litre or more.

---

40 Ibid., p. 164; Coggon et al., 'Coal mining and chronic obstructive pulmonary disease', p. 403.

41 A. Cockcroft et al., 'Post-mortem study of emphysema in coal workers and non-coal workers', *Lancet*, vol. 2 (1982), pp. 600–603.

42 V.A. Ruckley et al., 'Emphysema and dust exposure in a group of coal workers', *American Review of Respiratory Disease*, vol. 129 (1984), pp. 528–32.

43 Turner, p. 273.

2. Evidence of sufficient exposure to coal dust for this to be the probable cause of the reduction in FEV1. We recommend the criteria to be used for sufficient exposure to be both:
3. A minimum of 20 years underground exposure to coal dust and,
4. Definite evidence of coal dust retention on a chest radiograph which would be interpreted as at least Category 1/1.[44]

As a consequence of these recommendations, in September 1993 emphysema and bronchitis were added to the list of prescribed occupational diseases, with the understanding that the qualifying conditions be reviewed when the scheme had run for a year. This decision immediately resulted in a large number of claims, with 4,000 cases being assessed by the end of 1994 alone.[45]

In January 1995, a review of the scheme was conducted, and a report was published in February 1996. By now it had become clear that some of the requirements of the 1993 legislation were unfair. In particular, the necessity for claimants to have x-ray evidence of at least Category 1 pneumoconiosis was seen as excessive.[46] Research conducted since 1991 suggested to the IIAC that the requirement for Category 1 pneumoconiosis to be shown up under x-ray before compensation was paid was discriminating unfairly against miners in certain parts of the UK, as the diagnosis of pneumoconiosis was less problematic in some areas that in others. This was made clearer by an important study by Coggon et al. which found that although proportional mortality from pneumoconiosis varied quite markedly across the country, deaths for COAD were uniformly elevated.[47] The IIAC acknowledged, then, that far too many claimants had been unable to secure compensation because their x-rays had failed to reveal pneumoconiosis, while their post-mortems had later revealed they had been suffering from the disease all along.[48] In view of the general dissatisfaction with the state of affairs, combined with the strength of the evidence brought forth by the new research, the IIAC decided that the necessity for claimants to have radiographic evidence of coal dust retention be dropped.

However, some clinicians were dismayed at this decision, in particular Seaton, who had initially recommended to the IIAC that bronchitis and emphysema could in certain circumstances be classed as an occupational disease. Seaton was concerned that such changes to the legislation would lead to smokers being compensated for their habit, and he argued that an incentive for the coal industry to control dust exposure was being removed:

---

44 Ibid.

45 HSE National Statistics, 2004: http://www.hse.gov.uk/statistics/index.htm.

46 *Hansard* (18 January 1996), pt 32, col. 984.

47 D. Coggon et al., 'Contrasting geographical distribution of mortality from pneumoconiosis and chronic bronchitis and emphysema in British coal miners', *Occupational and Environmental Medicine*, vol. 52 (1995), pp. 554–5.

48 A. Newman-Taylor, 'Industrial injuries benefits for coal miners with obstructive lung disease', Letters to the Editor, *Thorax*, vol. 54, no. 282 (March 1999), p. 1; Turner, p. 105.

Even if dust concentrations were reduced to a theoretical zero, 20 years' service and smoking would automatically qualify a disabled miner for compensation for an 'occupational disease'. The industry does not now have the opportunity of preventing 'coal dust disease' except by preventing smokers from working in mines or by preventing men working for as long as 20 years. The latter provides an obvious means of reducing the figures since a mine owner needs only to institute a programme of spirometric tests and to retire on the grounds of ill health anyone who shows early evidence of a reduction in FEV1 before the 20 year period is achieved ... Now radiological dust retention is off the agenda, the immediate pressure is off the mine owners to continue their programme of progressive dust reduction below the legal standard.[49]

Despite opposition, though, the legislation was changed to near enough what the trade unions had been advocating for many years. Coal workers who suffered from emphysema and bronchitis and who had worked for at least twenty years underground were now entitled to compensation, regardless of whether they had smoked or not. Those who worked on the surface, though, were excluded from the legislation as it was assumed that they would not be exposed to the necessary volume of dust.[50] In comparison to those with pneumoconiosis, before they could qualify to be assessed for chronic bronchitis and emphysema, claimants had to prove they were suffering a reduction in their lung capacity of over one third. This reduction of FEV1 of around a litre correlated with a level of disability in which the sufferer would have difficulty keeping up with others on level ground.[51] Moreover, in the common law litigation which followed the IIAC scheduling of bronchitis and emphysema, the important adverse influence of smoking habits was explicitly recognised. The resulting scheme – from which half a million miners and their dependants benefited – was based on an innovatory computer model which awarded amounts of compensation dependent upon a series of causal variables, including cigarette consumption. This is examined in more depth in Chapter 7.

Into the Twenty-first Century and the Return of Black Lung

Research into miners' lung disease continued apace, and several of the old certainties were debunked by rigorous re-examination. This was certainly the case with silica/quartz. From the 1980s, the IOM investigated the relationship between exposure to respirable quartz and the risk of developing silicosis and pneumoconiosis. For this research, the IOM once again studied PFR data, this time from a Scottish colliery which had closed in 1981. On account of adverse geological conditions at this particular mine, workers had been exposed to higher levels of quartz dust than other mines included in the PFR programme. The PFR's conclusions in 1970 regarding

---

49 A. Seaton, 'The new prescription: Industrial injuries benefits for smokers?', *Thorax*, vol. 53 (May 1998), pp. 335–6.

50 By 2004, the IIAC were still reviewing this omission; IIAC, *Proceedings of the Second Annual Public Meeting, Glasgow, 18 March 2004*, p. 23.

51 Ibid., p. 13.

the importance of quartz had been ambiguous. However, the IOM researchers concluded: 'Quartz exposure may be an important factor in the development and rapid progression of coal workers' pneumoconiosis.'[52] Further research illustrated that this was indeed the case.[53]

In the late 1990s, preparations were under way for a major review of the 1975 Coal Mines (Respirable Dust) Regulations (RDR), and the HSE commissioned a number of research projects as part of this review. One of these saw the IOM undertaking an occupational hygiene assessment of miners' exposure to respirable dust. This involved IOM researchers and HSE scientists visiting several coal mines with the following mandate:

- Provide a summary of the personal exposure data available for different occupations and environments in underground coalmines;
- Develop a picture of the mean, range and distribution of personal exposures in underground coalmines;
- Understand the factors that affect the magnitude or intensity of exposures to respirable dust;
- Advise on suitable sampling strategy to be adopted within the new regulations;
- Advise on suitable sampling methods for use in confined spaces;
- Advise on a proposal for the numerical value for the new Maximum Exposure Limit (MEL) which is reasonable practicable.[54]

The HSE undertook a review of static and personal (that is, attached to the miner) dust sampling equipment, and in 1999 began field trials at ten mines to assess the capabilities of the various instruments. Interestingly, and somewhat belatedly, as part of this research the HSE was asked to identify individuals whose work exposed them to significant dust inhalation and who would especially benefit from carrying such devices.[55] It was now quite clear that fixed-point sampling was inadequate, and that personal dust sampling was the way forward – indeed, Britain was by now the only country that continued to use fixed-point sampling. The result of the survey saw the development of this kind of personal protection, and in particular the CIP10

52 A. Seaton et al., 'Quartz and pneumoconiosis in coal miners', *Lancet*, vol. 2 (1981), pp. 1,272–5.

53 See, for example, B.G. Miller et al., 'Risks of silicosis in coal workers exposed to unusual concentrations of respirable quartz', *Occupational and Environmental Medicine*, vol. 55 (1998), pp. 52–8; J.F. Hurley et al., 'Coal workers' pneumoconiosis and exposure to dust at 10 British coalmines', *British Journal of Industrial Medicine*, vol. 39 (1982), pp. 120–27; M. Jacobsen and W.M. Maclaren, 'Unusual pulmonary observations and exposure to coalmine dust: A case-control study', *Annals of Occupational Hygiene*, vol. 26 (1982), pp. 753–65.

54 Safety and Health in Mines Research Advisory Board, *Annual Review* (1999), p. 3.

55 Ibid., p. 2; L.C. Kenny et al., 'Evaluation of instruments for dust monitoring in United Kingdom coal mines', *Mining Technology*, vol. 110 (August 2001), pp. 97–106.

dust sampler which was small enough to be carried by the miner in a mobile phone harness.[56]

Notwithstanding the progress made on CWP, emphysema and bronchitis, and the clearer understanding of the hazards of quartz, the upward curve was suddenly reversed at the beginning of the twenty-first century. In the summer of 2000, the BBC's news Website reported the following story under the headline 'Miners refuse safety masks':

> Workers at a Fife colliery are refusing to use safety equipment which protects against a serious lung disease. Last month, BBC Scotland revealed that nine men at the Longannet site had been diagnosed as suffering from pneumoconiosis. The condition, which is most commonly known as black spit, was virtually eradicated with the introduction of new safety rules in the mid-1970s. But x-ray tests on workers at the pit found abnormalities in the lungs of 20 of the men, with nine suffering the most serious form of the disease … A recent Health and Safety investigation suggested the re-emergence of pneumoconiosis at the site could have been prevented by using the equipment …[57]

Longannet was developed in the 1960s to provide fuel for nearby Longannet power station. With the closure of the mine in 2002, after millions of gallons of water flooded the underground workings, deep coal mining in Scotland came to an end.

However, tragically and ironically, at the very end of the long history of the coal industry, the disease which everyone thought had been wiped out returned. The revelation caused consternation and surprise, with an NUM official declaring: 'we thought that the disease had disappeared. As a union we are concerned and it is our intention to take stock of the situation.'[58] It wasn't just in Longannet that the old nightmare disease of the coal industry reappeared. When the Coal Mines (Respirable Dust) Regulations were introduced in 1975, 10.2% of miners in the UK developed pneumoconiosis during their working lives, with 0.9% developing PMF. By the mid-1990s it looked as though the regulations were effective, as the prevalence of all forms of pneumoconiosis amongst miners had fallen to just 0.2%. For four years there were no cases of the disease reported beyond the lowest three classifications. However, by the end of 2001 the rate suddenly jumped to 0.6%, the same as it had been in the 1980s, with 40 miners – including the 20 at Longannet – showing evidence of pneumoconiosis, including 2 with PMF. The HSC suggested that this reversal may have been brought about by the changed age structure of a coal industry, which had an increased number of older miners and had practically ceased recruiting new workers. However, there was also the point that the earlier encouraging decline of

---

56 Ibid., p. 105.

57 BBC News Online, 15 August 2000: http://news.bbc.co.uk/1/hi/scotland/880675. stm.

58 *Guardian Unlimited*, 18 July 2000: http://www.guardian.co.uk/uk_news/ story/0,3604,344457,00.html.

pneumoconiosis had been underpinned by widespread redundancies amongst older miners as the pits closed up and down the country.[59]

There were other factors. For one thing, HSE investigators had found that although most pits tended to comply with the 1975 Regulations, many miners were being exposed to longer periods of dusty work because they worked longer shifts than had been the case in the mid-1970s – certainly, most of the men with the disease at Longannet had been working overtime. Consequently, as there was no time-weighted element to the exposure limits built into the 1975 regulations, men's health was being affected by increased periods of exposure. There had also been a change in the nature of the mining workforce, with a tendency to employ more contractors for specific tasks; and it was telling that the overall prevalence of the disease amongst contractors' employees was 1.8%, compared to only 0.5% amongst directly employed miners.[60] On top of all that, though, was the simple fact that a less than rigorous approach had been taken to the routine x-raying which had done so much to reduce pneumoconiosis rates from the 1950s onwards. At Longannet, 30% of miners had failed to take part in the most recent round of x-rays. The Chief Inspector of Mines certainly thought that this was one of the reasons for the outbreak:

> It was unusual to have found such an outbreak. But certainly in recent years the number of workers in mines attending for x-ray has been falling. It's not as good as it used to be and we only know about the prevalence of the disease from the people who are x-rayed.[61]

This was a trend apparent throughout what was left of the British coal industry, with attendance rates for x-rays dropping from 90% in the mid-1970s to 72% over the 1994–97 period. Tellingly, all the men diagnosed with PMF in the year 2000 were found to have missed at least one medical.[62]

The reappearance of pneumoconiosis quickly convinced the HSC that new regulations needed to be put in force as soon as possible, and in January 2004 its Consultative Document entitled *Proposals for the Control of Inhalable Dust in Coal Mines* was issued. The use of the phrase 'inhalable dust' in the title was significant, as for the first time a differentiation was being made between respirable and inhalable dust. This reflected the most recent knowledge that the larger non-respirable dust particles – previously thought to be less dangerous – could contribute towards bronchitis, and it was for this reason that new portable dust monitoring devices needed to be introduced.[63] Under the new regulations, managers were required to control inhalable dust – meaning dust which includes larger particles normally trapped by the nose, mouth and throat, and subsequently cleared from the body – and

---

59 HSC, *Consultative Document* (2004), p. 6.

60 Ibid., p. 7.

61 *Guardian Unlimited* (18 July, 2000): http://www.guardian.co.uk/uk_news/story/0,3604,344457,00.html.

62 HSC, *Consultative Document* (2004), pp. 7 and 10.

63 L.C. Kenny et al., 'Evaluation of instruments for dust monitoring in United Kingdom coal mines', *Mining Technology*, vol. 110 (August 2001), p. 97.

had to comply with exposure limits for respirable dust – dust which is small enough to reach the gas exchange region of the lungs.

It is expected that by the time new dust regulations come into effect, there will only be 10 large mines and 10 small mines in operation in the UK, with a total underground workforce of around 4,500. However, the HSC estimated that the introduction of its amended Regulations would still amount to a cost benefit to society of £5.3 million, relating to the number of cases of pneumoconiosis, emphysema and bronchitis which the new Regulations would prevent:

> Of this £79,000 relates to preventing 5 cases of pneumoconiosis, with a further £5,267,000 from preventing 27 cases of chronic bronchitis per annum. These benefits take into account the costs of contracting the disease: ill health, lost output, medical treatment and an allowance for pain, grief and suffering … Even if the new regulations were to prevent only one case a year of chronic bronchitis instead of the expected 27, the benefits, which would amount to £274,000 per annum, would still comfortably exceed the costs.[64]

The HSC also acknowledged that, thanks to the work of the IOM, the knowledge of the risks associated with exposure to quartz had advanced since the mid-1970s, when public enemy number one was thought to be coal dust:

> Unlike other constituents of coal mine dust, brief exposures to high quartz concentrations can substantially increase the risk …. We ought to have an exposure limit on quartz whatever its source and that exposure limit should take account of the health risks as well as what is achievable today.[65]

Consequently, it was decided that the exposure limit for the new twenty-first-century regulations would be set at $3mg/m^3$ for respirable coal mine dust and $0.3mg/m^3$ for respirable crystalline silica.[66] However, even more recently, in 2005, as medical knowledge of the dangers of silica continued to grow, the exposure level was dropped to 0.1%.[67]

The twenty-first-century coal dust regulations will also bring to an end the practice of mine management ensuring that dust levels fell within 'approved' conditions, and no more. Much more rigid risk assessments will be required before men are allowed to go anywhere near mine dust. A section from the guidance notes of the HSC's Consultative Document deserves to be quoted at length:

---

64 HSC, *Consultative Document* (2004), p. 18.

65 Ibid., p. 8.

66 Ibid., p. 17.

67 HSC, *Consultative Document, Control of Substances Hazardous to Health Regulations 2002 (as amended 2005): Proposals for a Workable Exposure Limit for Respirable Crystalline Silica* (2005); see also D. Buchanan et al., *Quantitative Relationships Between Exposure to Respirable Quartz and Risk of Silicosis at one Scottish Colliery*, IOM Research Report TM/01/03 (February 2001).

These regulations require workers' exposure to respirable dust and quartz to be controlled so that it is as low as it reasonably practicable; they also require certain action if exposure limits are breached; this could include stopping work until additional control measures can be put in place. Exposure depends of both the concentration of dust in the workplace air and on the length of time spent there. The exposure limits are therefore time-weighted i.e. the longer the period that the workers are exposed, the lower the maximum permitted concentration of dust in the air ... The regulations therefore require managers to consider not only measures to control dust concentrations in the workplace, but also the potential impact of working hours and shift patterns on exposure ... The regulations do not simply require the manager to ensure exposure limits are not exceeded; they require the manager to reduce exposure so far as it is reasonably practicable below the exposure limits.[68]

Conclusion

The struggle to have emphysema and bronchitis scheduled as industrial diseases was a long one, and success was only achieved towards the end of the twentieth century, when the British coal mining industry was in its death throes. Dembe suggests that several inter-related factors underpin the contested tussle over the recognition of occupational ill-health.[69] Certainly, as far as coal mining was concerned, the idea of exploitation by a capitalist-oriented state, and a concomitant deep reluctance of the state to acknowledge that a disease was compensatable, cannot be discounted. However, over and above the difficulties of explaining exploitation in a nationalised industry, this line of argument can only be accepted when the nature of medical orthodoxy aligned with state power is factored in. What emerges, then, is a complex picture of conflict and consensus between employers, workers and their trade unions, clinicians and the state within the contested terrain of the workplace.

There were several important differences between the struggle over coal workers' pneumoconiosis and the fight to get bronchitis and emphysema recognised. Firstly, and most importantly, CWP's occupational causation was never seriously disputed from the 1930s. The clear evidence which emerged from the South Wales coal fields before the Second World War was proof enough that this was an industrial disease, and not prevalent in the general population. Consequently, prescription – although costly – was not problematic. This contrasted sharply with emphysema and bronchitis, which were very common amongst miners and non-miners alike. Secondly, as the extent of CWP began to be realised, the British coal industry was, despite its inter-war atrophy, still the most important heavy industry in the UK. Therefore, any substantial threat to the industry's future – and especially regarding recruitment – had to be addressed effectively in the 1940s and 1950s. We also saw in Chapter 4 how the determination to address the issue of CWP coincided with the development of social medicine in the UK and the deployment of occupational

---

68 HSC, *Consultative Document* (2004), p. 34.

69 A.E. Dembe, *Occupation and Disease: How Social Factors Affect the Conception of Work-related Disorders* (New Haven, CT, 1996), pp. 3–21 and *passim*.

epidemiology. Consequently, medical intransigence to acknowledge the existence of CWP was quickly broken down from *within* the medical profession.

A different set of circumstances surrounded emphysema and bronchitis. Firstly, despite the fact that medical orthodoxy had for a long time accepted that miners suffered from respiratory diseases other than CWP, the inclusion of bronchitis and emphysema was constantly challenged on the grounds that these were diseases prevalent in the population at large, therefore totally at odds with the principles of state industrial compensation. Despite the fact that the TUC campaigned strongly for bronchitis to be accepted as industrial in the early 1950s, and for emphysema to be similarly accepted from the mid-1950s (see Chapter 7), the barrier was simply too large to scale. At the same time, the amount of attention being paid to CWP clearly overshadowed the need to broaden the scope of the research to include other respiratory diseases. Most importantly, though, by the time it became apparent that a broader approach to miners' respiratory health was needed – in that CWP was only one in a range of mine dust-related diseases – the mining industry was in serious decline, and the NUM was losing membership and was preoccupied with pit closures. When all this was coupled to the increasing acceptance of smoking as being the number one cause of respiratory ill health in UK, then it is understandable that the clash over scheduling bronchitis and emphysema was prolonged. Tellingly, perhaps, bronchitis and emphysema were only accepted as being compensatable diseases of coal miners when the number of coal miners had been drastically reduced. However, the sting in the tale was the reappearance of coal workers' pneumoconiosis in 2000. Perhaps this more than anything else should remind us to constantly question historical upward curves of progress, and especially those concerning occupational health and safety. For despite the intensity of research into the understanding of the causation and elimination of miners' respiratory disease throughout the twentieth century, a lack of balance between occupational health and productivity, combined perhaps with a sense of complacency on the part of management and workers, resulted in the most serious of coal workers' respiratory diseases returning.

PART III
The Industrial Politics of Miners' Lung

Chapter 6

'Enlightened Management'?
The NCB, the State and Dust

As highlighted in Chapter 1, although much has been written about the nationalised coal industry from several perspectives, the occupational health strategies of this important nationalised industry have been given sparse attention. Nationalisation of the coal industry coincided with a shift in the nature of British politics, and occurred at a time when many were hoping for the realisation of the more egalitarian order promised in the Beveridge Report. Certainly, nationalisation of the coal industry was something which the miners' trade unions had been pushing for throughout the inter-war period.[1] The introduction of the Coal Industry Nationalisation Act of 1946, then, was for many the fulfilment of a long held ambition in which miners were to have a stake in the future of their industry. Come Vesting Day, the first of January 1947, the patchwork pattern of private ownership which had characterised the British coal industry for so long disappeared. Suddenly 700,000 workers (5% of the working male population) found themselves working in a nationalised industry for which the Secretary of State had the power to appoint a Chairman and a Board made up of between 8 to 15 members. The principal obligations and priorities of the new NCB were clearly laid out in the act which brought it into being. These included:

a. working and getting coal in Great Britain …;
b. securing the efficient development of the coal-mining industry; and
c. making supplies of coal available, of such qualities and sizes, in such quantities and at such prices, as may seem to them best calculated to further the public interest in all respects …[2]

Some fifty years later, when the post-war coal industry was under trial in the High Court for exposing workers to dangerous levels of coal dust, it was suggested that the NCB's prioritising of production over health and safety was clearly apparent at its initiation, because the Board's duties regarding workers' health did not appear until Section 1 (4) of the Act:

---

1   See A. Campbell (ed.), *Miners, Unions and Politics, 1910–47* (Aldershot, 1996).
2   Coal Industry Nationalisation Act, 1946, c. 59, clause 1 (1).

The policy of the NCB shall be directed to securing, consistently with the proper discharge of their duties under subsection (1) of this section: (a) the safety, health and welfare of persons in their employment ...[3]

We will come back to the legal judgment in a later section. However, it could be argued that it would have been unrealistic to expect a corporation in this period (even one as idealistically motivated as the nascent NCB) to prioritise health and safety over production.

The aim of this chapter is to try to determine the extent to which the NCB effectively utilised its resources to protect its workforce from coal dust disease. How well did it try to strike a balance between supplying the nation's coal and caring for the health of its workers? Here we try to isolate Coal Board policy regarding dust, while in the following chapter we examine in some detail the role of the miners' trade unions regarding the dust disease problem. The relationship between the NCB and the National Union of Mineworkers (NUM) regarding occupational health and safety is a complex one. Taylor points out that although the structure of the nationalised coal industry suggested equal input by the state, the NCB and the NUM, the reality was a 'bifurcated tripartism' in which pricing policy, planning and the industry's restructuring remained very much the responsibility of the Board and the state, with the unions playing a consultative and legitimising role. It was also the case that although the NCB was a tripartite structure, there was no tripartite forum in which its segments could meet.[4] The evidence presented in this chapter points to a similar demarcation of responsibility regarding the dust problem, with dust suppression and dust monitoring lying very firmly within the NCB's jurisdiction, and the NUM playing a predominantly subordinate role.

The relationship between the NCB and the government is also difficult to pin down, with the Ministry of Fuel and Power determined that it would not become directly involved with the coal industry's industrial relations.[5] Initially, the Minister of Fuel and Power, Manny Shinwell, took a great interest in the new Board, and became involved with some of its day-to-day decisions. However, a policy decision in 1947 brought a loosening of this association, and from then on the Minister was only expected to deal with general issues affecting the coal industry. Notwithstanding this, though, when it came to any programmes of reorganisation which would involve substantial capital expenditure, the NCB was compelled to act along lines approved by the Secretary of State. The Board's borrowing power was initially limited to £10 million, with the understanding that any further expenditure could only be raised by Act of Parliament.[6] This was what happened in 1951 when the Coal Industry Act was passed to allow the NCB's borrowing capacity to be pushed up to £300 million

---

3   Judgment of Mr Justice Turner, 'The British Coal Respiratory Disease Litigation' (1998), p. 10; henceforth Turner.

4   A. Taylor, *The NUM and British Politics* (Aldershot, 2003), p. 35.

5   Ibid., Chapter 2.

6   NCB, *Annual Report* (1947), p. 81.

to finance its reconstruction plans; similarly, in 1956 another Act had to be passed to allow the Board to have another £650 million.[7]

The reasons for the substantial government subsidies which the NCB received in its early years lay in the economic turmoil which it immediately found itself in. Many collieries were in an archaic state – especially so in the Scottish Division – and were short of materials, as well as mine managers and other mining professionals. It was also the case that many colliery managers were ill equipped for the demands of nationalisation, and, indeed, opposed the very principle.[8] Heavy industrial demand had been draining coal stocks since 1946, and the situation was made much worse by appalling weather conditions throughout January and February 1947. Such bad weather further increased the demand for coal, made it difficult to transport coal to where it was urgently required, made it hard for many miners to get to work, and with a high incidence of flooding, made underground conditions difficult to work in. Compounding the coal shortage crisis, the NCB had to also deal with a serious labour shortage, and this also had its roots during the war. In 1946, 700,000 men were employed in the coal industry, compared to 800,000 before the war, and by 1947 the NCB also faced the prospect of the imminent loss of thousands of 'Bevin Boys'. As a way of helping the industry out of this predicament, the government prohibited the release of the 'Bevin Boys' until they had all completed their full term of national service, and prohibited any other men from leaving the coal industry until permission was granted by the Ministry of Labour. At the same time, the National Union of Miners (NUM) struck a deal with the NCB which allowed the Board to employ foreign workers.[9] In the initial stages of nationalisation, the NUM, which like the NCB had only just come into being, was fully committed to maintaining consensual relations with the Board and fully endorsed the drive to maximise production to deal with the coal emergency.

Therefore, it was within a maelstrom in which maximum productivity was the number one priority that the NCB (and to some extent the NUM) had to also deal with the additional problem of employing miners who had previously been barred from the industry because they had been diagnosed as suffering from pneumoconiosis.

The Re-employment of Pneumoconiotics

In Chapter 3, we illustrated how the introduction of legislation in 1948, the *Employment of Pneumoconiosis Cases* (Cd 354), demanded that a standard needed to be adopted with which 'approved dust conditions' could be determined. This was essential because of the need to re-employ miners who had lost their jobs in 1943

---

7   Ibid., p. 89.

8   A. Perchard, 'The Mine Management Professionals in the Scottish Coal Industry, 1930–1966' (PhD Thesis, University of Strathclyde, 2005), p. 166; See also A. Perchard, 'The Mine Management Professions and the Dust Problem in the Scottish Coal Mining Industry, c. 1930–1966', *Scottish Labour History*, vol. 40 (2005), pp. 87–110.

9   M.P. Jackson, *The Price of Coal* (London, 1974), pp. 75–6.

when diagnosed with CWP, but who could now, under the terms of Cd 354, return to work, providing that dust levels were kept within certain limits. However, as we illustrated in Chapter 3, due to the fact that the only scientific approximation of what safe dust levels might be was tentatively suggested by Bedford and Warner of the MRC in 1943, their arbitrary scale was adopted as a standard by default – although setting a standard had never been the intention of these researchers. What has to be understood, though, is that although the NCB was clutching at straws by adopting the only dust datum available, the 650 p.p.c.c. maximum for working in anthracite, the 850 p.p.c.c. limit for working in other coal, and the 450 p.p.c.c. maximum for exposure to rock dust would have offered miners some degree of protection from respiratory damage if this scale had been stringently enforced.

However, the only *statutory* compulsion on the NCB at this time was that imposed on it by the 1911 Coal Mines Act, which only required that dust levels should not be allowed to become excessive. Crucially, though, there was nothing binding the NCB to adhere to any specific standards of dustiness, and no such compulsion emerged in the new legislation. On the contrary, Cd 354 was quite explicit on this matter:

> It should be emphasised that these standards have no legal backing and that there is no question of the law being broken if a man returning to work is given a job in which the standards may occasionally be exceeded. In fact, even under the best systems of dust prevention, they may occasionally be exceeded. The standards are not meant to be peak measurements. They are meant to show the conditions as determined by several measurements made at representative times and points. The measurements from which the averages are calculated are, therefore, not to be made in abnormal conditions ...[10]

Therefore, when the NCB issued a policy document in 1949 (*Employment of Pneumokoniosis Cases: The Sampling of Air-borne Dust for the Testing of 'Approved Conditions'*), all of its Divisions were informed that although they had now to focus attention on keeping coal dust levels below recommended targets:

> The Regulations which came into force on 5th July 1948, do not confer legal status on the standards in the sense that the law would be broken if, momentarily, the permitted concentration were exceeded. The Board have accepted that the standards are to be interpreted, not as defining the allowable average concentration of dust over the whole period of the working shift but the average dustiness during periods of maximum dust production.[11]

However, the re-employment of pneumoconiotics into this labour-starved industry was made possible, and by 1960 there were almost 20,000 pneumoconiotic miners

---

10 Turner, p. 30.

11 NCB, *Employment of Pneuomokoniosis Cases: The Sampling of Air-borne Dust for the Testing of 'Approved Conditions'* (1949), pp. 1–2.

working throughout the UK.[12] The experience of such workers is explored in more depth in Chapter 9.

The 1949 NCB policy document betrayed a certain amount of 'fumbling in the dark' as the NCB struggled to implement the requirements of Cd. 354. At this time, the sampling of airborne dust in mines was in a tentative state, and the problem presented to the NCB by the employment of pneumoconiotic miners was 'one for which existing experience [was] insufficient to provide an immediate solution'.[13] Notwithstanding this, though, and despite the fact that no guidance was given on how 'periods of maximum dust production' as described in the document were to be identified, the NCB became committed to tackling the coal dust problem using 'approved conditions' as its principal yardstick. This was to be the criterion by which every UK colliery's attempts to reduce dust levels would be assessed. The toothless nature of the new protective measures was further exacerbated by the fact that incapacitated men to whom the NCB was unable to provide 'dust-approved' conditions were allowed, if they wished, to work in non-approved conditions. Such a man was '… not to be disallowed from continuing in his former work by reason only of the fact that the dust conditions fail to comply with the approved conditions'.[14] It does appear, then, that because instant action was required to deal with an unexpected and novel set of circumstances, a rather lame compromise emerged.

Therefore, the NCB's strategy for dealing with the re-employment of men suffering form pneumoconiosis rested on shaky foundations. More importantly, though, what initially emerged as a special contingency designed to allow for the employment of dust-damaged miners would be taken up as the NCB's main strategy regarding the coal dust problem in general for some time to come.

Production versus Protection: Mechanisation and the Dust Problem

It is important to contextualise the NCB's handling of the coal dust issue within the changing economic imperatives which the Board and its workers encountered. Initially, the biggest problem facing the industry was simply keeping up with demand for coal. Consumption of coal rose from 190 million tons in 1947 to 230 million tons by 1955, mostly from industrial customers, and the NCB struggled to meet this demand.[15] It was primarily for this reason that a decision was taken to bring about a reconstruction of the industry, with the assumption that consumption of coal would continue to grow throughout the 1960s and beyond. The reconstruction plans involved an investment in 250 existing collieries and opening new larger ones,

---

12 *Colliery Guardian* (30 June 1960), p. 732. Note that according to the NCB *Annual Report* (1955), the number was 12,347. For anthracite, the level was 650 particles per cc with a dust size of 1–5, and for stone dusts, 450 particles per cc, dust size 0.5–5; *Digest of Pneumoconiosis Statistics* (1955), NAS/HH 104/1 HOS/15/15.

13 NCB, *Employment of Pneumokonisis Cases*, p. 7.

14 Turner, p. 31.

15 Jackson, *The Price of Coal*, p. 74.

but also closing 300–400 of the less viable pits. Therefore, the Board's 1950 Plan for Coal, followed by its 1956 revised plan, 'Investing in Coal', were strategies to take the industry out of its inability to supply enough coal. However, in 1957 the economic imperatives suddenly changed and UK coal consumption began to fall. Although this decline was believed at the time to be temporary, this was not to be the case, and between 1956 and 1959 total coal consumption dropped by 33 million tons. This decline continued into the 1960s, and the main reason was the widespread exodus of consumers from coal to alternative fuels, in particular oil and natural gas.

In response to this shrinking market, the NCB initiated a revised plan for coal in 1959. In contrast to the early expansionist schemes, the 1959 plan was geared to a contracting industry in which pit closures were to play a role in ensuring the industry's long-term survival. The contraction of the industry under the new policy began in the early 1960s, and between 1957 and 1965 about three hundred collieries were closed, causing labour power to fall from 703,800 to 465,600.[16] This, though, was only the top of a slippery slope. The desertion of domestic coal consumers continued as more and more of the population turned to simpler to use, cleaner and easier to store fuels, and this was accompanied by a decline in export markets too. At the same time, the introduction of Clean Air Acts in the mid-1950s meant many customers had to change to either smokeless coal – which the NCB was unable to produce in large quantities until the 1960s – or find an alternative form of fuel. In the face of deepening uncertainty about its future, then, the NCB was forced in the mid-1960s to accelerate its pit closure programme within a rationalisation plan which involved the closure of another two hundred pits, with the intention of eventually concentrating coal production in 320 'long-life' pits.[17] The NCB's closure programme, which was at its height under the chairmanship of Lord Robens, hit mining communities hard, causing uncertainty, hardship and social dislocation. However, at this time the NUM fully concurred with the strategy and agreed with the NCB that radical rationalisation was the only way for the industry to have any kind of future.[18]

The second aspect of the NCB's stratagem was to have serious implications for miners' respiratory health. This was the drive towards increased mechanisation of coal production. In 1944, a Technical Advisory Committee appointed by the Ministry of Fuel and Power had examined the coal production process with a view to increasing its technical efficiency. This committee fully realised that although increased technology could improve safety in the pits – for example, hydraulic propping, ventilation and so on – one of the downsides would be an increase in dust levels.[19] However, technical change was seen as the way ahead. An editorial in the *Colliery Guardian* in 1963 retrospectively hailed the new production methods in glowing terms:

---

16 Ibid., p. 108.
17 Ibid., p. 109.
18 Taylor, *The NUM and British Politics*, Chapter 5.
19 Ibid., p. 15.

Mechanisation is the password to better environmental conditions at the coal face, higher productivity, and, it follows, increased prosperity for the Coal Board's 'ship' and all who sail in her.[20]

As we discussed in Chapter 2, there were several aspects to mechanisation of coal mining, but one of the most important during the nationalisation era was power loading. Between 1947 and 1957, the proportion of power-loaded coal in the UK rose from 2% to 23%, and by the end of the next ten years the figure had jumped to 86%, with 90% of British coal being power-loaded by the 1970s.[21] However, as production soared, so too did dust levels, and as we will see, machines such as the Anderton shearer were to prove to be very problematic when it came to suppressing the dust which they gave off.

Therefore, just as it was important to contextualise the NCB's initial strategy towards dusty conditions in the light of the problems which the new organisation had to face from Vesting Day, so too do we need to locate the NCB's programme to protect miners from dust against the background of an industry fighting for its survival and utilising increased levels of mechanisation to force up productivity. On the one hand the NCB was genuinely committed to protecting miners from coal dust – and clear evidence for this was its investment in high-quality epidemiological research – but on the other, its policy to mechanise as much as possible drastically increased dust levels. In 1969, Gilson of the PRU referred to this dynamic:

> There are powerful forces operating to perpetuate the risk. Increased output uses more power and with it the dust levels tend to rise ... Also, as production increases, work occurs on more shifts so that the total hours of higher dust levels tend to rise and this tends to offset, to some extent, fewer men exposed per shift as a result of mechanisation or automation.[22]

In a similar way, Sir Andrew Bryan, an ex-Chief Inspector of Mines, in his *The Evolution of Health and Safety in Mines* published in 1975, referred to the unequal contest between dust suppression and dust generation:

> Because of the big increase during the past decade of the make of dust brought about by the increased mechanization of coal getting, the concentration of working in high production long-wall faces, the adoption of multi-shift production, the full extraction of dirt banded seams, the mechanisation of ripping and so forth, in some instances the dust suppression specialist is, like *Alice in Wonderland*, 'having to run faster to stand still'.[23]

---

20 *Colliery Guardian* (30 May 1963), p. 635.

21 N.K. Buxton, *The Economic Development of the British Coal Industry* (London, 1978), p. 248.

22 J.C. Gilson, *The First Wade Lecture: 'The Changing Pattern of Pneumoconiosis'* (1969), PRU Collected Papers no. 450.

23 Sir Andrew Bryan, *The Evolution of Health and Safety in Mines* (Letchworth, 1975), p. 112.

Therefore, to summarise briefly, there were flaws in the NCB's strategy forged in the late 1940s aimed at addressing the dust disease problem. First of all, safe levels of dust in the mine air were determined by an inappropriate scale. This scale had initially been adopted as a measure designed to facilitate the re-employment of discharged pneumoconiotics, but was immediately used across the coal fields to determine maximum dust exposure levels for all underground workers. On top of this was the fact that the NCB was under no statutory compulsion to rigidly enforce the 'approved faces' scheme. None the less, the NCB did plough considerable resources into controlling dust levels, employing a large number of personnel to try to ensure that dust in the mine air was kept within the stipulated safe range, notwithstanding increased mechanisation. In the following sections, we scrutinise in some detail the dust measuring and dust suppression measures used by the NCB.

Gauging the Problem: Measuring the Dust

The idea of measuring the amount of coal dust in mines was not new by the time of nationalisation of the coal industry, and the NCB and the Ministry of Fuel and Power were able to draw from a knowledge base which had its roots in the era of private ownership. In the early twentieth century, it was assumed that the main problem posed by mine dust was its explosive potential, and it was primarily to conduct research on this that an experimental station was set up in Yorkshire by the Mining Association in 1908. In 1924, a new facility was opened near Buxton where experiments into fire damp, shot blasting and the nature of dust explosions were conducted.[24] In 1928, similar laboratories were opened at Sheffield, and here airborne dust samples – gathered by mines inspectors – were inspected to determine their silica content, while research was also undertaken on dust prevention and suppression. With the coming of nationalisation, the work of the research stations and laboratories at Sheffield and Buxton were brought together and became known as the Safety in Mines Research Establishment (SMRE).

By the mid-1940s, one of the most common dust samplers was the Konimeter. This machine had been developed in South Africa, and had been used in the UK since the 1930s. Dust particles were deposited on a glass slide coated with an adhesive jelly. The main drawback of the Konimeter was its inability to record very fine dust particles, which meant it was only useful for working in low-dust conditions. From the earliest years of nationalisation, those involved with dust measuring in the NCB were convinced that the thermal precipitator was the best device for sampling mine dust. The Standard Period Thermal Precipitator (SPTP) was developed in the 1930s and was utilised by the MRC researchers in the pre-Second World War South Wales research. Dusty air was drawn through a gap across a heated wire, and this caused the particles to move away from the heat and onto a glass slide. Sampling took 10–20 minutes, depending upon the dustiness of the conditions, and the slides were

---

24 *The Times* (10 June 1927), p. 15.

then examined under a microscope to determine a count/size ratio. Compared to the Konimeter, the SPTP collected fine dust particles. However, the downside was the laborious particle counting process which had to be undertaken, and the frustrating task of trying to count particles which overlapped with each other. This overlapping problem became more acute whenever working conditions became dustier, and this meant that the dustier the conditions, the less accurate was the reading.

Another device in use at this time was the Pneumoconiosis Research Unit Hand Pump. This was developed by the PRU at Llandough Hospital when it was thought there would be a shortage of SPTPs to carry out the PRU's field sampling. With the Hand Pump, the dust-laden air was drawn through a paper disc which produced a stain on the paper; the density of this stain could be related to the degree of dust in the air. This method removed the need for counting dust particles under a microscope. However, the Hand Pump could only measure total dust concentrations – as opposed to the SPTP which could gauge the amount of the finer respirable dust – and this meant that any correlation of the two machines was problematic.

What was realised very early, though, was that a device was required which could – unlike these 'snap samplers' – accurately measure dust levels throughout the miner's shift.[25] However, the ensuing race to produce the first pit-worthy Long Running Thermal Precipitator (LRTP) cast a shadow over an important technical and medical issue regarding dust counting which had been known for some time. This was that the best way to determine the risk posed to miners by coal dust was not to count the number of particles, but to determine the overall *mass* of the dust. The shortcomings of particle counting had been expressed in 1943 in the MRC report published by Bedford and Warner, who lamented that a machine capable of determining the mass of mine dust was not available.[26] The NCB was well informed about the need for such a device, and set up a Dust Sampling and Analysis Committee in October 1947. The recommendations of this committee also pointed to the need for a form of sampling instrument which would provide qualitative as well as quantitative assessment of the air which the miners breathed:

> There was some doubt … as to whether the present methods of sampling, in conjunction with the appropriate methods of size measurement, represented effectively the finer and most important sizes of dust. For this reason, it was agreed that the problem required investigation as a whole …[27]

Not only that, when the NJPC set up its Field Research Steering Committee in 1952, it also expressed its deep concern that a gravimetric form of sampling could not be implemented under the proposed 25-pit Scheme:

> There is still a gap in the sampling plan in that initially no gravimetric samples will be taken, from which the composition of the dust can be determined. Such sampling,

---

25 MFP, *Annual Report* (1953), p. 52.

26 NCB, *Annual Report* (1961), p. 32.

27 Turner, p. 29.

will however, be started in due course ... Much more sampling could be done than is practicable under present conditions if there were a reliable automatic sampling device.[28]

However, the impetus was directed into ways to progress, not from particle counting to mass estimation, but from snap sampling to continuous sampling over a whole shift. Consequently, particle counting, despite its shortcomings, would continue for a long time to come. More and more men were being trained in how to use thermal precipitators, and in 1949, 400,000 dust samples were taken in South Wales alone using this method. Experts from the South Wales coal field also began training men in other NCB Divisions in these dust sampling techniques.[29] The Board also distributed to every colliery manager in 1949 a comprehensive guide on dust suppression entitled *Dust Control in Mines*.[30]

The NJPC's Dust Sub-Committee fully realised the limitations of snap sampling, which could 'only purport to represent the conditions obtaining when that sample was taken and cannot be said to represent conditions which may vary greatly from day to day or even hourly'.[31] The Ministry for Fuel and Power also expressed concern.[32] But progress continued to be slow, and in 1959 the NJPC was complaining again about the delay over the development of the LRTP which had been 'tested and found satisfactory' by the NCB four years earlier.[33] Clearly, then, moves were being made by the NCB to develop and utilise a more refined method of dust counting, but the pace was far too sluggish, and – because of the lack of attention being focused on refining gravimetric techniques – largely misdirected.

A further clouding of the issues was caused by interpreting what was meant by 'periods of maximum dustiness'. The NJPC noted in 1950 that dust conditions varied so much over time and from place to place that a precise definition along these lines was very difficult. To a great extent, then, it was left up to the individual NCB Divisions to interpret as best they could what these periods were. The South Western Division (South Wales), an early leader in the fight against the dust problem, decided to adopt a system of dust surveying known as 'face efficiency', in which 100% face efficiency meant every measurement at any time or place was below the agreed limit, while 90% face efficiency implied 90% were below the agreed limit, and so on. Throughout the rest of the coal fields, though, with the exception of Scotland (which followed the Welsh method), dust measurements amounted to the average of all measurements, whether taken at times of maximum dustiness or not. So impressed was the NCB by the 'face efficiency' idea that a decision was taken to extend this

---

28 *First Report of the NJPC Field Research Steering Committee*, NJPC no. 52, NA/PIN 20/351.

29 NCB, *Annual Report* (1949).

30 NUM, *South Wales Area Council, Annual Conference Report* (1953), p. 12.

31 Turner, p. 28.

32 Ministry of Fuel and Power, *Annual Report* (1950), pp. 22–3.

33 *National Joint Pneumoconiosis Committee Sixth Report of the Field Research Steering Committee* (January 1955), NJPC 61, NAS/PIN 20/235; NJPC, *20th Report of the Field Research Steering Committee* (1959), NAS/PIN 20/351.

to all coal fields, and to aim for at least 80% face efficiency across the UK by 1951.[34] The NJPC's Dust Suppression Sub-Committee did not hesitate to reprimand Divisions if they strayed too far from correct dust sampling procedure. For example, the normally exemplary South Western Division was ticked off in 1953 when its Dust Prevention Committee introduced a system of 'incremental sampling' of faces, in which sampling machines operated for only 2 minutes followed by breaks of up to 6 minutes – normal practice was to run dust sampling machines for 10–15 minutes. The Chief Inspector of Mines was quick to condemn this 'departure from standard procedure', and insisted that the Division fell in with the rest of the UK.[35]

In 1956, the NCB adopted a new protocol regarding coal dust. The main aspect of this change was that the thermal precipitator was to become the standard sampling instrument throughout the UK – although the PRU Hand Pump was used alongside this for some time to come. However, the new protocol also decreed that to gain a clearer insight into the degree of dustiness of working places, a *series* of samples had to be taken. With this, then, the ambiguous 'periods of maximum dustiness' disappeared and average dust concentrations were measured periodically throughout an entire shift.[36] The 1998 legal case against British Coal found there were still serious flaws in the new 1956 protocol. For one thing, the system still allowed for local interpretation. Also, each face was only required to be certified every 12 months. Concern was also expressed at the time by the Ministry of Fuel and Power, and by the NUM, that the change from 'periods of maximum dustiness' to 'periods of active work' would bring about a relaxations of standards.[37] However, underpinning all the flaws in the new protocol of 1956 was the simple fact that dust exposure standards were not tightened, and that the mantra of the 450/650/850 p.p.c.c. to determine approved conditions remained.

By 1956, the SMRE finally managed to produce a commercially viable long-running dust measuring instrument which could operate over periods of up to 8 hours – the equivalent of a working shift. This machine became available to the coal industry in the spring of 1957, and as mentioned earlier, was known as the LRTP. The machine incorporated an elutriator which selected only respirable dust from the mine by filtering out the larger, faster-falling particles – simulating the human nose and the upper respiratory passages – and required only one slide per shift. To operate the machine, all that was required was for it to be hung in position, and once switched on, it would draw in dust-laden air via a small clockwork breathing pump.

However, despite this development, the Ministry of Fuel and Power was still pessimistic, and noted that 'considerable progress remains to be made before the industry is adequately equipped for dust sampling'.[38] Moreover, two years later the

---

34 *NCB Report on Dust Suppression as at 30 September 1950*, NJPC no. 35, NAS/PIN 20/18.

35 MFP, Memo from Chief Inspector of Mines, dated 15 April 1953, POWE8/420.

36 Turner, p. 37.

37 Ibid., p. 38; *The Miner* (November/December 1964), p. 16.

38 Ministry of Fuel and Power, *Annual Report* (1956), p. 41.

Ministry criticised the NCB for its adhesion to the concept of approved and non-approved conditions as a gauge of dustiness in the pits:

> The verdict on Approved or Not Approved may serve a useful purpose in classifying where men may work without undue exposure to risk, but as a criterion of the effectiveness of dust suppression measures it is surely insufficiently refined to serve much purpose.[39]

At the same time, the Ministry of Fuel and Power suggested that the NCB should produce an updated instructional booklet along the lines of *Dust Control in Mines*. However, no new guidance booklet emerged.[40]

The relationship between the government and the NCB over the dust problem was becoming strained by the mid-1950s – and we'll see that this was to continue when the Ministry was replaced by the Department of Trade and Industry in the 1970s. This was reflected in the reports of the Chief Inspector of Mines regarding how dust suppression was being addressed throughout the UK, which, as we shall see in the following section, became much more critical from the mid-1950s onwards. In short, though, the Mines Inspectorate was displeased at the NCB's use of 'approved conditions' as a blanket measurement for working conditions generally. For example, in 1959:

> The fact that the amount of dust on some power loader faces may be within the approved standards does not relieve managements of their statutory obligations to minimise dust production by using every known dust prevention measure.[41]

And in the *Annual Report* of 1964:

> Approval standards for the dustiness of mine atmospheres which were devised initially for places where pneumoconiotics could be allowed to work, have now become accepted standards of dustiness for all working places.[42]

There was also some abrasion between the NCB and the PRU over dust measuring strategy. For while the NCB was extolling the virtues of its new LRTP, research by the PRU drew attention to the problem of thermal precipitators underestimating the degree of dustiness due to dust particles overlapping. The Board, though, did not take kindly to the accusation that it was minimising the extent of the dust problem, and its scientific branch wrote to the PRU researcher concerned (S.A. Roach) strongly advising him to conduct more investigations before publishing his research, 'not only from the point of view of your scientific reputation, but also to avoid causing unjustified doubt on well established techniques …'.[43] However, despite this Roach published his paper in 1959 in the *British Journal of Industrial Medicine*, and its

---

39 Turner, p. 43.
40 Ibid.
41 *Report by the Chief Inspector of Mines* (1959), p. 18.
42 *Report by the Chief Inspector of Mines* (1964), p. 45.
43 Turner, p. 38.

summary highlighted what the PRU saw as a very significant flaw: 'A more important source of error is the bias, due to overlapping among the particles on the cover glasses. The count may give a serious underestimating of the number of airborne particles if high sample densities are used.'[44] This, then, was another nudge to the NCB that it should be developing and utilising gravimetric sampling – suggested over ten years earlier by the NCB's Dust Sampling Analysis Committee, and earlier still by Bedford and Warner in their 1943 MRC report. Even more criticism of the state of affairs came in 1961, this time in a Memorandum by the NCB's Chief Medical Officer, John Rogan. Here, though, the blame was laid at the door of the MRE for its slow progress at developing the much-needed machinery:

> We believe that in the long run mass standards ought to replace the present concentration standards ... we would press on you [the MRE] most strongly that ways and means should be found to continue this work which, has had to be abandoned, as a matter of high priority.[45]

As all this was going on, the NCB was also coming under increasing criticism from the NUM. In the years following nationalisation, relations between the NUM (which was determined to make nationalisation work) and the NCB were fairly consensual, with only a few hard-line areas remaining dedicated to pursuing workers' control of the industry.[46] However, the dust issue became one which the NUM could not ignore, and, as we examine in more detail in Chapter 7, the NUM continually pushed the NCB to tighten up on dust standards throughout the whole of the UK. Driving this was a sound understanding by the NUM of the unevenness of effort in tackling the dust problem across the coal fields.

In 1965, the NCB introduced another protocol, which replaced the 1949 and the 1956 protocols. The new aims were set out in a new publication, *The Sampling of Airborne Dust for the Testing of Approved Dust Conditions*. This booklet contained a clear statement of policy, of which paragraphs 1 and 3 are worth quoting in full:

1. It is the aim of the NCB to attain 'Approved Dust Conditions' generally. These conditions also have special application in relation to the employment of pneumoconiotic cases.

   ...

3. The classifications 'Approved and 'Not Approved' given to working places will remain in force for a period which is limited to six months for power loaded faces and to one year for working places other than power loaded faces. These approval periods are the maximum permitted; more frequent sampling should be carried out where possible.[47]

---

44 S.A. Roach, 'Measuring Dust Exposure with the Thermal Precipitator in Collieries and Foundries', *British Journal of Industrial Medicine* (1959), p. 104.

45 Turner, p. 39.

46 See Jackson, *The Price of Coal*, pp. 90–96.

47 *The Sampling of Airborne Dust for Testing of 'Approved Dust Conditions'*, NCB publication F3837 (1 October, 1965), p. 3.

The main difference was that dust samples were, at last, now to be taken using the LRTP. However, to implement the change from sequential to continuous sampling, a conversion factor was required. This changed the permissible limits of dust in the mine air. However, the NCB did not take the opportunity to introduce a stricter standard at this juncture, and care was taken to ensure that the conversion factor equated to the long-criticised 850/650/450 p.p.c.c. scale – despite the fact that the NUM was calling for a general adoption of a 450 p.p.c.c. maximum.[48]

The NCB's 1965 Protocol and the move to full shift sampling was a significant development. However, there were still holes in the protective shield which the protocol was supposed to provide. For one thing, it became common practice for the sampling of faces to be delayed until dust suppression measures were put in place. Subsequently, such 'belatedly bolting the stable door' tactics failed to provide a true picture of the dangerous conditions which the men were having to endure.[49] Secondly, miners were frequently allowed to work on what were termed 'Provisionally Approved' faces – a designation which could last for up to three months – while dust suppression measures were being improved on these faces. Thirdly, it was also the case, as it had been since 1949, that because only a minimum number of samples were required to be taken, dust conditions could vary considerably between samples.[50] Fourthly, further compounding the difficulties was the simple fact that many of the men who were employed to sample the dust were part of the NCB's *production* department. Given the furious productivity drive of the time, it is small wonder that reports of tinkering with the dust measurements were rife, and we examine oral history evidence of this in Chapter 8.

However, by far the main drawback of the 1965 Protocol was that it did not represent a change from determining the amount of harmful dust in the air by counting particles to assessing its overall mass. By this time, a pit-worthy gravimetric sampler had at last been developed by the MRE – in 1963.[51] What was holding things up now, though, was the problem of correlating the old particle count method to the new gravimetric system. Uncertainty and dithering over how to resolve this issue was to cause another five years' delay in the implementation of gravimetric sampling. Judge Turner pulled no punches regarding these delays during his summing up in the 1998 legal case, and suggested that a lack of commitment was the main factor: '… had the will been there, in the upper management of British Coal, a pit-worthy gravimetric sampler both could and should have been introduced ten years earlier than in fact it was'.[52]

As we saw earlier, the NCB had been criticised over its adherence to 'approved conditions'. However, to some degree the Board's long adherence to its initial dust

---

48   The new dust datum was as follows: 700 p.p.c.c. for anthracite, 500 p.p.c.c. for other coal and 250 p.p.c.c. for stone.

49   Turner, p. 40.

50   Ibid.

51   Ibid., p. 41.

52   Ibid., p. 48.

datum of 850/650/450 – and, indeed, to the concept of 'approved conditions' – can be partly explained. As we examined in Chapter 4, from the early 1950s the NCB was awaiting the results of the Pneumoconiosis Field Research. Therefore, the adoption of any new standard in advance of this – without hard evidence to back it up – would have been just as arbitrary as the implementation of Bedford and Warner's scale had been back in 1948. Following the PFR's Interim Standards Study in 1969, the NCB voluntarily adopted the more stringent metric-based dust datum recommended by Jacobsen et al. in their 1970 article, in which dust levels had to fall below 8–7 mg/m^3, with an even more stringent standard for working in stone. It was also the case that the incidence of pneumoconiosis was falling across the UK. In 1954, a survey conducted by the NUM found progression of the disease in around a third of pneumoconiotic men working in 'approved dust conditions'. However, the Board denied that this trade union study had any credibility.[53] On the contrary, as far as the NCB was concerned, the decline of the potentially deadly dust disease across the coal fields was clear proof that it was pursuing the best course of action. If we refer to Figures 2.1, 2.2 and 4.1, we can see that this was indeed the case. The number of newly diagnosed cases of pneumoconiosis fell sharply from the mid-1950s, and CWP rates per 1,000 miners employed were steadily falling. However, the deceleration in the rate of improvement for several years from the mid-1960s caused some concern. In 1972, the NCB's Chief Medical Officer stated:

> The overall deduction is that dust exposure has been greatly reduced in British collieries in the past twenty years, but in fact in the last few years the situation has been more or less static and may possibly be deteriorating. More intensive mechanisation and longer running times of coal face machinery have probably contributed to this trend.[54]

Whilst the NCB policy does need to be carefully contextualised, on balance the evidence indicates that a stricter adherence by the NCB to reducing dust levels across the coal fields would have saved lives.

Certainly, as far as the approved dust conditions policy was concerned, the Department of Trade and Industry was losing its patience, and conveyed this in a letter to the NCB in 1971:

> We have serious doubts about the effectiveness of the 'Approved/Not Approved' classifications as a management tool, for it can be of use only to the minority of faces 'not approved', as it is equally important to contain or reduce dust levels on 'approved' faces. Even 100% 'approved' conditions under the present interim standard would not necessarily mean any reduction in the incidence of pneumoconiosis … we feel it should go sooner than later.[55]

---

53 *The Miner*, vol. 8, no. 3 (May/June 1960), p. 13.

54 J.S. McLintock, 'The changing prevalence of coal workers' pneumoconiosis in Great Britain', *Annals of the New York Academy of Sciences* (1972), pp. 278–91, p. 290.

55 Turner, p. 46.

The same year as the DTI expressed its concern to the NCB, the Board published *Approved Conditions for Airborne Dust in Mines: Standards and Procedures for Sampling* (F4040). This document contained yet another statement of policy regarding dust – although much of this was really the NCB's statutory duty under the 1954 Mines and Quarries: 'It is the aim of the National Coal Board to minimise dust and to attain Approved Dust Conditions in every working place ...'.[56] This publication was a comprehensive attempt to tighten up on the fairly loose approach to dust sampling. But most importantly, at long last, mine dust was to be measured by its mass:

> Dust conditions at a working place will be classified as 'Approved' or as 'Not Approved'. They will be 'Approved' when the mean mass concentration of dust as defined below does not exceed:
>   (I) 3.0 mg/m^3 in stone drivages.
>   (II) 8.0 mg/m^3 in all other locations.[57]

As we have seen, the reason for this lay with the evidence produced by the Interim Standards Study (ISS) of the PFR. The ISS revealed a much closer correlation between the progression of pneumoconiosis and the mass of dust compared to particle counting – something that had been predicted by experts for some time. Consequently, the gravimetric sampler was to become from 1971 the dust measuring instrument of choice. Also clearly apparent in the new scale was the debunking of the 'rank of coal' thesis regarding CWP causation, as there was no longer a separate standard for anthracite coal, the dust of which was initially thought to be the most dangerous. The results of the ISS were published in 1970, and as noted earlier, the NCB immediately adopted the recommendations as its voluntary standard in April 1971. Under this new voluntary code, the period of sampling was to be the working shift, dust samplers were to be distributed amongst working places in relation to their dust conditions, and clear guidance was to be given regarding the positioning of samplers and the procedures to be implemented if places fell into the 'Not Approved' category. There were also minimum routine sampling frequencies which had to be adhered to. For example, coal faces on production shifts, coal drivages and stone drivages had to be sampled every month, loading and transfer points every quarter, coal face cutting shifts every half-year, and preparation shifts were to be sampled annually. Immediately these new stipulations created difficulties for a number of collieries which found it difficult to comply with the much more stringent requirements. However – and this was to be a particularly damning observation during the 1998 legal case – when such problematic collieries realised they were not meeting the standards, dust prevention schemes were implemented which *utilised existing technology* to ensure that they fell into line. Clearly, then, if the NCB had

---

56 *Approved Conditions for Airborne Dust, Standards and Procedures for Sampling*, F4040 (1970). pp. 1–4.

57 Ibid.

– as the NUM had demanded for some time – forced the issue, such technology could have been used to the same effect many years before.[58]

By the late 1960s, the NCB was well aware that the government was planning to introduce coal dust regulations which would impose a statutory duty upon the industry to enforce a more rigorous standard of dustiness than it had adhered to since 1949. Therefore, to a great extent, anticipation of the 1975 regulations lay behind the Board's adoption of its 1970 voluntary standard – which came into force in 1971. The NCB also published a comprehensive 85-page guidance booklet in 1973 on how to deal with dust in the pits. However, as we have seen, the Ministry of Fuel and Power suggested this was required sixteen years earlier.[59] Once again, then, the threat of statutory obligation seemed to lie behind the publication of a potentially life-saving code of good practice.

The new Coal Mines Respirable Dust Regulations (RDR) came into effect in 1975, with the NCB's 1970 voluntary standard set as the measurement of safe working conditions – although further regulations in 1977 reduced the maximum for coal from 8 to $7mg/m^3$.[60] The Mines Inspectorate now had the power to require more frequent sampling of faces, and to close coal faces or other working places if these failed to meet the approved limits. With the introduction of the RDR, a new page in the history of state intervention in coal mining had been turned, although it had taken a very long time for it to happen. A note to the new regulations clearly set them in context:

> These Regulations impose requirements with respect to the sampling of air for respirable dust in coal mines at which more than 30 persons are employed below ground and the evaluation of the samples at approved laboratories. They require the appointment of persons to take and supervise the taking of samples, the keeping of records and the making of a scheme relating to the taking of samples. They also regulate or prohibit the carrying on of operations where the respirable dust content in the air is excessive and require dust respirators to be made available. Further requirements relate to the medical supervision of employees liable to injury by inhaling respirable dust and the making of a scheme for the prevention and suppression of dust.[61]

There was now a legal obligation on mine management to go beyond the approval principle and ensure that coal dust levels were reduced in general. Coinciding with the adoption of its new dust datum in 1971, the NCB initiated a 'Destroy Dust' campaign. Posters throughout the Divisions projected slick slogans designed to eliminate dust, including 'Sharp Tools Cut Cleanly', 'Seal Belt Joints', 'Spray Dust Away', and 'Keep Sprays Working'.[62] For its part, the NUM – which, as we know, had been campaigning for stricter dust limits for some time – was pleased with

---

58 Turner, p. 45.

59 The new publication was *Control of Harmful Dust in Coal Mines* (London, 1973).

60 Turner, p. 51.

61 Ibid., p. 49.

62 *Colliery Guardian* (June 1971), p. 253.

the new regulations, noting immediately how 'the general level of protection aimed for by these statutory provisions represented a notable advance on that presently obtaining'. However, the union also noted that numerous working places throughout the UK would fail to meet the new standards.[63] Clearly, then, in these mines workers had been exposed to dangerous working practices for a long time.

Therefore, thanks in great measure to the evidence gathered by the PFR, the early 1970s saw concerted efforts being taken to combat dust, based on new standards. A more determined attitude was apparent at pit level. For example, when dust levels at Highhouse Colliery in Ayrshire were found to be too high in 1972, a Dust Combat Team was formed, a full airborne dust survey was conducted 'from pit bottom to coal face', and action was immediately taken. This included reducing the number of joints on conveyor belts, correcting a misaligned belt, erecting shrouds at conveyor belt transfer points, adjusting the height of coal chutes, and attaching water sprays to all the bottom belts.[64] Consequently, dust levels were brought down.

However, despite their sharper focus, amazingly the new 1970s dust regulations still did not entail any requirements regarding the shutting down of any faces which failed to comply with the new stricter dust datum. On the contrary, procedures became even more tuned towards maintaining production. If a face fell into the non-approved category, the area Dust Suppression Engineer and the Area Chief Scientist would be called in to find out why. However, the guidelines did not direct personnel to shut down the face, only to ensure: 'Dust production along the face should be carefully examined and the dust concentration at particular sources measured and reported …'.[65] Therefore, despite the new crusade and the sophistication of the new dust measuring equipment being deployed, production continued to take precedence over workers' health. There is no doubt that the mid-1970s regulations were a step in the right direction, and that the NCB tackled the dust problem much more assiduously when the shadow of statutory regulations loomed – although it is worth repeating that much of this was achieved using existing dust suppression technology. From the 1970s, standards of dustiness were no longer arbitrary; sampling techniques were perfected; and an instrument capable of continuously measuring the mass of dust was at last in service. But there is little doubt that the NCB could have pushed for this to be in use much earlier, and that its 'leisurely approach to the introduction of the gravimetric sampler', combined with an almost manic attachment to the notion of 'approved' and 'non-approved' conditions, proved seriously detrimental to the health and well-being of a great many coal workers.[66] Certainly, once the 1975 Regulations were in place, dust concentrations fell across the coal fields. However, this should have happened ten years earlier.

---

63 NUM, *Annual Report and Proceedings* (1974), p. 13.

64 NCB Scottish South Area, *Airborne Dust Prevention and Suppression Report, Second Quarter* (1972/73), CB/099/03/6.

65 NCB, *Approved Conditions for Airborne Dust, Standards and Procedures for Sampling*, F 4040 (1969), p. 14.

66 Turner, p. 46.

We should also note that although a major step was taken in 1975 to protect coal miners from dust, twenty years later, when the HSC completed another reassessment, significant shortcomings were revealed. One of the most serious flaws was the adherence of the 1975 RDR to fixed-point sampling of faces. Studies subsequently found that the representativeness of fixed-point sampling varied widely between faces, and – more importantly – between individuals within face teams. Consequently, it was realised that *personal* sampling was the only way to assess whether conditions were dangerous or not. However, the principal weakness of the 1975 RDR was that men's exposure limits to dust were not time-weighted, in that the amount of time miners were exposed to respirable dust during their shifts was not factored in to any protective matrix. In short, the longer the miners were exposed, then the lower should have been the permitted concentration of dust. Therefore, although standards improved in 1975 and risks from dust exposure declined, miners were still exposed to dangerous dust levels thereafter, as the high rates of bronchitis and emphysema in the pits and the revival of pneumoconiosis in the early twenty-first century illustrated.[67]

Dealing with the Problem: Suppressing the Dust

> The amount of effort put into solving the problems of dust measurement may seem to some observers to have overshadowed the more difficult but essential problem of controlling the dust itself.[68]

This comment was made in a paper by the Chief Inspector of Factories and the Deputy Senior Medical Inspector of Factories entitled 'The Problems of Dust in Industry', incorporated into the Chief Inspector's 1966 *Annual Report*. This should remind us that the problem of dust at work was by no means confined to the coal mines, and that although the quest to find the best methods of eradication and measurement of respirable dust was concentrated in the coal industry, these efforts would have important repercussions for workers in other industries too, such as in iron and steel, foundries and quarries.[69]

As was the case with dust measuring, dust suppression had a history which pre-dated the NCB. Some of the techniques that had proved successful before 1947 included water infusion, the systematic wetting of cut coal or rock before it was filled, the use of ventilation to carry harmful dust away from miners, spraying of faces prior to working, using wet cutting techniques on jib machines, and fitting percussive drills for wet cutting. Therefore, as early as 1948 the NCB had a significant matrix of expertise, research, monitoring and technical know-how, all dedicated to addressing the dust problem. At colliery level, managers were advised and assisted on all aspects of dust suppression by Safety Officers and by the NCB's Divisional

---

67 HSC, 'Proposals for the Control', p. 7.

68 *Annual Report or the Chief Inspector of Factories* (1966), p. 78.

69 Ibid., p. 79.

Scientific Service, which at that time was responsible for dust sampling and analysis. Each Division had its own advisory Dust Suppression Committee comprising members of the Board and the NUM, and chaired by a local Inspector of Mines. Dust count figures were collated by these committees and sent annually to the NJPC, where they were assessed by the Chief Inspector of Mines. Procedures were also initiated in which Annual National Dust Progress Reports for Dust Suppression were introduced, the first presented for the year September 1950–September 1951.

At this time, the only state regulations which empowered Divisional Mines Inspectors to *enforce* the application of dust control measures were in South Wales, under the Coal Mines (South Wales) (Pneumoconiosis) Order of 1943.[70] The NCB, though, fully realised that to stave off the introduction of broader national regulations it had to prove to the government that it had the dust problem under control. However, the first Annual National Dust Progress Report in 1951 revealed that this was not the case, and especially so regarding the fitting of dust suppression to percussive drills. Indeed, so disappointed was the NJPC with the number of non-approved faces that it threatened to recommend to the government that the 1943 South Wales regulations be taken up nationally.[71] Disappointment was also expressed at this time by the Chief Inspector of Mines, Sir Harold Roberts, at the slow and patchy nature of dust prevention measures across the UK. His summary found that much remained to be done, especially in Scotland where many faces had dust concentrations well above the minimum standard. Progress in the North Eastern Division, though, was, he noted, outstanding, while Yorkshire was the most unsatisfactory.[72] As we will see in Chapter 7, the NUM was fully aware of this patchwork situation which needed to be addressed, and pressed the NCB to ensure that all regions achieved acceptable dust standards.

The NJPC took its role very seriously, and – well aware of the approach of the 1954 Mines and Quarries Act – its reaction to the poor run of returns from the Divisional Committees was to immediately get tough.[73] A special inquiry was initiated in December 1954 in which every Divisional Dust Suppression Committee received a memo from the Chief Inspector of Mines demanding that they record the exact location of each coal cutter operating without dust suppression equipment, include a written explanation from colliery managers why this was the case, and explain what steps were being taken to rectify the situation.[74] This resulted in a flurry of memos from the Divisions to the NJPC which illuminated the state of play regarding dust suppression across the coal fields at this time. Some reported, as was the case in the North East and in some of the Scottish collieries, that men were reluctant to use

---

70 *The Miner* (December 1944), pp. 12–13.

71 Turner, p. 36.

72 *Colliery Engineering* (December 1953), p. 490.

73 Memo from Chief Inspector of Mines to Divisional Dust Suppression Committees, dated 15 December 1954, POWE8/420.

74 Ibid.

water because of the discomfort this caused.[75] There were cases in the East Midlands of miners shying away from using water while working with electrical machinery.[76] The East Midlands Division had been slow to become motivated regarding the dust problem, and in 1954 its dust figures for working in rock were the worst in the UK.[77] From Durham came accounts of problems encountered when routing water hoses over very rough ground.[78] However, an important characteristic of the Durham coal field was that the NCB always looked upon it as having a short life span. This might go some way to explaining why its attention to dust suppression measures was not as dedicated as some other NCB regions.[79]

In 1954, a report from the Northern Division highlighted how a 'wet cutting agreement' with men in some of its pits was being negotiated.[80] The problem of miners refusing to use water jets fitted to machines to damp down dust was a persistent one in some areas – and we highlight some oral testimony related to this in Chapter 8. In late 1958 and early 1959 in the Central East Area of the Scottish Division, 39 coal cutters fitted out for wet cutting in eight collieries were lying idle because men refused to operate them. Indeed, at one pit (Kingshill) the men walked out in protest at the amount of dust they were being asked to work in; then, after water was utilised to suppress the dust, they walked out because they didn't like working in the water.[81] Ironically, the region in which these men worked had the highest pneumoconiosis rates in the Scottish Division, with around 55% of Scottish cases of CWP coming from this area in 1959.[82] However, we need to keep the issue of the men's refusal to operate dust suppression in perspective, as working in excessive wet could be perceived to be just as unpleasant as working in excessive dust. This was fully realised by Charles Fletcher of the PRU in 1948 when he commented on the need to get the balance right:

> A further role of the doctor as a human biologist is to insist that dust-suppression measures should not only be mechanically and physically effective, but that the men who have to operate them should find them convenient and acceptable to use … Sprays that are ill-

---

75 Ministry of Fuel and Power, Divisional Inspector of Mines, North East Division, dated January 1955; Ministry of Fuel and Power, HM Divisional Inspector of Mines Scottish Division, 17 May 1955, POWE8/420.

76 Ministry of Fuel and Power, *East Midlands Divisional Dust Suppression Committee Progress Report*, Appendix A (2 May 1955), POWE8/420.

77 Turner, p. 455.

78 NCB *Durham Division Report: Percussive Drills being Operated in Rippings Without Dust Suppression Measures* (April 1955), POWE8/420.

79 Turner, p. 428.

80 NCB Northern Division, *Dust Suppression, Information Requested by the NJPC* (15 May 1955), POWE8/420.

81 Divisional Dust Prevention and Suppression Advisory Committee (henceforth DDPSAC), Minutes of Meeting, 13 October 1959, SNA/CB/099/61/1.

82 Ibid.

adjusted may wet the men more than the coal and will be turned off. Excessive use of water in any method may cause unpleasant working conditions.[83]

The Mines Inspectorate provided a valuable lens through which the NCB's attempts to honour its commitment to reduce dust levels could be viewed. The number of mines inspectors grew steadily, from 93 in 1921 to 158 by the early 1950s.[84] The Chief Inspector based in London was kept informed by a chain of Divisional Inspectors in each of the NCB's Divisions, and these were assisted by District Inspectors and Inspectors in various areas. Visits to mines were, in theory at least, unannounced, and could take place at any time, day or night. The fact that the NCB's efforts at suppressing the dust got off to a pretty poor start was certainly reflected in the comments of the Chief Inspector of Mines in his annual reports. The 1949 Annual Report of the Chief Inspector noted that there was 'slow progress in the extension of water supply to faces', and that only a quarter of conveyor transfer points and less than half of conveyor loading points had sprays fitted.[85] In 1950, there had been some progress, but not enough: 'wet picks should be used but progress demands the fullest co-operation between workmen and management'.[86] In 1951, the main complaints were that only two-thirds of coal faces requiring dust suppression were receiving such treatment, and that there was slow progress fitting dust suppression measures to machines which were drilling in stone.[87] The 1952 report was even more scathing – 'the number of cases where dust suppression equipment had not been used and the officials claimed to be unaware of the failure is even more unsatisfactory' – and this provoked the Chief Inspector to circulate to all Divisions asking mine managers to ensure their Deputies reported to them on any breakdowns of dust suppression equipment.[88] However, the following year it was reported: 'Of stone drilling ... there has been some improvement, but the rate of progress still does not meet the urgency of the problem.'[89]

More intense pressure was put on the NCB to improve the situation from 1954 with the passage of the Mines and Quarries Act, which came into effect in January 1957. The Mines and Quarries Act made important stipulations regarding a multitude of mining issues, including shafts, roadways winding, transport, ventilation and lighting, and required that the NCB had to issue formal written instructions defining

---

83 Quoted in D. Hunter, *The Diseases of Occupation* (London, 1975), p. 1,011.

84 Ibid., p. 214.

85 North Western Division, *Dust Control Inspector's Report* (April 1949), POWE 8/420.

86 North Western Division, *Dust Control Inspector's Report* (December 1950), POWE 8/420.

87 North Western Division, *Dust Control Inspector's Report* (December 1951), POWE 8/420.

88 North Western Division, *Dust Control Inspector's Report* (October 1952), POWE 8/421.

89 North Western Division, *Dust Control Inspector's Report* (October 1953), POWE 8/421.

the duties and responsibilities of workers concerned. There was also a shifting of responsibility for dust control. Under the 1911 Coal Mines Act it had been the Pit Deputy's role to 'make such inspections and carry out such other duties with regard to the presence of gas, ventilation, supports of roofs and sides and general safety – including the health of persons working in the district – as are required of the Act and the regulations of the mine'. However, the Mines and Quarries Act 1954 compelled the NCB to centre the responsibility for dust prevention squarely on the shoulders of the mine managers:

> It shall be the duty of the manager of every mine to ensure that, in connection with the getting, dressing and transportation of minerals below ground in the mine the giving off of … (b) dust of such a character and in such quantity as to be likely to be injurious to the persons employed is minimised.[90]

From now on, then, as far as dust suppression was concerned, the buck was to stop at the mine manager's door, and it was up to the managers to ensure that dust suppression methods were being used to their best advantage. We go on now to look closely at these methods.

Water Infusion and Improved Ventilation

Water infusion was first carried out successfully in 1944 in experiments in Staffordshire, and the technique was quickly adopted across the South Wales coal field.[91] The process involved injecting water into the slips or planes in the coal face, as it was within these geological faults that dust had been created by the action of coal under pressure grinding against coal. This was one reason why South Wales coals were so dusty, and why pneumoconiosis rates in South Wales were so high. Holes were cut into the coal seam – initially six feet deep at six-foot intervals – into which 20–30 gallons of water per hole were pumped into the seam every day at pressures ranging from 100 pounds per square inch (p.s.i.) to 600 p.s.i. By 1965, water infusion was being applied to 14% of the UK's coal faces – mainly the anthracite districts of South Wales, north-west Durham and the Kent coal fields. In 1958, some disappointing attempts were also made to infuse dirt bands in Scotland prior to machines cutting through them – this was after similar attempts in South Wales had proved to be successful.[92] High-pressure water was essential to the success of infusion, and in 1963 tests at two collieries found that for best results, infusion holes had to be no less than 30 feet deep, with 1,000 gallons of water needed to treat a 40 square yard area of coal.[93] The problem in Scotland, though, was that the coal

---

90 L.R. James, *The Control of Dust in Mines* (Cardiff, 1959), p. 3.

91 Turner, p. 69.

92 NCB Divisional Dust Prevention and Suppression Advisory Committee, Minutes of Meeting of 15 April 1958, CB/099/61/1.

93 *Colliery Guardian* (17 October 1963), p. 492.

seams were not suited to such treatment as they had fewer cleavages, and solid coal faces would not accept pumped water even when pressures as high as 5,000 p.s.i. were tried.[94]

A Dust Suppression Officer who worked in South Wales in 1949 recalled how miners welcomed water infusion because the pressure of the water tended to make the coal easier to get:

> They were always glad to see me because they realized that what I was doing would at the end of the day help them ... it would assist them to get the coal because the pressure of the water would ease the coal out and made their task easier. So, that was another reason why it was accepted without any prejudice or malice at all.[95]

This observation ties in to some extent with that of Dai Dan Evans, the General Secretary of the NUM, who suggested in 1960 that from the outset the NCB was more interested in the potential productivity increases made possible by water infusion than by the suppression of dust which the process was originally intended to bring about.[96] Other miners from South Wales have suggested that water infusion worked if it was done properly, although in many cases it was not, and this is supported by the testimony of a Dust Suppression Officer from Wales whose trained eye could detect when management had not given enough attention to the process.[97]

As we have seen, the respiratory coal dust problem was initially perceived to be confined to South Wales. Indeed, in 1948 the NCB *Annual Report* stated that in comparison with South Wales, the problem of dust disease in the other coal fields was small.[98] South Wales continued to receive the lion's share of dust suppression equipment and personnel until 1948. That year, though, the NCB decided that dust suppression should be utilised throughout its Divisions.[99] However, due primarily to the initial Welsh-centred focus of the problem, other regions were slow off the starting blocks. For example, in 1956 an article in the *Edinburgh Evening News* drew attention to the lack of effort in Scotland:

> No matter what has been done in the past there are many coal cutting machines without the equipment to suppress dust. Hundreds of rotary drilling machines have not been equipped for wet drilling. Water infusion has been applied only on a limited scale due to neglect in the past and failure to provide an adequate water supply to the coal face.[100]

If properly carried out, infusion of the coal seams did keep dust levels down. However, the problem was that the process demanded a certain amount of time for the water to percolate adequately into the seam. However, as the pace of coal

---

94 *Colliery Guardian* (25 June 1965), p. 840.
95 Interview with Thomas Thomas, SWCC AUD/149, 6/2/80.
96 *The Miner* vol. 8, no. 3 (May/June 1960), p. 13.
97 Interview with Thomas Thomas, SWCC AUD/149, 6/2/80.
98 NCB, *Annual Report* (1948), p. 19.
99 Ibid., p. 16.
100 *Edinburgh Evening News* (2 March 1956), p. 8.

production increased, time became a commodity in increasingly short supply. Certainly, the Mines Inspectorate and the Dust Suppression Sub-Committee of the NJPC became more and more concerned at the reduction in the use of short-hole water infusion from the late 1950s onwards, and one of the prime reasons for this was the increasing number of rapidly advancing power-loaded faces, compounded by an increase in three-shift working.[101] The committee urged the NCB to increase its use of deep-hole infusion, which, although taking longer, had the potential of keeping ahead of production.[102] Experiments with infusing a face with holes around 60 feet in length were first carried out in the Northern Division in 1951, and the technique was cited in the NUM publication *The Control of Dust in Mines in 1959*. In 1961, the Ministry of Fuel and Power expressed its concern, and pointed out to the NCB that 'water infusion on rapidly advancing power loaded faces does not always present insuperable difficulties and that more use could be made of this method of dust suppression'.[103] Mines inspectors were also far from pleased with the lack of enthusiasm for water infusion, as this was a form of dust suppression which they knew worked. The reports of the Chief Inspector of Mines make this quite clear. In 1950, he noted that as far as water infusion was concerned, 'progress was possible if there was perseverance'.[104] In 1952, the Chief Inspector drew attention to the fact that the East Midland Division was regularly infusing 5,000 square yards of face, and that in one pit this had reduced dust levels by 75%, despite the fact that it had been previously assumed that these faces were not suitable for infusion. He commented: 'it shows how pre-conceived notions, based on a few inadequate tests, can be an effective bar to progress'.[105] By 1959, he noted that there was 'a decline of water infusion where power loaders were working',[106] and by 1962 a note of despair was beginning to creep in regarding the unequal contest between dust suppression and coal production:

> The cycle of power loading operations often preclude the application of short-hole water infusion, because there is insufficient time available provided between operations to enable the work to be carried out. The main hope of success, therefore, lies in deep-hole infusion, which can be carried out at the weekends. It is disappointing to record that its application has not yet extended beyond the experimental stage.[107]

---

101 *Report of Chief Inspector of Mines* (1958).

102 Ministry of Fuel and Power, National Joint Pneumoconiosis Committee, *Report of the Dust Prevention Sub-Committee*, NJPC no. 109 (30 January 1960).

103 National Joint Pneumoconiosis Committee, *Report of the Dust Prevention Sub-Committee*, NJPC no. 11 (1962).

104 *Report by the Chief Inspector of Mines* (1950), p. 19.

105 *Report by the Chief Inspector of Mines* (1952), p. 11.

106 *Report by the Chief Inspector of Mines* (1959), p. 24.

107 *Report by the Chief Inspector of Mines* (1962), p. 18.

By the mid-1960s, then, at the height of the NCB's production drive, deep-hole infusion had still not progressed very far.[108] Therefore, the intensifying pace of coal production was rendering a proven method of coal dust suppression obsolete.

By this time, mining engineers had a broad range of dust suppression and dust gathering techniques at their disposal. For example, there were screens made of woven cloth designed to trap the airborne dust, although the downside of this method was the labour costs involved in continually having to clean or change the fabric when it became clogged. There were Cyclone filters which used the principle of centrifugal force to settle dust particles; and there were dust collectors, such as the Microdyne collector, which soaked the collected dust and expelled it as harmless slurry.[109] The flow of air through the mine could also be used as a dust suppression tool. However, the velocity of the air had to be delicately balanced, and this proved to be an especially difficult problem on longer coal faces. The ideal was to achieve an air velocity of at least 150 feet per minute, but it was understood that velocities in excess of 400 feet per minute were liable to *increase* dust concentrations.[110] If the fine balance could be achieved, though, concentrations of dust in the mine air could be halved by using ventilation alone. But here again, rapid production was to cause problems, because as mechanisation was pushed to greater heights, any improvements in air quality struggled to cope with the ever-increasing levels of dust.

Water Jets and Sprays

While water infusion was targeted at coal dust caused by compression within the seams, water jets fitted to coal cutting machines were intended to deal with the dust thrown up when coal was disintegrated by the mechanical cutters. Initially, the Mines Inspectorate was pleased with the efforts which the NCB were making in this respect. However, it was less pleased with the attitude of the workers, as a serious problem which inspectors became increasingly concerned with was that many colliers refused to use dust damping equipment. In 1952, for example, one Scottish Inspector mentioned in his report that 'trivial excuses are used by some workmen to explain, or attempt to explain, their failure to use the appliances when they have been provided'. And two years later, he noted:

> The Divisional Coal Board are doing their utmost to press forward with suppression measures wherever there is a problem, and the higher officials of the National Union of Mineworkers too, lend their support, but it is regrettable that there are cases where dust

---

108 *Report of the Chief Inspector of Mines* (1966), p. 20.

109 NCB Mining Department, *The Control of Harmful Dust in Coal Mines* (London, 1973), pp. 21–4.

110 *Colliery Guardian* (17 October 1963); NCB Production Department, 'Dust Suppression on Power Loaded Faces', Working Group Minutes of meeting, 9 July 1968, CB 120/03/2.

suppression is urgently required yet the local workmen (the very men who in the future may be victims to the dust disease) flatly refuse to operate the equipment.[111]

There were other problems. In some cases, too much water was found to damage the roadways and make the coal harder to clean, and it was for this reason that experiments using foam and other wetting agents were tried out.[112] It was also the case – as reported by some of our oral history respondents in Chapter 8 – that water nozzles frequently clogged due to the sheer amount of dust in the air, and this was a problem which the NCB's Central Engineering Establishment was investigating in 1965.[113]

Another serious problem was dealing with the large amounts of dust that were generated when machines cut through stone – or dirt bands, as they were known. Mines Inspectors frequently drew attention to this, and the following statement from a report by an Inspector relating to conditions on one Yorkshire face is not atypical:

> It will be seen that in many cases working conditions are unsatisfactory, particularly on faces where dirt bands are present since the hazard to health is substantially increased in high counts of stone in the 1–5 microns range. This is a feature which appears to be completely overlooked in the National Coal Board assessment of dust counts …[114]

Dr J.M. Rogan, the Chief Medical Officer of the NCB, also drew attention to these dangers in his Annual Report for 1968–69:

> When coal was hand-got, if the coal seam was narrowed by an intrusion of stone – or 'dirt' – from the roof or floor, it was possible to work around the dirt or remove it in large lumps. However, with machine-got coal the machine simply cuts through the dirt, grinding it into fine pieces, and adding substantially to the amount of airborne dusts.[115]

Scottish NCB records reveal a frenzy of activity from the 1950s regarding efforts to suppress dust on the most common coal cutter used in the Scottish Division at this time, the Anderton shearer. These efforts included installing water jets on machines, fitting cowls around shearer drums, as well as attaching exhaust fans to scrubber units to soak up the dust and convert it into slurry.[116] By 1960, the problem was persisting, and two Workmen's Inspectors noted that the dust thrown up by the Anderton shearers was so intense that it was difficult for them to see.[117] Other

---

111 *Report of H.M. Inspector of Mines, Scottish Division* (1954), p. 21.

112 NCB, *Annual Report* (1947).

113 NCB, Scottish Division, Production Deptartment, 'Dust Suppression – Recent Developments', 15 October 1965, p. 2, CB 53/10.

114 Turner, p. 445.

115 *Colliery Guardian* (March 1970), p. 106.

116 See, for example, Minutes of 13th Meeting of Area Ventilation Engineers, 17 September, 1964, in CB53/4.

117 Divisional Dust Prevention and Suppression Advisory Committee, Minutes of Meeting, 7 July 1960, SNA/CB/099/61/1.

evidence suggests that the problem posed by the Anderton shearers was compounded in some instances by machines being run at excessive speeds so as to increase production rates. In 1961, for example, a Mines Inspector visiting Frances Colliery in Scotland found Anderton shearers being run at around 1,200 feet per minute (500 feet per minute over their optimum speed of 700 feet per minute), resulting in a sharp increase in airborne dust. What is not completely clear is the degree to which men and management *colluded* in these rapid rates of mechanised coal production, and we will come back to this in Chapter 8. What is evident is that, as was the case with water infusion, the speed-up of production was nullifying the best efforts of dust suppression. In 1964, the Scottish Division made its first operational profit for thirteen years; and by this time Killoch Colliery in Ayrshire had become Scotland's first million-tons-a-year pit. Unfortunately, though, much of this success had been achieved by a mechanisation drive with which dust suppression personnel were desperately trying to keep pace.[118]

The Anderton shearers caused problems in other regions too. For example, the NUM South Wales 1959 publication *The Control of Dust in Mines* noted how increased levels of dust were being generated because many Anderton shearers were cutting from floor to roof, rather than from roof to floor. In the opinion of the author, L.R. James, a combination of cutting from roof to floor and properly placed sprays within cowls should have been enough to reduce dust levels considerably on the most obstinately dusty of coal cutting machines.[119] The situation was so bad that in 1963 a joint NCB/MRE report, *The Production of Dust by Anderton Shearers*, was produced for the Board. The investigators examined Anderton shearers on 25 coal faces, and found that in only 7 cases were dust counts below the recommended 850 p.p.c.c. The researchers also expressed concern at the amount of non-coal dust being generated when the machines cut through dirt bands. Of even more concern, an experiment with Anderton shearers operating in the Durham coal field found there was no difference in the amount of dust generated by one machine cutting dry and one on which dust suppression equipment was in full flow. Therefore, not only were these machines creating lethal amounts of dust, but in some cases water jets were making little difference to the volume of dust.[120]

By 1967 – two years before the PFR's Interim Standards Study – there were 140 power loaders working in unapproved conditions throughout the UK.[121] By this time the NCB had its own Power Loading and Cutting in Dirt Working Group, and its investigation had revealed several problems. These included having to constantly adapt machines to suit local geological conditions, not having machines fitted out

---

118 *Colliery Guardian* (30 April 1965), p. 522.

119 James, *The Control of Dust in Mines*, pp. 39–40.

120 NCB Production Department, Mining Research Establishment Report 2227, G.C. Evans and R.J. Hamilton, *The Production of Dust by Anderton Shearers* (1963), NA Coal 74/7621.

121 9.2% of power-loaded faces in the East Midlands Division were 'not approved'; Turner, p. 458.

for dust suppression available as replacements in the event of breakdowns, and water getting into the motors of the machines, causing them to fail.[122] The bottom line, though, was that while the Working Group deliberated, production was being maintained to the detriment of miners' health. The High Court judge's comments in 1998 are apposite:

> The more difficult the conditions, the more thought and care had to be devoted to devising, implementing and maintaining methods which would minimise the extent to which dust was created and released into the atmosphere.[123]

One of the initial problems was that newly purchased machines needed to have dust suppression equipment fitted on site, because they did not come kitted out for suppression by the manufacturers – this was a state of affairs which Charles Fletcher drew attention to in 1948.[124] Further, it was also the case that any breakdown of dust suppression equipment meant that sprays and machinery needed to be dismantled and rebuilt, resulting in the loss of output and earnings for the face workers.[125] In 1952, the International Labour Office organised a meeting specifically to look into the problem of suppressing dust in mines, and one of its recommendations was that 'all coal getting machines should be supplied by the manufacturers equipped with devices for suppressing dust'.[126] However, despite the logic of this, it was not until the 1960s that the NCB began insisting that manufacturers fitted effective dust suppression equipment.[127] Once again, then, a serious time lag occurred, and by 1962 the Chief Inspector of Mines still felt it necessary to stress in his report that no machine should be allowed underground unless it was pre-fitted with dust suppression equipment.[128] In 1961, the NCB's Production Department issued guidelines on how engineers could best adapt Anderton shearers for dust suppression to suit a range of local conditions – indicating that it was still seen as normal at this time to adapt such machines in an *ad hoc* manner.[129] Further, in 1964 the MRE published a report entitled *Proposals for Improving Dust Suppression*, which recommended that machines should utilise fewer, larger and more slowly moving cutting tools which took deeper bites at the face, that mining using remote control should be developed, that more use should be made of water infusion and exhaust ventilation, and that cutting into dirt bands should be avoided. The report acknowledged, though, that using water in many cases did not solve the problem because the water tended to simply push the finer airborne particles aside. To be effective, then, water had to 'be applied to bind the points of the

122 Scottish NCB, Minutes of Meeting of Power Loading/Cutting in Dirt Working Group, 13 October 1967, CB/120/03/02.

123 Turner, p. 378.

124 Hunter, *The Diseases of Occupation*, p. 1011.

125 Perchard, 'The Mine Management Professionals', pp. 372–4.

126 Turner, p. 65.

127 Ibid.

128 *Report of the Chief Inspector of Mines* (1962), p. 31.

129 Turner, p. 66.

cutting tools', and several experiments were under way along these lines. Along with a host of other recommendations – including an increase of the number of specialist dust suppression staff – the report also recommended that all new machines should be approved by the MRE before going underground.[130]

For far too long, then, it was left up to individual colliery mechanics to do what they could with Anderton shearers regarding dust suppression. Clearly, the amazing production potential of the machines was prioritised. Research into dust suppression methods on Anderton shearers should have been conducted at the design stage, not after machines had been delivered to their respective pits. It was not until the coming of the 1975 RDR that the problem was given the consideration which it had demanded since power loaders were first installed. By the early 1970s – in advance of the new regulations – two-speed gearboxes were being fitted to ranging shearers so that slower speeds could be used on their return runs. Also, pick face flushing had at last been perfected, in which water was applied through hollow shafts directly to the pick points. This system was now being installed to all new shearers, and the Board was refusing to purchase any shearers which were not fitted with hollow shafts. Moreover, by this time there were 159 full-time dust suppression officers in the collieries. Clearly, then, as was the case with the problem of dust measuring and standards of dustiness, the approach of the 1975 RDR removed the drag anchor which had been impeding progress for so long. Tellingly, the July 1971 figures for approved faces and drivages across the UK were the best ever recorded.[131]

As well as the dust raised by power loaders such as Anderton shearers, another major source of dust was from the conveyor belts which took the coal from the faces to the shafts, as dust tended to gather in the conveyor belt seams and spill off the return belt. High dust levels were also common when coal had to fall from a height at the belts' transfer points. By the early 1960s it was acknowledged that to address the dust problem on the belts, water jets needed to be directed on to the belt at certain points; that chutes at transfer points needed to be designed to contain dust, and that efforts had to be directed at cleaning dust from the bottom belts with a cleaning unit.[132] Once again, though, progress was slow, and – like the dust issue in general – it was really from the early 1970s that the problem was addressed adequately by the NCB as part of its 'Destroy Dust' campaign.

To keep things in perspective, despite the NCB's mechanisation drive, many faces not suited to the application of machinery continued to be advanced by blasting and cutting with pneumatic picks. A great deal of dust was generated by these methods, and especially when picks were operated without water. Merthyr Vale was known to be one of the dustiest pits in South Wales (by 1965, the mine had the highest rate of pneumoconiosis in the whole of South Wales), with work at the coal seams generating large quantities of dust and fumes. Pneumatic picks were used frequently, although it was only after 1958 that an attempt was made to fit them out with water to

130 MRE, *Proposals for Improving Dust Suppression* (11 November 1963), pp. 1–2.

131 Turner, pp. 74–5.

132 *Colliery Guardian* (17 October 1963), p. 491.

suppress the dust. Many of the miners at Merthyr Vale, though, did not like using the so-called 'wet picks'. For one thing, the machines were heavier and more ungainly than the older type; and it was also the case that cutting wet was an uncomfortable process, especially when picks had to be held above head height.[133] As was the case in many other mines throughout the UK, though, when dust suppression measures were put in place at Merthyr Vale, management only aimed at bringing faces into the approved range, and did not try to reduce dust levels to as low a level as possible. One miner who gave evidence to the 1998 British Coal court case worked at Lady Windsor Colliery in South Wales, where the most common system of mining involved the use of pneumatic picks and shot firing. In this particular mine there were frequent problems getting water to the picks, as well as maintaining a supply of sharp pick points.[134] Therefore, the combination of cutting dry with blunt tools meant dust levels in the pit were very high.

Dust and fumes produced by shot firing also continued to be a problem into the era of mechanised mining. In pits such as Merthyr Vale and Lady Windsor, boring and firing were utilised as the foremost method of coal face advance. Miners, then, were continually exposed to nitrous fumes and dust generated by shot firing.[135] Men working in hand-got faces were also exposed to dust from filling what in some regions was know as 'gummings' – the cut coal lying ready for loading onto face conveyors or pans. In many cases, even although the gummings had been water-infused before being blasted or cut from the seam, by the time loading took place they had dried out, and this was especially the case in warmer mines.[136]

As was the case with measuring mine dust, there was great variability across the coal fields when it came to suppressing dust. For example, in the Durham coal field in the run up to the 1975 Regulations, the situation was particularly grim, as a memo from the North East Division made clear:

> The airborne dust conditions in the area are not under control, this is borne out by the reports of the Area Dust Combat Team … It is evident that where the Undermanagers and Engineers are interested in dust problems, progress can be made to improve the situation that at the present moment seems insurmountable.[137]

To be sure, an important factor acting upon the relative enthusiasm for dust suppression across the coal fields was that power loading also drastically shortened the lifespan of individual collieries. In a late 1950s survey of the Scottish Division, it was found that around half the coal faces surveyed had an average life of only six months. Such short-termism, then, added another disincentive towards directing resources to dust prevention.[138] Some collieries also had very active safety committees dedicated

---

133 Turner, p. 340.
134 Ibid., p. 381.
135 Ibid., p. 343.
136 Ibid., p. 443.
137 Ibid., p. 428.
138 Perchard, 'The Mine Management Professions' p. 235.

to dealing with dust, while others only paid lip service to the problem. Andrew Perchard's survey of Scottish mine management in the era of nationalisation certainly finds this to be the case.[139] Also, in South Wales, where it was originally assumed the respiratory dust problem in mining was confined, dust suppression measures were initially targeted only at the anthracite pits, because they were thought to be the most dangerous.[140] Finally, the influence of geology meant that dust suppression techniques which worked in some faces were totally ineffective in others.

It is sad and somewhat ironic to reflect that the NCB's most significant contribution to protecting miners from respiratory disease may have been its closure programme. As it turned out, preventing men from going underground was the only guarantee that their respiratory health was not going to be damaged by mine dust. In the early 1960s an attempt was made to introduce a system of fully automated coal mining using the Remotely Operated Long-wall Face (ROLF) system. This method required no men to be at the coal face at all. ROLF was trialled at a Nottingham colliery in 1965. However, it was soon withdrawn because of geological and technical problems. Reintroduced in 1971, ROLF proved to be too problematic to control. This, combined with its £500,000 price tag – compared to £150,000 for a standard power loader – meant its use was discontinued.[141]

Dealing with the Problem: Dust Respirators

> I have tried just walking around a coalmine wearing the latest dust respirator. I soon dropped it below my chin and was glad to breathe freely again. Miners want to shout to each other. You will never get them all to wear masks, expect perhaps for short periods on special jobs which are particularly dusty.[142]

This piece of testimony comes from a 1950 radio broadcast by Charles Fletcher of the PRU. Although respirators were available in the pre-nationalisation period, they were very uncomfortable to wear and their efficiency was questionable. However, as we will see, despite, and to some extent *because* of, the intensity of the effort that was being put into dust suppression, any focus on developing an effective mask and educating workers to wear it was seen as the wrong course of action, and indeed, by some, as an admission of failure. In 1959, for example, the Medical Officer of the Scottish Division of the NCB stated that although masks had improved and were better than nothing, 'it was admitting defeat to resort to that method'.[143] Clearly, then – to continue with his military metaphor – in the war against coal dust disease,

---

139 Ibid., p. 237.

140 Ibid., p. 57.

141 Buxton, *The Economic Development of the British Coal Industry*, p. 248; Jackson, *The Price of Coal*, p. 110.

142 Charles Fletcher , 'Fighting the "Modern Black Death"', *The Listener* (28 September 1950), p. 407.

143 NCB Divisional Dust Prevention and Suppression Advisory Committee, Minutes of Meeting, 8 July 1958, SNA/CB/099/61/1.

everything was being staked on dust suppression measures, and not enough on the development of an effective and comfortable personal dust defence measure.

The NCB took this line from Vesting Day onwards, as a memo to the Board's Head of Scientific Control in September 1948 illustrates:

> Where collection and suppression methods are practicable they are obviously preferable, because they attack the evil at source, to any method that aims at enabling persons to work in dust laden atmospheres.[144]

Around the same time, Dr John Rogan – the Head of the NCB Medical Branch – voiced the same opinion: masks had a place in mines, but only for exceptional circumstances, and not as a routine measure. Indeed, Rogan was so dedicated to suppressing dust at source that in 1954 he expressed his concern that if Divisions began resorting to issuing dust masks, they might become too distracted from dust suppression efforts.[145] Only a few individuals questioned this line of approach. For example, in 1962 the NCB's Group Manager for the Scottish Central Area expressed his surprise that masks were not being used in coal mining, and presumed that one of the main reasons 'might be due to the increased attention that was being given to dust suppression at collieries in the area'.[146] Certainly, in the early 1960s dust masks were few and far between, and only issued to machine-men or to those working in close proximity of machines. At this time, the Scottish Division issued around 2,500 masks every year. However, there was a great variation of demand, with some Scottish areas requisitioning much more than others. Somewhat tragically, Central Area – which for some time would be the black spot of Scotland's pneumoconiosis problem – did not request any masks at all, and this was primarily because the men found them too uncomfortable to wear.[147] The notion that the extent of pneumoconiosis in an area had little correlation with the use of dust respirators in that area is backed up by the fact that the use of respirators in South Wales was also very low.[148] The problem was that a situation had been allowed to develop in which efforts to suppress dust at source cultivated an anti-respirator culture amongst miners. The NCB's own reluctance in the 1950s and 1960s to encourage the wearing of respirators compounded this.

This is not to say that efforts were not being made to improve respirators over the period. The SMRE was conducting tests on respirators in the early 1950s, but held to the notion that they would only be used as a 'last line of defence'.[149] In 1955, a Glasgow company, Mine Safety Appliances, introduced its Dustfoe 55 light-weight respirator. According to the manufacturers, this mask weighed less than 3 ounces,

---

144 Memorandum from NCB Coordinating Secretary to Dr Skinner, Head of Scientific Control, dated 22 September 1948, cited in Turner, p. 77.

145 Turner, p. 77.

146 Scottish NCB, Minutes of the 63rd meeting of the Divisional Dust Prevention and Suppression Advisory Committee, 23 November 1962, CB/099/61/1.

147 Ibid.

148 Turner, p. 81.

149 MFP, *Annual Report* (1952), p. 44.

had a low breathing resistance, was designed for comfort, and was easy to clean.[150] Six years later, the Draeger Dust Respirator, approved by HM Chief Inspector of Factories, was advertised in the *Colliery Guardian*:

> Deadly mineral dust particles less than 5 microns can wreck the health of your workers. Protect them from this invisible danger with the light, comfortable easy-to-wear Draeger Dust Respirator which stops all injurious dust particles down to 0.5 microns.[151]

However, although this particular respirator was approved by the NCB for use in the pits, an advert in the *Colliery Guardian* showed a masked worker dressed in a white shirt and joiners' bib-and-brace overalls, clearly indicating that the manufacturers assumed that most of their customers would be non-miners. Also available at this time was the Martindale Heavy Duty Dust Respirator, triangular in shape, weighing 4½ ounces with a plastic face piece designed to be moulded with the fingers 'to effect a comfortable seal of any shape and size of face'.[152] Moreover, in 1966 trials of disposable respirators were first carried out – and it was these which were to be eventually made widely available to miners from the early 1970s onwards.[153] From 1969 (as we saw in Chapter 4), the Institute of Occupational Medicine in Edinburgh undertook valuable research on behalf of the NCB, and in 1972 it prepared a memorandum for the Board's National Dust Prevention Committee. This also suggested that resources had been misdirected:

> A greater use of dust respirators could probably do more to eliminate dust disease among coal miners than any other course that is technically feasible at the present time – and at a fraction of the cost.[154]

Once again, it was the impending 1975 RDR which brought a reassessment of policy as, crucially, the new regulations stipulated that respirators had to made available.[155] However, despite the fact that the NCB now had to ensure that respirators were accessible to those who wanted to use them, they were still seen as second best to tackling dust at source, as this comment in the *Colliery Guardian* of 1971 illustrates: 'Protection must not take the place of prevention but the latest dust masks are extremely effective dust filters if the men can be encouraged to wear them more in very dusty conditions.'[156] The following year, though, the same journal also noted: 'Dust respirators are now worn by an increasing number of miners, and that this practice will grow should be in no doubt once they have seen what happens to the lungs when their working is impaired by pneumoconiosis.'[157] But perhaps the clearest evidence

---

150 *Colliery Guardian* (January 1955), p. 38.
151 *Colliery Guardian* (18 May 1961), p. 21.
152 *Colliery Guardian* (June 1961), p. 750.
153 Turner, p. 69.
154 Ibid., p. 79.
155 Ibid., p. 49.
156 *Colliery Guardian* (June 1971), p. 253.
157 *Colliery Guardian* (November 1972), p. 498.

that the NCB was now conceding that it had got it wrong regarding respirators is contained in a note by Dr Skinner of the Scientific Department in 1971 entitled 'The Application of Dust Respirators in the British Coal Industry'. In Skinner's summing up, he stated that although dust respirators were still to be regarded as a 'last line of defence', their use had become much more important due to the increasing use of power loading, 'which may make it more difficult to maintain approved conditions on a face at all times'. He also went on to say that thanks to the NCB's Medical Service, respirators were now available which were much easier to breathe through than their predecessors.[158] By the early 1970s, then, miners were being urged to wear the newest type of respirator, although the Board acknowledged that a long legacy had to be overcome. Not only that, though, it was also realised that younger miners were resisting wearing respirators, as well as the older workers:

> There is a disinclination, especially amongst younger men, to wear these respirators, but it is to be hoped that a better realization of the long term dangers will help wear down this resistance.[159]

By this time, the NCB's Assistant Chief Medical Officer was of the opinion that 'dust suppression must remain the basic measure in the control of occupational pulmonary disease'. However – no doubt fully informed of the nature of the impending statutory regulations – he was also advocating that masks should be made available for working in places where dust suppression was not effective, and that they should be well maintained and easily accessible:

> Depending on the number of masks in use at a mine a full-time or part-time attendant will be needed to carry out daily inspection and servicing ... A register should be kept to record the daily issue, return and maintenance of the masks in use ... mechanical methods of servicing are being developed ... These arrangements should ensure that this costly and relatively sophisticated protective equipment is used most effectively.[160]

The difficulty remained, though – as much of our oral testimony in Chapter 8 illustrates – that expecting men to work underground with uncomfortable masks strapped to their faces was unrealistic. In 1974, the IOM surveyed the use of respirators throughout the UK, and found that only 5% of underground workers *carried one* on a day-to-day basis.[161] The survey also found that most men found such masks uncomfortable to wear and difficult to breathe through while working. In 1977, the IOM went so far as to suggest that research needed to be carried out on the production of a more comfortable respirator, even if this meant reducing the efficiency of the filter for the sake of the mask's wearability – and the idea here was that getting miners to wear a mask *sometimes* would be better than not at all.[162]

---

158 Turner, p. 78.
159 *Colliery Guardian* (March 1970), p. 106.
160 J. Rogan (ed.), *Medicine in the Mining Industry* (London,1972), p. 315.
161 Turner, p. 81.
162 Ibid.

From 1975 onwards, the coal industry was under statutory compulsion to provide dust respirators to miners. Moreover, in the 1980s, British Coal had began to issue workers with disposable respirators. According to miners, though, these masks quickly became soggy and unusable – and we highlight this testimony in Chapter 8. Another innovation in 1975 was the new, radical Racal Airstream helmet, developed by the SMRE – this incorporated a face visor and a flow of air at the mouth and nose. The NUM had been pushing for the development of this kind of sophisticated personal dust protection since the 1960s, and in the face of rank-and-file criticism that such equipment would be too restrictive to wear. Over the 1982–85 period, an NUM survey found that the use of the new helmets varied across the coal fields, with – as predicted – widespread objection to either their bulk, and in some areas, to their lack of availability. What was missing, though, was stringent regulations that would have compelled the NCB to ensure that miners took advantage of the new protective equipment. As one area NUM secretary remarked: 'If there had been a Mines and Quarries regulation to wear them, the men would have adjusted accordingly.'[163] Finally, it is worth noting British Coal's closing admission to the 1998 legal case regarding the provision of respirators:

> Greater attention could have been paid to the training and education of the work force in relation to the wearing of respirators … By the early 1960s respirators were available which could have been used by men during periods of high dust concentration … [and] that more effort should have been made to supply men with these respirators and to encourage their use. Nevertheless it remains the case that these respirators were clumsy and uncomfortable to wear during arduous activity and the contribution which they would have made to reducing dust exposure was therefore limited.[164]

Judgment: The British Coal Industry on Trial

> Thousands of former miners jammed telephone hotlines after the judgment by Mr Justice Turner in six test cases, which the judge described as the 'tip of the iceberg.' The ruling is the culmination of a long legal battle by the pit deputies union NACODS to pin the blame for emphysema, bronchitis, and other respiratory illnesses on the failure by British Coal and its predecessor, the National Coal Board, to control the levels of coal dust in mines. The payouts are expected to amount to the largest industrial injury compensation package in British legal history.[165]

By the end of March 2004, a staggering 547,342 bronchitis/emphysema claims had been lodged across the UK – 303,000 of which represented claims of miners who had already died. The cases stretched back to men who had been employed in the mining

---

163 Labour Research Department, *The Hazards of Coal Mining* (London, 1989), p. 9.

164 Turner, p. 89.

165 C. Dyer, 'Miners win historic battle for compensation', *BMJ*, vol. 316 (31 January 1998), pp. 316–27.

industry in England and Wales from 1954, and in Scotland from 1949.[166] Years of pent-up frustration by the coal industry workforce had suddenly erupted into the biggest industrial compensation claim the UK had ever experienced. However, the landmark High Court ruling of 1998 was not the first time that miners had attempted to claim damages for lung diseases other than pneumoconiosis. In December 1989, a case was brought to the High Court against British Coal on behalf of John Charles Tanner, who had died of lung disease after having worked for British Coal for some time. However, in this instance the court decided that Mr Tanner's legal team had failed to prove his death had been caused by coal workers' pneumoconiosis, PMF or from emphysema as the result of exposure to mine dust. When the case was taken to the Court of Appeal two years later, though, the judge decided that the plaintiffs should have been awarded damages for the chronic bronchitis which Mr Tanner had suffered from, even although this had not been a cause of his death. Consequently, damages of around £3,000 were recovered.[167] It was this which cleared the way for future claims from dust-damaged miners.

After a trial lasting 119 days, in 1998 the judge, Justice Turner, found that British Coal – and the National Coal Board before it – had been negligent under common law, and in breach of duties under the Mines and Quarries Act, for failing to protect workers from the harmful effects of respirable dust. There was 'abundant evidence', according to the judge, that NCB officials interpreted their duties as 'requiring the production of coal first and the taking of precautions in respect of health second'. Therefore, British Coal had failed to take all reasonable steps to minimise the effects of dust by using known and available dust suppression techniques 'from about 1949 to 1970 and to a lesser extent thereafter'. He found that British Coal had taken a 'leisurely approach' to measuring the extent of dust in its coal mines. He found that suitable respirators which the miners could have worn for at least part of their shift could have been provided from the mid-1960s. During their closing submission, British Coal conceded that that they had been in breach of the Coal Mines Act of 1911 and the Mines and Quarries Act of 1954, as they had not done all they should have done to minimise dust.[168]

For several complex legal reasons, it was decided that compensation could only be paid to miners relating to damage over a certain period. This 'date of guilty knowledge' was set from 4 June 1954 in England and Wales, and 4 June 1949 in Scotland.[169] Before these dates, it was assumed that the NCB could not have been expected to be aware of the risks of exposure. However, after this time there was no excuse, and the NCB should have been perfectly capable of taking steps towards protecting its employees from the effects of coal dust. On the medical side, British

---

166 Figures kindly provided by Mick Antoniw, Thompsons Solicitors, Cardiff, interviewed 14 May 2004.

167 Turner, p. 93.

168 Ibid., p. 354.

169 Miners also won a court case for damages for Vibration White Finger, and here the date of guilty knowledge was set at 1 January 1975.

Coal's legal team tried to argue that emphysema caused by mine dust was only related to CWP, and even attacked the validity of the PFR evidence by suggesting that such epidemiological research presented a 'blurred picture'.[170] However, the argument failed to convince the judge. Damages were awarded to six of the original eight plaintiffs – with two cases rejected because the link between ill health and coal dust had not been proved. Damages for pain and suffering and for loss of amenity ranged from £3,200 to £10,500, although most of the men received reduced awards because their illnesses were also deemed to have been caused by smoking as well as dust. The findings of the High Court case against British coal were as follows:

1.   Coal mine dust (coal and stone) is a cause of centriacinar emphysema;
2.   Such emphysema may, and usually does, lead to a loss of ventilatory capacity most easily demonstrated by loss of FEV1;
3.   Confirmation that the causes and effects of tobacco smoke are as in findings 1 and 2 above;
4.   It is probable, but not certain, that there is a common causal pathway to both cigarette and mine dust-induced emphysema which usually gives rise to breathlessness;
5.   Whether 4 is established or not, the effects are generally the same in that there is a spectrum of effect which in the majority is not clinically detectable but in the minority does produce a range of effects from simple impairment, frank disability and occasionally death;
6.   In the individual smoker it is not possible to attribute the cause of breathlessness either to the one insult or the other, this is so whether or not there is a common pathway.[171]

The government immediately accepted the judge's recommendations and prepared to pay out an estimated £1 billion to former miners.

Conclusion

Nationalisation of the coal industry in 1947 represented a watershed in the history of coal mining in the UK. From its inception, the NCB placed a much higher priority on health and safety than had previously been the case with the private owners, and by the mid-1950s had established a comprehensive health and safety infrastructure which included the Mines Medical Service, the x-raying of all new miners, and the Pneumoconiosis Field Research, while important links were established between the NCB, the Safety in Mines Research Board and the National Joint Pneumoconiosis Committee.

The coal dust problem was certainly given a high priority by the NCB, and significant resources were directed at the issue. Initially, this was driven by the urgency of having to re-employ pneumoconiotic miners. This resulted in the notion of approved conditions, determined by the only standard available at the time. NCB policy on dust control from 1947 did have positive results, reflected in the declining

170 Turner, p. 96.
171 Ibid., p. 257.

rates of pneumoconiosis incidence per 1,000 miners employed and newly diagnosed cases of CWP a decade or so later. However, the evidence is compelling that until the 1970s the NCB never seriously directed resources towards bringing dust levels down to levels significantly *below* those which determined the approved conditions. There was also a long reluctance by the NCB to encourage miners exposed to dust to wear masks. Certainly, the wearing of masks was accepted as impractical and uncomfortable by management and men alike. However, an anti-mask culture in the pits was compounded by the NCB's insistence that only dust suppression at source would solve the dust problem. It was only the approach of statutory regulations in the 1970s which stimulated a more comprehensive effort by the NCB to bring dust levels down, and this applied to the provision of dust respirators too.

As we saw in Chapter 4, a great deal of attention was being devoted by occupational health experts from the 1950s onwards to better understand the nature of pneumoconiosis, and to determine exactly how much dust was dangerous to miners' health – and the most significant element of this was the PRU. To a great extent, then, the NCB's disinclination to keep dust levels at lower limits over the 1950s– 1970 period, was underpinned by an expectation that scientifically determined safe maximums would become available. However, while the PFR progressed, the NCB was failing to strike a balance between coal production and effective dust control. Increasingly, the need to mechanise production in this declining industry meant that in many cases, efforts to reduce dust levels amounted to tokenism. What developed in many instances was a priority of production over dust control. A prime example to illustrate this point was the fact that although water infusion was known to be an effective dust suppression technique under certain geological conditions, this method was increasingly rendered inappropriate because it was simply too slow a process to keep up with the intensifying production frenzy.

That said, though, we also need to appreciate that despite the NCB's lack of dedication towards initiating and enforcing a more stringent anti-coal dust regime, the effort which it did deploy was one of the reasons that rates of CWP fell. However, the much steeper trajectory of CWP decline from 1970 onwards, when new standards were adhered to – but using technology which could have been deployed ten years earlier – illustrates that many more miners could have been protected from CWP, as well as from bronchitis and emphysema, in the years before statutory dust regulations were introduced. An underlying reason for this was the chasm between intention and execution of coal dust policy, and we examine this in Chapter 8. Before that, however, we turn our attention to the role played by the miners' trade unions.

Chapter 7

The Trade Unions and Dust

Historical interpretations of the role of the trade unions in generating medical knowledge, challenging 'orthodox' medical opinion, undertaking research and health education, and campaigning to regulate occupational hazards and compensate victims vary quite widely. Studies of occupational health tragedies in the USA have invariably cited a strong British trade union movement as a key player in earlier regulation of hazards.[1] Whilst states such as Massachusetts were the exceptions in that they mirrored the UK labour code quite closely, typically safety regulations with statutory authority were embedded within the Factory and Mines legislation in Britain long before the USA. Moreover, asbestosis, lead poisoning, silicosis, coal workers' pneumoconiosis and byssinosis (brown lung) are all pertinent examples of earlier and somewhat more effective regulation of chronic occupational health problems in the UK than in the USA. Collective pressure from the organised labour movement may well have played a key role in this, though judgment must be reserved because this is still a markedly under-researched area (we still await a systematic historical research project on the trade unions and occupational health). However, as we noted in Chapter 1, much of the UK literature on this topic is critical of the historical role of the trade unions on occupational health. The indictment is that British trade unions invariably failed to *prioritise* occupational health, to develop their own 'alternative' body of scientific knowledge, or to lead a sustained and effective critique of 'orthodox' medical expertise. Such orthodox medical knowledge tended to minimise risks and promote the view that hazardous products and toxins could be controlled by science and technological fixes – such as improved ventilation and medical monitoring. As one Scottish occupational hygienist put it:

> There are unions which are the exception to the rule, but in my own experience trade unions have not been as concerned about things like health and safety as they are about the fact the job is still there and what the wage rates are.[2]

---

1   See D. Rosner and G Markowitz (eds), *Deadly Dust* (Princeton, NJ, 1994); A. Derickson, *Black Lung* (Ithaca, NY, 1998); C. Levenstein and J. Wooding, *Work, Health and Environment* (New York, 1997); C. Levenstein, G. DeLaurier and M.L. Dunn, *The Cotton Dust Papers* (New York, 2002), p. 50.

2   Robin Howie, Interview C45 (SOHC). Howie added this point about union priorities in the 1970s: 'I blame the trade unions to a large extent … During the 1970s we had a series of wage freezes, that's when the unions should have been going for better conditions. They couldn't go for money, they could have gone for better conditions, for better safety in the workplace, and they chose not to.'

Hence, from one point of view the unions failed to act as an effective 'countervailing' force, prioritising compensation over systematically developed preventative policies, or, for some, were constrained by their close association with employer health and safety strategies and state compensation procedure.[3] Thus it was only from the late 1960s that victim and activist pressure groups emerged which pioneered knowledge accumulation and research, campaigned vigorously and ensured wider and more effective dissemination of information about workplace hazards. The Society for the Prevention of Asbestosis and Industrial Disease and Clydeside Action on Asbestos are examples. Such organisations were created – at least in part – by individuals frustrated at the slow pace of action and progress achieved by the trade unions and the political process. What is revealing, moreover, is the marked lack of industrial conflict on occupational health issues in general in the UK. Strikes and protests did occur, but they were extremely rare. Revealingly, neither Church and Outram's detailed analysis of strike activity in coal mining nor Taylor's recent two-volume history of the NUM and British politics have anything of substance to say about the coal unions and occupational health and safety policy after 1945.[4] One might deduce from the relative silence on this issue within such secondary sources that health and safety was not a priority for the main mining trade union in the decades following the Second World War.

Our argument here accepts that this critique of the unions has some validity, but we try to understand the choices unions made within the prevailing context, and argue that the relationship between trade unions and occupational health was far more complex. The 'orthodox' negative interpretation fits the asbestos experience in the UK rather better than other industries, including coal mining. In part, this is because asbestos manufacture and use was scattered across many industries and occupations, where, in the main, the trade union presence was weak.[5] Moreover, in many workplaces, such as construction sites and shipyards, exposure to asbestos only affected a relatively small proportion of the total workforce. Here more workers faced the possibility of traumatic injury, so accident avoidance and control were prioritised by workgroups and their collective organisations. Generally, though, it appears that a range of positions were taken by the trade unions on health issues, and much strategic choice was in evidence across the labour movement. At one level,

3   P.B. Beaumont, *Safety at Work and the Unions* (London, 1983), p. 42; p. 62; T. Dwyer, *Life and Death at Work: Industrial Accidents as a Case of Socially Produced Error* (New York, 1991); pp. 74–8.

4   See R. Church and Q. Outram, *Strikes and Solidarity: Coalfield Conflict in Britain, 1889–1966* (Cambridge, 1998); A. Taylor, *The NUM and British Politics, Volume 1. 1944–1968* (Aldershot, 2003); A. Taylor, *The NUM and British Politics, Volume 2. 1969–1995* (Aldershot, 2005).

5   R. Johnston and A. McIvor, *Lethal Work* (East Linton, 2000); G. Tweedale, *From Magic Mineral to Killer Dust* (Oxford, 1999); P.W.J. Bartrip, *The Way from Dusty Death* (London, 2001); M. Greenberg, 'Knowledge of the Health Hazards of Asbestos Prior to the Merewether and Price Report of 1930', *Social History of Medicine*, vol. 7 (1994), pp. 493–516.

with the appointment of a Medical Adviser to the TUC, the trade union movement in Britain did develop a quite innovatory process of knowledge-gathering on health issues from the early 1930s. The first incumbent, Sir Thomas Legge, was previously Chief Medical Inspector of Factories in the Home Office.[6] Furthermore, research by Wyke, and Bowden and Tweedale suggests a different picture for the cotton industry compared to asbestos, as in cotton textiles the unions were more powerful and very progressive in campaigning to recognise and regulate spinners' cancer and byssinosis (brown lung) throughout the twentieth century.[7] This was also the case with the British coal miners' unions and dust disease, where there was a sustained campaign to challenge medical orthodoxies, generate 'alternative' knowledge and use lay knowledge in campaigns to regulate hazards and control risks. However, the strategies of the miners' unions on dust differed markedly across the coal fields, depending, in part, on both objective and subjective judgements about the dust risk and incidence of respiratory impairment. This created tensions and conflicts within the MFGB and the NUM. Coal mining thus provides a revealing case study, not only for what it tells us about the process of 'expert' and 'lay' knowledge-accumulation on the dust problem in this industry, but also the prevailing structures of power, the distinctive work culture of the miners and their efforts to collectivise responses to the unhealthy work environment and the threat to their bodies that inhaling dust at work constituted.

The Miners' Unions and the Recognition of CWP

In marked contrast to what occurred with asbestos, from the 1920s the miners' unions in the UK energetically contested the prevailing 'orthodox' medical knowledge on miners' lung, drawing upon lay knowledge of disability and mortality in mining communities, caused by coal dust, especially in mechanised work processes. As the work of Melling and Bufton, and Bloor has shown, the miners' unions in the inter-war period challenged the notions that coal dust was innocuous, and that only silica was the problem, whilst pressing for coal miners to be included within compensation schemes.[8] By the 1930s, there were several elements to this strategy. The South Wales

---

6   However, further research is required to determine the extent to which the TUC Medical Advisers challenged medical orthodoxy on dust disease. See, for example, the conservative position of Robert Murray on asbestos-related diseases; Johnston and McIvor, *Lethal Work*, pp. 167–8.

7   S. Bowden and G. Tweedale, 'Mondays without Dread: The Trade Union Response to Byssinosis in the Lancashire Cotton Industry in the Twentieth Century', *Social History of Medicine,* vol. 16, no. 1 (2003), pp. 79–95. See also S. Bowden and G. Tweedale, 'Poisoned by the Fluff: Compensation and Litigation for Byssinosis in the Lancashire Cotton Industry', *Journal of Law and Society,* vol. 29, no. 4 (December 2002), pp. 560–79; T. Wyke, 'Spinners' Cancer', in A. Fowler and T. Wyke (eds), *The Barefoot Aristocrats* (Littleborough, 1987).

8   J. Melling and M. Bufton, '"A Mere Matter of Rock": Organized Labour, Scientific Evidence and British Government Schemes for Compensation of Silicosis and Pneumoconiosis

Miners' Federation (SWMF) was particularly active in exerting political pressure to redirect epidemiological research into the dust problem and to reform compensation legislation. The interest of this organisation was prompted by the severity of the dust problem in the region, especially in the anthracite, hard coal area to the west of the South Wales coal field. Around 80% of all prescribed pneumoconiotics in the UK in the 1940s were located in South Wales.[9] The South Wales 'Fed' thus generated its own knowledge base through independent epidemiological studies and engaged directly with the dominant medical discourse. This involved challenging the influential view held by J.S. Haldane and others that coal dust was not only harmless, but positively beneficial in protecting the lungs against TB (see Chapter 3). In this process, the union employed its own medical and geological experts, supported 'independent' expertise that pushed the union cause and contradicted opposing evidence, including, in some cases, fabricating geological evidence. In the period before coal was officially recognised as the causal agent in lung disease, this involved clandestinely sprinkling silica dust underground.[10] One South Wales union lodge official, Howard Jones, described this:

> It was not uncommon for them to come down to his place of work to find out if silica was present, and these pieces of silica were sprinkled around the roadway and they were collected, *reusable* (laughs). There was no doubt about it that silica is present in the anthracite coalfield, but you made it obvious by putting a little bit into position here and there so that it could be seen.[11]

The Miners' Federation of Great Britain (MFGB) had a prolonged campaign to get silicosis classified and made compensatable in mining (1929) and, thereafter, to improve the scheme and to get 'anthracosis' or coal workers' pneumoconiosis (CWP) officially prescribed as an occupational disease, which, as we have seen, was achieved in 1943. In the early 1930s, efforts were directed towards the extension of compensation rights and the replacement of the practice of scheduling specific mining processes (such as hewing) with the scheduling of the entire industry instead.[12] This involved liaison with the General Council of the TUC and discussion with the Labour government. A.J. Cook, who played a part in the negotiations, commented that the political *milieu* was significant in the passage of the 1931 reform (Various Industries Silicosis Scheme 1931), noting 'whilst we sometimes criticize our own people, had

---

among Coalminers, 1926–1940', *Medical History*, vol. 49, no. 2 (April 2005), pp. 155–78; M. Bufton and J. Melling, 'Coming Up for Air: Experts, Employers and Workers in Campaigns to Compensate Silicosis Sufferers in Britain, 1918–39', *Social History of Medicine*, vol. 18, no. 1 (2005), pp. 63–86; M. Bloor, 'The South Wales Miners' Federation, Miners' Lung and the Instrumental Use of Expertise, 1900–1950', *Social Studies of Science*, vol. 30, no. 1 (February 2000), pp. 125–40.

  9   *Report of the Chief Inspector of Mines and Quarries for 1967* (London, 1968), table 7.

  10   Bloor, 'The South Wales Miners' Federation', p. 133.

  11   Howard Jones, Interview C25 (SOHC).

  12   MFGB, *Annual Volume of Proceedings* (1931), pp. 14–15, 321–4, 395–99.

it been a Conservative Home Secretary we should not have got the improvements which have been obtained for our silicosis men'.[13] Cook described the 1931 Scheme as 'a godsend to our men. It has opened a door which we thought had been closed.' This was achieved in the face of stonewall opposition by the Mining Association of Great Britain, which rejected any amendment to the 1928 scheme.[14] There remained severe limitations in the 1931 Scheme, however. It was not retrospective, and it still included the need to define the rock worked on as silicaceous. Critically, moreover, there was no recognition of anthracosis. J. Bettney, one of the MFGB South Wales delegates, commented:

> In the anthracite coalfield of South Wales we have a very large number of men suffering acutely from anthracosis. We are powerless to do anything on their behalf. The reports and evidence that has been gathered proves conclusively that men are slowly dying as a result of anthracosis ... Men on the surface; men working on the screens; men underground. They are simply dying; some are partially disabled, some are totally disabled. We are in a precarious position, having to admit that these poor fellows are unable to perform work in any sense of the term whatever.[15]

As we discussed in Chapter 3, it was partly in response to this pressure from the union that the Mines Department initiated an enquiry focusing on the surface workers, and the Home Office referred the issue of anthracosis to the Industrial Pulmonary Diseases Committee (IPDC) of the MRC in 1931. However, the Home Office noted that progress was likely to be slow because 'there are serious technical difficulties in the way of prosecuting the necessary research'.[16] This may have been a reference to the potential cost of such an exercise, though the union suspected 'vested interests'.[17] At this stage, as we've seen, medical opinion was sharply divided. The MFGB, however, was co-operating in the research, providing to the IPDC the names of 50 men employed solely for the previous twenty-five years in coal getting and filling. J. Griffiths of the SWMF commented on the outcome:

> It was found that every one of those 50 men were suffering from anthracosis. The examinations revealed that the dust of a hard, gritty nature from anthracite produces anthracosis. We have come to the conclusion that every man employed in the anthracite coal, cutting and filling, is suffering from this disease ... every miner over 50 is suffering from the germs of anthracosis.[18]

The Home Office, however, wanted more hard evidence to justify any 'sweeping change in the law involving a tremendous widening of the liabilities to be undertaken

---

13 Ibid., p. 322.

14 Ibid., p. 396.

15 Ibid., p. 324.

16 MFGB, *Annual Volume of Proceedings* (1932), p. 20.

17 Ibid., p. 234.

18 Ibid. This belief in the harmful effect of anthracite compared to other grades of coal was later discredited (see Chapter 3).

by the industry'.[19] They insisted on the union providing more cases. The SWMF responded by supplying 23 individual cases of miners who had been diagnosed or certified with silicosis, but had failed to get compensation. The Home Office interpretation of this evidence, however, was that 14 of the 23 had been engaged in processes covered by the scheme, and 3 of the remaining 9 had not been officially certified. The Home Office refused to proceed without further evidence of certified cases with full employment histories to prove they had just worked in coal and not in the scheduled processes exposed to rock dust.[20]

The MFGB endorsed the South Wales miners' plea to have anthracosis scheduled as an industrial disease under the Workmen's Compensation Act and officially represented the men's case in meetings with the Home Office. Their initial position was that the Scheme should be amended to make it applicable to all processes underground (rather than just those scheduled such as drilling and blasting) and irrespective of the silica content of the rock or any other restriction. This was achieved in the Various Industries (Silicosis) Amendment Scheme in 1934. The 50% silica clause remained, and the legislation had other severe limitations (it was not retrospective, and nobody who had been out of the industry for more than three years was eligible). Meanwhile, the miners' unions were continuing to employ chemists and geologists, in what Bloor has referred to as an 'instrumental use of expertise' to prove contact had been made with rocks of 50% silica underground and support miners' compensation claims.[21] This was taking up a considerably amount of union time and resources. F. Swift, an MFGB representative for Somerset, commented on one such case in 1934:

> The owners disputed the fact that the man had been working in silica rock. They disputed that he was working under the conditions as laid down by the scheme. I went into the pit and got a sample of the rock and had it analyzed by a geologist. We had to take this man to court to give evidence. The owners had a geologist there who had analyzed 30 samples. In the thirty samples the owners' geologist submitted there was no sandstone. Our geologist said it was sandstone. We had to fight for two days on the matter, and eventually we succeeded in convincing the Judge that he did come within the process, but it was a touch and go question.[22]

What was increasingly evident was the rising number of cases of respiratory disease from coal mines where miners had little or no exposure to silica (see Chapter 3). The crucial point here is that these were being identified by the miners' unions, sometimes going against the views of local GPs (who diagnosed what were then perceived to be 'non-occupational' ailments such as pneumonia or bronchitis). The unions were paying for preliminary medical examinations, then sending the affected miners to the Silicosis Medical Panels. Increasingly, the Panels were certifying

---

19 MFGB, *Annual Volume of Proceedings* (1933), p. 94.

20 Ibid., p. 95. For more detail, see Melling and Bufton, '"A Mere Matter of Rock"'.

21 See Bloor, 'The South Wales Miners' Federation'.

22 MFGB, *Annual Volume of Proceedings* (1934), p. 106.

that these miners had silicosis. However, they continued to be unable to get any workmen's compensation because the mine owners and the courts stuck rigidly to the legal definition of the disease, especially the 50% silica ruling. Whilst there were occasional *ex gratia* payments by the more welfarist collieries, the mine owners routinely rejected liability. Most of those affected were not only disabled and suspended from the industry, but were also forced upon the local Public Assistance Committees for relief.[23] Nor was the issue solely confined to South Wales. In Somerset, it was reported to be common for local doctors to continue to wrongly diagnose the problem as bronchitis. The union challenged this, sent the men to the Silicosis Medical Board, and apparently in all cases got them certified as silicotic.[24] In another case in the Midlands, one of the horse-keepers (termed an ostler) was certified as silicotic by the Medical Board, but compensation was refused because the man had not worked in any of the scheduled processes.[25] In North Staffs, the union lawyers were more aware of the silicosis problem because of its prevalence in the potteries, but relatively few cases could be proven where the silica content of the rocks was 50% or above. In this litigation, the employers were advantaged by being able to employ eminent geologists and analysts to support their case, whilst the unions struggled to find experts and meet the costs. The Midland Federation, for example, had to go to South Wales because they could not find a geologist who would support their case in the Midlands.[26]

As we saw in Chapter 3, medical evidence was accumulating that coal dust was the causal agent, as well as silica, and the unions played a key role in pressing this case from the early 1930s. From 1931 to 1933, it was estimated that there were about 250–300 men certified as silicotic by the Medical Boards in South Wales, and of those 130 were totally disabled, suspended from the industry and unable to claim any compensation because they could not prove work had taken place on rock of 50% or more silica content. In one of the worst anthracite collieries, Tirbach Colliery in Ystalyfera, there were 23 certified cases (14 of total disability), of which only two had been able to claim compensation. Eighteen of the 23 were coal hewers. The youngest of the Tirbach cases was just 29 years old. James Griffiths, MP for Llanelli, commented on the injustice and unequal struggle the mineworkers were involved in:

> We made ten different independent searches in these men's places looking for silica rock for evidence, for quartz, sandstone etc and we were able to find only one tiny piece of quartz or shales called lenticular. We entered into Court. What do we find. That the colliery company are employing men of considerable standing in scientific work to come and give evidence in order to deprive these men of any compensation ... It is a scandal

---

23 MFGB, *Annual Volume of Proceedings* (1933), p. 99; MFGB, *Annual Volume of Proceedings* (1934), p. 105.

24 Ibid., pp. 104–5, 106.

25 Ibid., p. 109.

26 MFGB, *Annual Volume of Proceedings* (1932), pp. 232–3.

that the Mining Association is spending money, buying brains and experts in order to confuse counsel and the Government.[27]

In November 1933, the SWMF submitted a list of 59 cases of certified silicosis where miners had been refused compensation to the Home Office in support of their case for legislative change. A few months later they added a detailed report from a University of Wales geologist whom the union had commissioned to investigate the causes of rising respiratory disease rates in the coal field. The report by A. Hubert Cox was a damning indictment of existing policy. He argued that frequently the coal measures in South Wales contained little silica, and that new cases of silicosis amongst the miners were 'constantly occurring' in such pits. On the other hand, high-silica pits which were at the same time wet pits produced few cases. He concluded:

> I am, therefore, driven to the conclusion that a dry and dusty mine is dangerous, quite
> irrespective of whether the rocks supplying the dust contain sufficient free silica to bring
> them within any of the specified characters of silica rocks.[28]

Cox went on to identify a relationship between silicosis and the nature of the coal, with the highest incidence of the disease in the anthracite region in the western part of the South Wales coal field: 'the higher the carbon content of the coals the greater appears to be the incidence of silicosis'. He posited: 'this excessive amount of coal dust produced in anthracite and steam coal working may, through its interference with the mechanism of the lungs, be a contributory or predisposing cause in relation to the incidence of silicosis'.[29] Interestingly, whilst the Home Office recognised that such expert evidence 'was undoubtedly favourable to their [the unions'] case, nevertheless, as evidence, it was not nearly so good as specific cases of men who had contracted the disease while working underground and whose employment record showed it could not have been contracted in any of the processes'.[30] It appears to have been the epidemiology that was critical rather than expert opinion, and in the manufacture of both, the unions' role was important. This was significant in raising awareness of a disease which was largely ignored by the local Medical Officers of Health (MOH) because they myopically regarded it as only an industrial illness. Hence, there was no mention of silicosis or anthracosis in the MOH Annual Reports in South Wales, or elsewhere. As Dr E. Colston Williams, MOH for Glamorganshire, put it: 'It is an industrial disease and as such does not interest those who work with

---

27 MFGB, *Annual Volume of Proceedings* (1934), p. 108.

28 Ibid., p. 214.

29 Ibid., pp. 214–15. Whilst the Cox study rightly drew attention to coal dust as the agent, the 'rank of coal' thesis was later discredited, whilst subsequent research indicated that the silica content of the dust generated at the coal face was indeed very important in the etiology of miners' respiratory diseases.

30 MFGB, *Annual Volume of Proceedings* (1933), p. 95. The comment is from R.R. Ballantyne of the Home Office.

the public health.'[31] This position was criticised by another report commissioned by the SWMF, this time from J.H. Davies, the Principal of the Mining and Research Institute at Pontardawe, which also outlined a range of practical, preventative measures to suppress the dust at source, including radical changes in labour processes, improvements in ventilation, systematic use of water and the wearing of dust masks.[32]

The government reacted to this escalating campaign by the unions and to the growing fissures in expert medical knowledge about the nature of silicosis and of anthracosis by referring the matter for a full scientific investigation by the Industrial Pulmonary Diseases Committee of the MRC (see Chapter 3).[33] One of the factors impinging upon the Home Office decision to establish the MRC investigation that eventually led to the scheduling of CWP was shifting public opinion, swayed by press reports.[34] Around this time, in February 1936, a series of articles appeared in the *News Chronicle*, penned by journalist Louise Morgan, exposing the dust problem in mining communities in South Wales and northern England. She reported graphically on case after case of miners wasting away at a very young age with pneumoconiosis, using lurid, attention-grabbing headlines such as 'Where young men grow old too soon', 'Death stalks behind shortness of breath' and 'Healthy men who gallop to death'. Communities, she reported, were decimated by respiratory disease, commonly, Morgan found, referred to as asthma, bronchitis or just 'shortness of breath'. 'This', she noted, 'is as familiar among them as the common cold.'[35] Most local doctors claimed ignorance of silicosis, though one commented: 'silicosis is very prevalent in Durham only we've been calling it by other names'.[36] Apart from exposing individual cases, Morgan marshalled an impressive array both of lay knowledge and of 'expert' medical evidence, citing medical journals and local epidemiological research, including studies of surface workers and a survey of

---

31 *News Chronicle* (17 February 1936), SWCC/MNA/NUM/G20; for a discussion on the lack of integration between occupational health and general health, see J. McEwen et al. 'The Interface between the OHS and the National Health Service', *Public Health*, vol. 96 (1982), pp. 155–63.

32 J.H. Davies, 'Methods of Preventing Miners' Silicosis and Some other Lung Diseases in the Anthracite District' (SWCC paper, n.d.), pp. 7–8.

33 'Industrial Pulmonary Disease in Coal Mines', IPDC Minutes, 19 March 1936 and 28 May 1936; Letter, Home Office to MRC, 23 May 1936; MRC to Home Office, 18 June 1936, NA/FD1/2884.

34 Letter, Home Office to MRC, 23 May 1936; MRC to HO, 18 June 1936, NA/FD1/2884. The Home Office noted adverse press reports and encouraged the MRC IPDC to produce results quickly. The Committee clearly resented this 'political pressure'. See Melling and Bufton, '"A Mere Matter of Rock"', for a full account of the complex background to CWP certification.

35 *News Chronicle* (24 February 1936). The full series of articles is copied in SWCC/MNA/NUM/G20.

36 *News Chronicle* (24 February 1936).

130 'healthy' miners by the Cardiff TB hospital in 1935–36. Morgan asserted that medical experts in South Wales:

> ... are unanimous in condemnation of the conditions responsible for the appalling toll of disease exacted from the miner by his occupation and of the present interpretation of the silicosis order by the mine owners. It is the conviction of 95 per cent of the medical profession that not only the 'new' disease of silicosis, but all the chest diseases to which miners are peculiarly susceptible, such as bronchitis, emphysema, tuberculosis, anthracosis, pneumonia etc., are directly traceable to the working conditions at the collieries. All should get compensation. And yet under the present order a miner receives compensation only on the grounds of silicosis ... All the experts with whom I have talked are agreed that mining dust, wherever found and of whatever type, whether coal or stone, leads to chest disease.[37]

This was an important piece of investigative journalism in which the trade unions played a significant part – especially Evan Williams and the SWMF – in supplying information, research leads and corroborative evidence.[38]

To sum up: in contrast to the campaign in the USA in the late 1960s, the recognition of CWP in the UK in 1943 was the product of a coalition of progressive forces in which the unions played an important, and perhaps even the *pivotal* role.[39] Sustained union pressure in the 1930s – remarkable given the relative weakness of the miners' unions with high levels of mass unemployment and an eroded membership base – preceded the creation of the crucially important government-sponsored MRC Pneumoconiosis Investigation of 1937–42, which led directly to the 1943 Regulations recognising CWP. During the course of the investigation, moreover, it was a union compensation secretary, Harry Finch, who suggested to the MRC investigators that they initiate the epidemiological study of coal trimmers (specialised dockers responsible for shovelling coal onto ships for export) in the South Wales ports, which – as noted in Chapter 3 – went a long way to proving that coal dust was a causal agent in fibrosis of the lungs, and not just silica.[40]

The miners' unions in South Wales were thus engaged through the 1920s and 1930s in a bitter and protracted campaign against the coal owners to achieve decent levels of financial compensation for their members. These related campaigns were pursued in very difficult circumstances, in the face of intense and well-organised opposition on the part of the coal owners, and in a context of high unemployment, defeat and demoralisation after the failure of the 1926 General Strike, and sharply falling trade union membership to the mid-1930s. In the courts, the miners' union in South Wales was particularly active in challenging the orthodox medical discourse and the prevailing 'silica fixation', fighting to expand compensation, and advocating

---

37 *News Chronicle* (17 February 1936).

38 See correspondence between Louise Morgan and Evan Williams, 22 February 1936 and 24 February 1936, SWCC/MNA/NUM/G20.

39 On the USA, see Derickson, *Black Lung*.

40 Bloor, 'The South Wales Miners' Federation', pp. 133–4.

on behalf of dust disease victims. By the mid-1930s, this also involved making representations to collieries which had refused to employ silicotics.[41] In 1939, a Silicosis Pageant was also organised by the SWMF in the Amman valley to bring the issue to the public's attention.[42]

Judging from the attention devoted to the dust issue in the records of the coal unions, getting the existing restrictive compensation scheme extended appears to have been an important priority of the unions in the 1920s and 1930s. Did this mean that the miners' unions placed financial recompense above tackling the cause of the problem head-on? Perhaps a case might be made for this. However, there is plenty of evidence to show that preventative policies were being promulgated, and especially on the key issue of dust suppression. By the mid-1930s, the SWMF was working with the Mines Inspectorate and the employers' associations to disseminate preventative knowledge and develop policies. This involved making representations to collieries to suggest improvements which would reduce levels of dust, including dust generated on the surface at the screening processes.[43] In 1935, the SWMF came up with a 'hit list' of six proposals to minimise dust in the pits, including water infusion, wet drilling and spraying, dust traps, road cleaning and restrictions on shot-firing.[44] The following year, the SWMF Compensation Secretary Evan Williams J.P. lambasted the mine owners in two press articles for ignoring preventative measures and being preoccupied with minimising compensation payments to victims of respiratory disease. Williams accused the employers of callous indifference and hypocrisy, and called for preventative measures to be made compulsory in the industry.[45] In a private letter to a journalist, Williams commented that in his view, 'except in isolated cases', the mine owners were doing nothing to control dust.[46]

At around the same time, the appointment of the Royal Commission on Safety in the Mines in 1935 provided the MFGB with an opportunity to identify preventative dust control measures. In its evidence, the MFGB campaigned for an extension of the statutory requirements under the 1911 Coal Mines Act. Section 78 of this Act laid down that no drilling by mechanical power could be used in siliceous rocks without a water jet or spray to damp down the dust. The MFGB argued that the risk was much wider that just those involved in drilling operations, positing: 'there can be no doubt that the development of machine mining with its rapid turnover of the face, its increase in shot-firing, and its greater use of the haulage roads per hour, has caused such greatly increased quantities of dust to be thrown into the air'.[47] The union went on to argue that experience indicated that 'new legislative measures

---

41 South Wales Miners' Federation (SWMF), *Minutes* (1935), p. 92.

42 H. Francis and D. Smith, *The Fed: A History of the South Wales Miners in the Twentieth Century* (London, 1980), p. 439.

43 SWMF, *Minutes* (1935), p. 92.

44 Ibid., p. 149.

45 *Western Mail* (n.d., *c.* January/February 1936), copies in SWCC/MNA/NUM/G20.

46 Letter, E. Williams to Louise Morgan, 22 February 1936, SWCC/MNA/NUM/G20.

47 MFGB, *Annual Volume of Proceedings* (1936), pp. 432–3.

should be passed to compel adoption of preventative measures on a comprehensive scale' and detailed their proposals:

1. action on dust suppression had to recognise the universal nature of the problem, with dust not confined to particular processes but dispersed throughout the pit – 'such dust may exist throughout the mine workings';
2. compulsory introduction of the necessary equipment – dust traps, water infused drilling, and respirators;
3. improved ventilation, including a prohibition on men returning after shot-firing 'until the air has been thoroughly cleared';
4. Mines Department to stop work in any mine or part of a mine where dust generation 'would be likely seriously to affect the health of the workmen'.[48]

As we saw in Chapter 3, although some action was taken by a few of the leading employers in South Wales (motivated partly by the need to ensure that mechanisation continued), in general, notwithstanding trade union pressure, the control of respiratory dust was not given a high degree of attention. Moreover, despite going some way to preparing a new Mines Act based on the recommendations of the Royal Commission on Safety (Cmd. 5890), new legislation was put on hold by the government when the war broke out.[49]

The War, the Mining Unions and Dust

During the war, the pressures impinging upon miners to produce coal to sustain the war effort led directly to an increase in risk, with higher recorded injury rates and a rising exposure to dust, especially in South Wales from 1939 to 1942.[50] The MFGB alerted the government to this:

> Under present circumstances there was an intensification of production, and while we did not blame the owners or Government for this we could not ignore the fact that risks were greater today than under normal circumstances.[51]

What also concerned the union was that with the rising costs of living, the real value of the Workmen's Compensation benefits for such disabled workers (and their dependants) had eroded sharply during wartime. According to the union's estimates,

---

48 Ibid., p. 433.

49 MFGB, *Annual Volume of Proceedings* (1943), p. 519.

50 For a discussion of how wartime conditions impacted on occupational health in Scotland, see R. Johnston and A. McIvor, 'The War and the Body at Work: Occupational Health and Safety in Scottish Industry, 1939–1945', *Journal of Scottish Historical Studies*, vol. 24, no. 2 (2004), pp. 113–36.

51 MFGB, *Annual Volume of Proceedings* (1942), p. 228. E. Edwards in a meeting between the MFGB and the Minister of Fuel and Power, 19 November 1942.

by 1942 such disability benefits averaged only 40% of the minimum wage (of £4 3s.) a face worker earned.[52]

None the less, the strategic importance of coal during the war, high demand and persistent trade union pressure led to a number of important developments regarding pneumoconiosis, including, as we've seen, the pivotal certification of CWP in 1943 and the passage of a new compensation scheme covering all mine workers. The legislation also established a scheme to provide compensation to 'old' cases employed from 1934. This was a retrospective recognition of the claims of those thousands of miners the unions had been fighting claims for who had been excluded from the restrictive Silicosis Scheme. It also included surface workers, for the first time.[53]

There were also significant developments on the preventative side during the war with the passage of the special regulations covering South Wales which enabled the Ministry of Fuel and Power (MFP) and the Mines Inspectors to force mine owners to introduce dust suppression measures including water infusion and spraying.[54] The SWMF Safety Committee considered dust control an integral part of its remit, and worked during wartime to extend statutory control, including the application of water to suppress dust, lobbying the MFGB and the MFP to these ends.[55] Statutory controls were initiated, moreover, after a deputation arguing this case from the MFGB had been heard.[56] This followed the creation by the MFP of a Joint Committee in South Wales, of the coal owners, the union and the Mines Inspectors to agree methods to prevent and suppress dust.[57] The 1943 Statutory Order replaced previous reliance upon voluntary action by the private coal owners. Alf Davies of the SWMF openly criticised some mine owners for failing to comply with dust suppression measures, commenting: 'there could be no complaint if compulsion were applied through lack of voluntary co-operation'.[58] The Chief Inspector of Mines, J.R. Felton, endorsed this in 1943 with a scathing letter addressed to the South Wales Coal Owners'

---

52 MFGB, *Annual Volume of Proceedings* (1942), p. 228.

53 Ibid., pp. 130–31; MFGB, *Annual Volume of Proceedings* (1943), pp. 159–60.

54 Statutory Rules and Orders 1943, no. 1,696, Coal Mines (South Wales) (Pneumoconiosis), Order 1943, Emergency Powers (Defence), NA/POWE26/1150. Again, this firmer action contrasts markedly with what occurred with asbestos dust around this time, when the hazards of using the product in insulation on ships was becoming apparent. The Factory Inspectorate issued a warning circular to shipbuilders, but there was never any compulsion or statutory control (until 1960).

55 SWMF, *Minutes of Safety Committee*, 20 August 1943, SWCC/MNA/NUM/K17J; MFGB *Annual Volume of Proceedings* (1943), pp. 486–7, 519.

56 MFGB, *Annual Volume of Proceedings* (1943), pp. 486–7.

57 MFGB, *Annual Volume of Proceedings* (1942), p. 145.

58 Meeting of the South Wales Pneumoconiosis Sub-Committee, 28 July 1943, SWCC/MNA/NUM/K175, p. 5. The Ocean Collieries group and the smaller individual collieries were identified as the worst offenders. Powell Duffryn and the Amalgamated Anthracite Company had gone furthest to implement dust suppression measures in 1942–43. See also MFGB, *Annual Volume of Proceedings* (1942), p. 515.

Association (SWCOA) threatening further compulsion because 'the position seems to us to be far from satisfactory'.[59] Thereafter, the union pressed the MFP for a further extension of these statutory powers to force all coal owners to implement dust suppression measures, rather than waiting for Mines Inspectors to issue orders to that effect on a colliery-by-colliery basis.[60] That the colliery companies failed to voluntarily implement preventative dust control measures to any significant extent constituted a further indictment upon private ownership. At the same time, by the end of the war the union was actively involved in the practical experiments taking place on dust suppression, feeding suggestions through the MFP on improved dust suppression in shot-firing and on surface screens. Reports on trials appear to have been routinely sent to the union by the Ministry for feedback and discussion. The minutes of the MFGB/NUM Safety and Health Sub-Committee show that this was no rubber-stamping exercise. Draft Regulations and reports from the Ministry were carefully scrutinised, and detailed responses and additional provisions passed back from the union. In November 1946, for example, the Committee responded to new draft regulations on dust suppression in stone drifts and shafts with six detailed recommendations, including water spraying on roadways, the removal of workmen by the colliery official where dust suppression failed, and a proviso that exemptions only be granted by Mines Inspectors after consultation with the NUM.[61] Tackling the dust at source was clearly the priority. Even amongst the wide-ranging activity of the miners' trade unions on dust at this time, there was no mention of respirators, though other protective clothing was campaigned for.[62]

Two other issues preoccupied the SWMF in this period. The first was the enormous number of miners requesting medical 'boarding' (to be sent to the Medical Panels) after the 1943 recognition of CWP. This swamped the procedure, leading to a massive waiting list for examinations. The union responded by pressing the government to send more doctors to the region to deal with the 2,000 or so backlog of Panels and by tightening up its own pre-selection procedure by refusing to endorse any boarding unless a preliminary x-ray at a local hospital or TB clinic showed 'reasonable evidence' of pneumoconiosis.[63] The latter was the customary procedure in the region, and the SWMF routinely paid the 30s. fee for the preliminary x-ray. One South Wales lodge official explained:

> The lodge had a fund, a medical fund. You were paying, I think it was three pence a week, and then you were selected on the basis of your service in the industry to go to the radiologist in Swansea. The radiologist was then paid by the lodge out of this particular fund. This is pre-national health mind, back in the 1940s. His report came back. I remember

---

59 Letter, J.R. Felton (Ministry of Fuel and Power) to Mr Carey, South Wales Coalowners' Association, 23 July 1943, SWCC/MNA/NUM/K175.

60 MFGB, *Annual Volume of Proceedings* (1945), p. 623.

61 MFGB, *Annual Volume of Proceedings* (1946), p. 625.

62 MFGB, *Annual Volume of Proceedings* (1945), p. 621.

63 SWMF Compensation Department, Memorandum, 20 June 1944; Letter to Lodge Secretaries, 21 July 1944, SWCC/MNA/NUM/K17J.

having a report in 1946 saying that there was a reticulation of the lungs and to send me back in a year's time. But of course Aneurin Bevan put a stop on that and he brought in the health service so the medical board then was just common place and you just filled in your form and waited to be called, and there was no need then to pay for the radiologist. But on the basis of his report the lodge was to send people to be, to the medical, the pneumoconiosis medical panel and they would decide it.[64]

At this time, about 40–50% of those sent by the union to the Medical Panels were rejected. Even as early as the mid-1940s, the miners' unions were in no doubt as to the cause of disablement of this large number of miners with respiratory disease who fell outside any compensation scheme. Ebby Edwards of the MFGB noted in 1946:

Of the members who did not succeed in obtaining certificates of disablement there is not the slightest doubt that they are suffering from a disabling chest condition caused or aggravated by coal dust. Many are suffering from emphysema, and the National Union is convinced that this disability is directly attributable to the nature of the members' employment.[65]

The other issue that the union campaigned vigorously on from 1943 was the provision of suitable work for those thousands of miners suspended from the industry as a result of the post-1943 Medical Panels. Numbers thrown out of work rose sharply, including those who had evidence of 'simple' pneumoconiosis but were not incapacitated and fully capable of working. These men were provided with half pay for just 13 weeks under the 1943 scheme. The MFGB Workmen's Compensation Sub-Committee regarded such treatment as 'worse than useless', commenting: 'the employers either cannot or will not find suitable employment'.[66] They campaigned for full compensation at 'loss of earning capacity' level for as long as pneumoconiotics remained unemployed, and an extension of re-training and employment opportunities. The extent of the problem became evident in 1945 when the SWMF initiated a lodge survey. It discovered that 2,875 certificates of suspension were issued at 79 collieries, of which 2,165 miners failed to find any alternative employment. Of those 710 who had found other work, only 64 were employed by the collieries on light employment at the surface. The finger was also pointed at the Ministry of Labour for failing to provide adequate alternative employment for these pneumoconiotics.[67] What the union identified as happening here was a significant shift from the pattern of diagnosis and certification in the 1930s. Before 1943, a high proportion of those certified were completely incapacitated, older miners whose working life was effectively finished. After 1943, men were being suspended in a relatively early stage of disability, hence the issue of rehabilitation and re-employment was more important. In one part of the South Wales anthracite

---

64 Howard Jones, Interview C25 (SOHC).

65 NUM, *Annual Report and Proceedings* (1946), p. 90.

66 MFGB, *Annual Volume of Proceedings* (1944), p. 616.

67 NUM (South Wales Area Council), Letter to Lodge Secretaries, 24 August 1945, SWCC/MNA/PP/127/C19 (D.J. Williams Collection).

collieries in 1932, 80% of the men certified in 1932 were designated totally disabled; in the same area in 1943–44, only 3 out of 312 suspensions were designated as totally disabled. Interestingly, the union also noted that about half those who applied to the Medical Panels were rejected, and 'most of these men are suffering from emphysema, which is not a scheduled industrial disease'. The same union report from the anthracite region in South Wales outlined the devastating social impact of this loss of employment:

> The difficulty in these valleys is that there are no suitable jobs for the bulk of these men. These mining villages have been built on coal and are dependant upon coal as the only industry. There are no other industries where the disabled miner could find employment after he is suspended from the coal industry. He finds himself economically at a dead end – suspended from the only industry in his community, fit for other work and anxious for it, but unable to get it owing to the complete absence of any other kind of industry in the area ... Thousands of men and their families are affected, in some parts there are whole streets with a victim in every house.[68]

This pressure from the union was significant in the newly established Pneumoconiosis Research Unit focusing upon the re-employment of pneumoconiotics as one of its first tasks in the aftermath of the Second World War. The experience of being disabled by dust is explored in more depth in Chapter 9.

The National Union of Miners (NUM) and the Struggle over Dust Disease

The war and nationalisation saw the activities of the mining unions on occupational health extended. At this time, high demand for labour provided a further catalyst. As the Welsh miners' leader Dai Dan Evans noted: 'The nationalisation of the coal industry gave a great impetus to the work of dust suppression. Somehow a new spirit became apparent.'[69] Union policy was enshrined in the Miners' Charter, drawn up by the newly formed NUM in December 1945. The Charter represented immediate demands in relation to working conditions, recruitment and the labour power 'crisis'. Taylor has noted how the campaign for a five-day working week became prioritised as a symbol of what the NUM regarded as 'the new order'.[70] An indication of the union's commitment to protecting miners from damage in the workplace is that 4 of the 12 clauses (nos 3, 4, 11 and 12) dealt with occupational health and safety, including demands for 'new safety laws to meet the conditions of modern mining and especially to suppress the development of industrial diseases

---

68 Memorandum of the Need for New Industries, Prepared by the Executive Committee of the Amalgamated Anthracite Combine Committee, August 1945, SWCC/MNA/PP/127/C19 (D.J. Williams Collection).

69 D.D. Evans, 'A Survey of the Incidence and Progression of Pneumoconiosis' (NUM, South Wales Area, April 1963), p. 12.

70 A. Taylor, *The NUM and British Politics, Volume 1. 1944–1968* (Aldershot, 2003), p. 44.

... the complete re-organisation of health and welfare services ... [and] compulsory medical examinations with training arrangements at full wages pending employment as a skilled workman in another industry if withdrawn from the coal mining on medical grounds'.[71] The damage inflicted upon the body from such toil may also have lain behind the union commitment in the Charter to a reduction in the pensionable retirement age of miners to 55. The Charter reflected a conscious step in the direction of prioritising prevention, whilst continuing to maintain a strong union interest in compensation, rehabilitation and re-employment for pneumoconiotics.

At a national pneumoconiosis conference, organised just 18 days after the creation of the NCB, Will Arthur expressed the collective anger of the mining community that so little had been done to address the dust problem for so long. By this stage the SWMF position had congealed into a demand for statutory controls in place of weak and ineffective voluntary regulation:

Dust should be treated in the same way as gas has been treated under the Coal Mines Act. Where an explosion occurs 10, 100 or 200 lives may be lost and public attention is at the same time focused on the occurrence and everything possible is done to deal with the dependants of the victims, but an Act of Parliament made it possible to supply some preventative measures to the gas content. ... We say that the tremendous effect of pneumoconiosis calls for as drastic an application of dust preventative measures and therefore these changes should be brought about at an early date. First we ask instead of allowing colliery managers to 'contract in' in accordance with the instructions given by the Mines department we are asking for it to be compulsory for colliery managers to apply dust suppression methods unless they have a right to 'contract out'.[72]

Whilst mining engineers and Mines Inspectors adopted a positive, self-congratulatory tone at this 1947 conference – one going so far as to posit, 'In South Wales, I venture to state that a miracle has happened. We have suppressed dust.' – Will Arthur was more circumspect and cautious, warning 'I am not yet convinced that the cause of the disease has yet been found.' He continued: 'we do deprecate the propaganda that implies that the collieries are now free from dust and therefore they have become suitable for the employment of youths and boys from school'.[73] Later in the conference, Lawther emphasised the transition in union thinking taking place, telling delegates: 'you can have the assurance so far as we are concerned in the NUM that it is no longer a question of looking after a man's compensation but rather of seeing that steps are taken ... to prevent these things taking place'.

Where the unions were also very active in this formative period was in exerting influence over the process of medical examination, diagnosis and certification of the disease. The SWMF Compensation Secretary, Harry Finch, stressed in his contribution to the Pneumoconiosis Conference that a vital element of the union's

---

71 NUM, *Annual Report and Proceedings* (1946), pp. 9–10, for full draft of the Charter.

72 Conference on Pneumoconiosis in Coal Mines, 18 January 1947, SWCC/MNA/NUM/ K17J.

73 Ibid.

preventative strategy was the demand for periodic, routine medical examinations for all miners. It was to be more than a decade before that particular reform came about. More important in the first years of nationalisation was the influence which the SWMF had upon policy-making in this area through the NJPC. Union submissions to this body could be detailed and persuasive. An example would be the five-page presentation by R.W. Williams in September 1947 which laid down union arguments about diagnosis and certification procedures. Whilst accepting that x-ray evidence of reticulation (initially thought to have been the first radiological signs of CWP) was vital, the principle that a miner could be disabled even where there was only clinical and not radiological evidence was adhered to, and the union case was that doctors should give 'the benefit of the doubt in the workman's favour' in such cases. The union endorsed some of the established practice in the Panels, including the policy that where focal emphysema was indicated by x-ray, this presupposed reticulation. They also argued that existing disabling conditions and illnesses could be 'aggravated' by pneumoconiosis, and that in such cases the whole disablement should be assigned to pneumoconiosis and the miner entitled to be so certified. This was a contentious issue, and many doctors regarded other illnesses, including heart disease, as more significant and 'apportioned' disability accordingly. Practice varied. For pneumoconiotics who died as a consequence of a bout of pneumonia, it was common for certification to be recorded as death from pneumoconiosis. The terrain was more contested with other life-threatening illnesses:

> It is not so easy to obtain a certificate in cases where apart from the pneumoconiosis there are conditions which of themselves could have caused the death. Even a small degree of pneumoconiosis may have a significant effect on the vitality of a man whose resistance has already been seriously reduced by non-industrial conditions.[74]

The SWMF interpretation of the 1943 legislation was that the expression 'caused' by pneumoconiosis should read 'caused and accelerated by'. Apart from aggressively campaigning to get their interpretation of the 1943 legislation accepted, the NUM were also concerned to maintain the system of certification through the state, via the established Pneumoconiosis and Silicosis Medical Panels. When it was mooted in 1946–47 (in the context of long delays in certification and a rising waiting list of cases) that the NCB's Mines Medical Service might take over this responsibility, the NUM argued vociferously against such a move. An underlying factor in this was that the old coal owners' doctors had been deeply mistrusted by the men, not least because of their partisan, pro-employer role in the workmen's compensation struggles of the 1920s and 1930s.[75] The union also noted continuing tensions between community GPs and the NCB Medical Advisors over assessments of fitness for disabled miners to return to work in the mid/late 1940s.[76]

---

74 Memorandum relating to Pneumoconiosis Cases, Prepared by R.W. Williams for the NJPC (1947), SWCC/MNA/NUM/K17J.

75 Ibid.

76 NUM (South Wales Area Council), *Annual Conference and Report for 1947–8*, p. 74.

Two other significant developments for the unions in the immediate post-war years were the passage of the National Insurance (Industrial Injuries) Act 1948, and the change in policy which led in 1948–49 to the continuation of employment of newly certified pneumoconiotics (rather than dismissal), in the so-called 'approved places' (examined in some detail in Chapters 5 and 6). The former substantially increased compensation payments compared to the old Workmen's Compensation Scheme. None the less, the NUM also negotiated a supplementary coal industry scheme with the NCB to add to the state benefit. The re-employment policy created its own problems and dilemmas, but was widely considered at the time to be the lesser of two evils enabling as it did miners with lower levels of simple pneumoconiosis to stay in work (subject to routine regular re-examination) rather than face unemployment (as occurred over 1943–48). Where the union had less success was in enforcing the policy embedded in the 1946 Miners' Charter that insisted on pneumoconiotic miners being trained for skilled work elsewhere. A proportion ended up in labouring work, some doing work that was clearly too heavy for their impaired respiratory function to cope with (see Chapter 9 for further discussion of this).

So the miners' unions had a very proactive role in occupational health policy, not just in compensation struggles, but also in prevention and rehabilitation. In 1952, Arthur Horner addressed the Second National Pneumoconiosis Conference in a much more confident mood than in 1947, quoting rapidly falling new certification rates and claiming '75% of the problem has been progressively solved … in spite of many weaknesses there has been remarkable improvement'. This he put down to 'the great pioneering work done in South Wales'.[77] However, the union did not operate in a vacuum, and it would be wrong to claim that ameliorative changes were just the consequence of union pressure. Other factors such as the empowering impact of war and of full employment, the favourable political climate and the emergence of social medicine were important (see Chapter 4 for more detail). But union activity and prioritisation of occupational health had a significant role too. Work in this area was undoubtedly made easier by the strength of the union – in the immediate post-war years, the NUM was virtually a closed shop with around 700,000 members. Moreover, in the early years of nationalisation, the NUM developed a supportive and co-operative relationship with the NCB and wielded considerable influence within this largely consensual relationship. Whilst unofficial strikes rose in some of the more militant coal fields, notably South Wales and Scotland, the NUM remained loyally committed to making nationalisation work. Facilitating good relations through to the mid-1950s was a sustained rise in real earnings, with wage increases in mining outstripping most other manual occupations by a considerable margin. Still, the more radical areas such as Scotland and Wales pressed to no avail for more workers' participation and control over the industry.[78]

---

77   Pneumoconioisis Conference, Porthcawl, 11 October 1952, SWCC/MNA/NUM/K17J.

78   See M. Jackson, *The Price of Coal* (London, 1974), pp. 90–96.

The union also continued to challenge what it perceived as the NCB's and the government researchers' tendency to underestimate the problem. In 1956, Arthur Horner scathingly attacked such complacency in the NJPC, dismissing 'miracle cures' and alerting the Committee to 'dramatic increases in some coal fields' in pneumoconiosis rates (singling out North Staffs and Scotland):

> Pneumoconiosis was originally thought to be an anthracite disease but it later appeared in the steam coal pits, then the bituminous pits and it was now diffused throughout the whole country … It was a pity the medical men had not found the disease in Scotland until lately … It would be difficult to maintain that current diagnoses were a relic of past conditions, if the disease continued in areas where dust suppression methods had been operating for some years.[79]

Horner went on to press the union's demand for regular x-ray examinations for all miners throughout the UK – which became a reality in 1959.

The NUM also tried to get conditions standardised throughout the country. As noted in Chapter 6, a key issue in the 1950s was the uneven application of dust control measures across the coal fields. In the mid–late 1950s it was the Northern Division of the NCB that was particularly lax. Whereas the national average of faces where dust suppression was applied was 80% in 1957, in the Northern Division only around 40% of faces were being treated in any way. The Board offered 'inertia' and the traditionally low incidence of pneumoconiosis in this region as explanations for this 'hard core' of inactivity on dust control. The NUM response was to call for tougher statutory controls over recalcitrant managers: 'all Divisions should be made to toe the line'. The NCB retort was to oppose a shift from voluntarism and to shunt the blame on to the men: 'some of the men working in cold and shallow mines objected to the use of water on amenity grounds and education and persuasion were the only methods possible'.[80]

The NUM insisted that the Board should be tougher with mine managers who showed insufficient dedication to the dust problem. The NCB, though, resisted this and instead put the blame for the higher dust levels on miners refusing to use water to suppress the dust. Moreover, as far as getting tough with the managers was concerned, the Board argued that an educative rather than a hard-line approach was the best tactic.[81] The NUM was also proactive in conducting its own pneumoconiosis survey in 1954 to highlight the tendency of CWP to progress after diagnosis and certification. The results indicated that over one third of pneumoconiotics certified in 1948 suffered further deterioration in lung function by 1951 *after* their diagnosis and certification.[82] This was influential in getting the notion of 'progression'

---

79 National Joint Pneumoconiosis Committee (NJPC), Minutes, 17 April 1956, NA/POWE8/422.

80 NJPC, Minutes, 17 January 1957, NA/POWE8/422.

81 Ibid.

82 D.D. Evans, 'A Survey of the Incidence and Progression of Pneumoconiosis', pp. 13–14; *The Miner*, vol. 8, no. 3 (May/June 1960), p. 13. This research was severely

accepted by the late 1950s (that is, the fact that the disease could advance and loss of lung function proceed, even after the patient had been removed from the dusty environment). Later, one Scottish study in the 1960s showed almost a quarter of retired miners in Scotland to be pneumoconiotics, challenging other evidence which tended to underestimate the extent of this social problem in mining communities. We also noted in Chapter 6 how the NUM was also initiating research into the design of dust masks and respirators, including the then (1960s) state-of-the-art Air Stream helmet, sometimes in the face of criticism from rank-and-file members that such equipment restricted productivity.[83] By this point, the routine utilisation of medical knowledge by the NUM was formalised further with the appointment of Dr Andrew Meiklejohn (Senior Lecturer in Industrial Health at the University of Glasgow and an expert on pneumoconiosis) as its honorary medical adviser.[84]

The NUM also made a vital contribution in energising the community to provide full support for the major epidemiological studies of pneumoconiosis in the 1950s. This was recognised by one of the medical experts, Julian Tudor Hart, who recalled that the support of the NUM was crucial to the success of the Rhondda Fach project:

> Archie [Cochrane] had got round the National Union of Miners (NUM) which was a very important force in South Wales at that time, and if Dai Dan Evans had not been persuaded that this was in the interests of the miners, and that it wasn't only for the cause of humanity – which he actually cared quite a lot about – but also that it met the immediate needs of the miners and their families, nothing ever would have happened. You would have had a 3 per cent response rate, instead of a 97 per cent response, or whatever it was.[85]

The same applied to the Pneumoconiosis Field Research (PFR). In Scotland, this was publicised by the NUM; miners were urged to co-operate; assurances were given that all x-ray reports and medical evidence were to be completely confidential, and the union lobbied successfully to have the notoriously dusty Northfield Colliery in Shotts in Lanarkshire (an anthracite mine) added to the original list of pits selected. As early as the 1920s, the Shotts pits were unpopular because of their reputation for intensively dusty coal seams. Hence the NUM endorsed the 1954 research project and played a significant role in the coverage of the epidemiological survey and its administration in the 1950s and 1960s. Pressure from the NUM also succeeded in getting some of the restrictive clauses of the 1943 legislation amended, including

criticised by the NCB, which claimed this could have been caused by the men's non-mining occupations after they left the industry.

83 Information supplied by Danny O'Connor, NUM member of the National Joint Pneumoconiosis Committee in the 1970s. We are grateful to Danny, and to Susan Morrison for this reference.

84 NUM (South Wales Area), Minutes of Executive Council Meeting, 22 December 1959, pp. 1,258–9.

85 Testimony of Dr Julian Hart, Wellcome Institute for the History of Medicine, Witness Seminar. *The MRC Epidemiology Unit (South Wales)*, vol. 13 (November 2002), p. 22; henceforth Wellcome Witness Seminar, 2002.

the controversial dismissal policy. From 1951, rather than being dismissed, pneumoconiotic miners could be re-employed either in 'approved' processes away from the face underground, or at the surface in designated 'non-dusty' jobs.

From very early on the NUM also campaigned for stricter dust exposure limits. In 1960, D.D. Evans, the then General Secretary of the South Wales NUM, suggested in *The Miner* that if the 300 p.p.c.c. standard was possible to achieve in haematite mines, then the same standard could and should be put into place throughout the whole coal industry.[86] At the 1960 Annual Conference of the South Wales NUM a resolution demanding a rejection of the 850/650/450 p.p.c.c. standard was carried unanimously. In its place, the union demanded that until 'a sound medical appraisal of safe conditions' became available, a standard of 450 p.p.c.c. from ½ to 5 microns for coal and 250 p.p.c.c. from ½ to 5 microns for stone should be adopted. The following year, the National Conference of the NUM carried this resolution unanimously. However, as we saw in Chapter 6, nothing was done by the NCB at this time, partly because it was awaiting the PFR producing evidence on which a new dust datum could be based.

The miners' unions kept the pressure up. In 1963, another article in *The Miner* reported on a recent survey undertaken by the NUM of ten collieries in South Wales in which it was found that 1,047 men had suffered a progression of their disease while working in the NCB's so-called 'dust-approved' conditions. This survey also found that 30 of these men were under the age of 34, indicating that they had been exposed to fairly recent unhealthy working conditions.[87] Moreover, the following year the head of the union's Safety Department suggested that a standard of 450 p.p.c.c. between 1 and 5 microns for all coal dusts should be adopted.[88] Clearly, then, when we evaluate the significance of the miners' trade union in protesting against the dust issue, it has to be acknowledged that sustained pressure was kept on the NCB for some time, notably by the South Wales district of the NUM.

However, on the negative side, in 1961 the NUM forged an agreement with the NCB that workers paid on a day wage basis, such as maintenance men, electricians and so on, would receive an extra 1s. 6d. a shift for working in non-approved conditions. Somewhat ironically, this 'dust money' was to be paid when conditions exceeded the safe limit agreed for approved working faces –850 p.p.c.c. between 1 and 5 microns in size.[89] Although this agreement was adopted nationally, the South Wales Division of the NUM did not accept the principle. Indeed, the Secretary of one union lodge in South Wales called for an immediate Area Conference to discuss what he saw as a move towards 'organized murder'.[90] A letter in *The Miner* also expressed dissatisfaction:

---

86 *The Miner* (November/December 1960), p. 5.

87 *The Miner* (May/June 1963), p. 6.

88 *The Miner* (November/December 1964), p. 16.

89 NUM, Annual Conference 1961, *Report of National Executive Committee*, pp. 48–9.

90 NUM (South Wales Area), Minutes of Area Executive Council Meeting, 15 August 1961, p. 659. This is indicative perhaps of the consensus politics of the NUM National

I am rather disgusted and shocked to read that an agreement has been signed for payment of an allowance for working in dust … I personally believe that by implementing this agreement a lot of miners will be going to their graves a lot earlier.[91]

Undoubtedly, the pneumoconiosis issue was tackled more vigorously by the mining unions in some districts than in others. South Wales and Scotland appear to have had a particularly high profile. Here, there was an entrenched tradition of militant collective action and more rigorous local activist surveillance of the work environment. Miners from these areas who moved to work in other coal fields were struck by the differences. The following dialogue between interviewer and two Scottish miners, George Bolton and David Carruthers, provides an example:

> GB: I think it's fair to say this. In Scotland, a different approach from the NUM in Scotland to safety and health and the rest of it. See down South, down South [gasps], unbelievable … *Much worse*. I mean, there were men cutting without water.
> NR: Why was it worse down there, do you think? Are you saying England generally, George, or are you saying certain areas?
> GB: No, I worked in Stoke-on-Trent, it was bloody awful.
> NR: Was that because the union was of a different culture or …?
> GB: Didn't exist properly, it really – it didn't exist in a certain sense, the men were on their own and men are very fearless on their own. Me, I worked on a stone mine with the blast borers for the drills – no water. Mining with dust often with a low boring machine – 'Keep going, Jock,' you know, 'Come on, come on, keep going, Jock.' Shocking stuff. Through a middle cut machine, no water. You imagine a machine up there throwing all the dust out.
> NR: Just what you said there about keeping on working, why was that part of the culture, do you think?
> GB: It was just the lack of good trade union, how things developed.
> DC: I would say money at the end of the day.
> GB: There was money, but there was also a bad culture. In Stoke-on-Trent, the men werenae, they were not union-conscious. I remember working on a road, went out on strike one day, see when the place turned – other men doing the job for us [laughs] … that wouldn't happen in Scotland, but it happened in Stoke-on-Trent and elsewhere in England. Different approach to trade unionism. That applies to Yorkshire too, apparently, they're not as clever as they thought they were. They're very clever in Scotland, and I think also in South Wales to some extent, from what I know of it, union-conscious, safety-conscious, dust-conscious – really, really conscious. So that difference applied.[92]

Apart from vigilance in the workplace to ensure preventative measures were applied, union support in compensation struggles, sponsorship of research and educative work, the miners' unions were active in extending treatment and

---

Executive Conference at this time. Because the policy was that only three resolutions could be forwarded from the Areas up to the Annual Conference, health and safety issues tended to get squeezed out of national policy, with wages and job preservation prioritised. See Taylor, *The NUM and British Politics*, p. 7.

91 *The Miner* (September/October 1961), p. 10.
92 George Bolton and David Carruthers, Interview C23 (SOHC).

rehabilitation facilities. There were problems in the mid-1950s with the lack of specialist medical expertise and the extent of misdiagnosis. For example, through 1956–58, the Scottish Area NUM lobbied the Department of Health for Scotland to increase specialist chest clinics, the number of trained physicians, and expand into undertaking research on lung disease in miners by establishing a pneumoconiosis research unit in Scotland. This campaign produced a number of positive results, including the creation of three main pneumoconiosis clinics in Bangour Hospital (West Lothian, 15 beds), Belvidere Hospital (Glasgow, 20 beds) and Bridge of Earn Hospital (Perthshire, for the Fife coal field, 5 beds). These were supported by 36 'preliminary' clinics located in the Scottish coal fields, where a chest physician specialising in pneumoconiosis was in attendance. Research was also developed in three Scottish teaching hospitals in Glasgow, Edinburgh and Dundee, though the Scottish miners never got the specialised research unit to rival the PRU at Cardiff that they hoped for.[93]

The miners' unions were also actively involved in rehabilitation, convalescence and therapy for disabled miners. The NUM pressed hard for the re-employment of partially disabled miners and the creation of alternative jobs for pneumoconiotics after the Second World War, resulting in ten special factories being erected in South Wales by 1948 especially for these disabled workers.[94] A number of convalescent homes and rehabilitation centres for injured miners also existed in the 1940s, run jointly by representatives of the NUM and the National Coal Board (NCB). In Scotland, there were eight such homes (interestingly, four catering for the convalescence of men, and four specifically for women) together with the Miners' Rehabilitation Centre at Uddingston, near Glasgow, which opened during the Second World War. In these centres, physiotherapists applied new medical knowledge on occupational therapy, and in an era when precise medical knowledge was often withheld from patients, some units played an important role in informing disabled miners about the nature of their impairment. The Mabon Club in South Wales – run by the social welfare arm of the Pneumoconiosis Research Unit (PRU) and supported by the South Wales NUM – would be the outstanding example. The NUM also provided financial assistance to support studies of the viability of drug combination treatments for pneumoconiotics.[95]

Recent accounts have stressed the consensual nature of mining trade union politics in the early years of nationalisation.[96] This is also evident in the politics of occupational health in coal mining. Beyond the shop floor, at the policy-making level, much of the union's activity on dust disease was directed through the National Joint Pneumoconiosis Committee. As we noted earlier (see Chapter 4), this body was formed just after the end of the Second World War to advise the newly created

---

   93 Report of meeting at Scottish NCB, Edinburgh, March 1956, NAS/HH104/46, p. 34 in file.
   94 NUM, South West Area Council, *Annual Conference Report* (1946–47), pp. 47–8.
   95 NJPC Minutes, 17 May 1961, NA/LAB 14/799.
   96 See Taylor, *The NUM and British Politics, Volume 1, 1944–1968.*

NCB (1947), and included representation from the NUM, the Ministry of Fuel and Power, the Mines Inspectorate and the PRU. This was a key committee through which medical knowledge and new research findings percolated to the member constituencies and through which the unions exerted influence on policy-making. Its work up to the 1970s suggests that much of what the union wanted was achieved through such consensual mechanisms, rather than confrontation with the NCB. The union view was brought in at all levels through the main NJPC and the various sub-committees established. This included representation and input into the working of the Medical Panels and medical treatment for pneumoconiosis and dust control (including the design of the 25-pit Field Research Scheme). Where the unions appear to have been most active, however, was in the Employment and Rehabilitation Sub-Committee. It had less influence on dust suppression, and appears to have played a largely reactive rather than proactive role. The minutes of the NJPC indicate that it was the government, the PRU and the NCB that played the most dynamic role in this pivotal forum. The NJPC was part of the coal industry consultative machinery on which the union represented the voice of labour. First and foremost, however, dust control was perceived to be the responsibility of the NCB. The dynamics operating within the NJPC were clearly indicated in 1957 when the NCB, as part of its new 1956 protocol, initiated a revised dust standard, based on average dust counts throughout a shift, as opposed to the existing system based on the average during periods of maximum dustiness on the face. The Ministry of Power accused the NCB of trying to lower the dust standard, and the NUM called for an emergency meeting of the Committee to examine the facts. Rogan of the NCB denied any reduction in the dust datum, revealed that the NCB and the Ministry were in discussions, and that the NUM and MRC would be consulted 'before any final documentation was prepared'.[97] This provides some support for Taylor's assertion that in the 1950s, 'the NCB retained control over major economic and technical decision making and although the NUM was consulted, its views were not accorded the same weight and status as "expert" opinion'.[98]

Brothers in Arms: The Trade Union Congress, the NUM and Dust Disease

The wider trade union movement represented by the British Trade Union Congress (TUC) played an important supportive role in the campaigns to control dust and compensate miners. By the early 1950s, the TUC was arguing strongly that failure to provide cover for bronchitis and emphysema was a major weakness of the National Insurance system. Within this system, the prime consideration regarding the scheduling of diseases was that they had to be clearly occupationally caused. This was a principle which rested on deep historical foundations, and stemmed from the inclusion of the first industrial diseases under the Workmen's Compensation Scheme. In 1905, the House of Lords decreed that if it was conclusively proven

---

97 NJPC Minutes, 17 December 1957, NA/POWE8/422.
98 Taylor, *The NUM and British Politics, Volume 1, 1944–1968*, p. 114.

that a disease had been contracted by an occurrence which could be classed as an *accident*, such a disease could be classified as an injury under the 1897 Workmen's Compensation Act. This led to the 1906 Workmen's Compensation Act, which included six industrial diseases, to which the Home Secretary had the power to add more. However, the question of how to decide whether further diseases were worthy of inclusion under the act remained problematic, and in 1907 a Committee was appointed under Herbert Samuel – eventually to become Lord Samuel – to examine this very issue. The conclusion of the Samuel Committee was that three tests were accepted as being rigid enough to underpin scheduling:

1. Was the disease outside the category of accidents and diseases already covered?
2. Did it incapacitate from work for more than the minimum period for which compensation was payable under the Act?
3. Was it so specific to the employment that causation by the employment could be established in individual cases?

The upshot of this was that diseases which were associated with occupation but which were also common in the general population could not be scheduled. Indeed, in the light of these three tests, the Samuel Committee went on to schedule only 18 of the 43 diseases it was asked to consider. However, for the duration of the Workmen's Compensation Scheme, workers could still obtain compensation for any disease – whether it was scheduled or not – if it could be demonstrated beyond doubt that it had been contracted by an accident. Therefore, diseases such as tetanus, cattle ringworm, yellow fever or blood poisoning caused by a cut or abrasion at work were all accepted as being industrial diseases.

In 1946, the Industrial Injuries Act replaced the Workmen's Compensation Scheme. This greatly extended the scope of the old industrial compensation scheme, and by the 1950s over 20 million workers were covered. The two main benefits paid out under the new system were Injury Benefit, paid to persons incapacitated by industrial injury or industrial disease for up to six months, and Disablement Benefit to workers who were so disabled for more than six months. Under the scheme, it was also possible for workers to claim a Special Hardship Allowance for periods in which their ailment prevented them pursuing their regular occupation or work of an equivalent standard.

However, as far as any addition to the list of industrial diseases was concerned, this was still to be determined by Samuel's three tests. In March 1947, a Departmental Committee was set up, chaired by E.T. Dale, to advise on the principles governing the selection of diseases for insurance under the National Insurance (Industrial Injuries) Act – this was the same judge who would later chair a committee to examine occupational health provision, discussed in Chapter 6. The TUC sent a Memorandum to the Dale Committee suggesting important changes to the system, and one of its main recommendations was that compensation should be paid, not only to those who could show their injury was caused by an accident, 'but equally to those who can show that they are suffering from a disease caused or aggravated by their employment'.[99] The TUC was especially concerned at the third of the Samuel Committee tests – that the disease is 'so specific to the employment that causation ... could be established in individual cases?' – and strongly recommended that this clause by abolished. Indeed, the TUC had fought against the principle of this test for some time: first of all in 1933, and then in 1939 when it gave evidence before the Royal Commission on Workmen's Compensation.[100]

The Dale Committee was also being pressurised by the TUC towards extending the system of compensation for dust disease. This had also been an issue with the TUC for some time. Indeed, in 1945 the TUC put a strong case to the Minister of Labour, the Home Office and the Ministry of National Insurance to extend the pneumoconiosis scheme to include all coal workers, and to introduce similar schemes to cover damage caused by other industrial dusts. Interestingly, the TUC was told by the government in 1945 that it would not be able to extend the scheme for at least two years, and that this was because the prevalence of pneumoconiosis in South Wales was so high that all available medical personnel were concentrated there.[101] The TUC's representation to the Dale Committee in 1947, then, was an opportunity to resume its campaign:

The following are the general criticisms which we [the TUC] have made against the scheme in the past:

1. The need for a single comprehensive scheme to cover industrial lung diseases generally. We regarded the Coal Mining Industry (Pneumoconiosis) Scheme, introduced in 1943, as a step in the right direction, but have constantly pressed for its extension to cover, not only all coal workers, but also all those exposed to other dust hazards.
2. The technical restrictions which confine the right to compensation to those engaged in particular processes.
3. The artificial time limits laid down in the Scheme ...

We wish ... to emphasise that in our view a drastic overhaul of the schemes is urgently needed... What is required is the abolition of the whole structure of separate schemes and extension of the existing Pneumoconiosis Scheme in such a way that it will cover all those exposed to dust hazards.

The Dale Committee rejected these recommendations. However, its conclusion did leave the door open for the future inclusion of diseases such as bronchitis, as its recommendation was that the primary consideration for the prescription of a disease should be:

Whether a disease is specific to the occupations of the persons concerned, or, if it is not so specific, whether the occupations of those persons cause special exposure to the risk of

---

99 TUC, *Congress Report* (1948), p. 130.
100 Ibid.
101 TUC, *Congress Report* (1945), p. 84.

the disease, such risks being inherent in the conditions under which the occupations are carried on.[102]

This at least was a chink of light in the usual pitch-black refusal to accept that diseases which were widespread throughout the population could not under any circumstances be accepted as industrial.

Undeterred by the government's failure to extend the pneumoconiosis scheme to include workers other than coal miners, the TUC set out to strengthen its case by generating its own knowledge base. This involved undertaking a large-scale survey of dust disease in non-prescribed occupations led by its medical adviser, Dr A. Meiklejohn. Five centres were set up throughout the UK to which trade unions were asked to refer suspected pneumoconiosis cases – the centres were in South Wales, Durham, South Staffordshire, Manchester and Glasgow.[103] The results of this survey verified that the problem was significant: 36 workers in non-scheduled occupations including fireclay processes, boiler scaling and coal handling, were found to be suffering from pneumoconiosis.[104] Following this revelation, the TUC issued a report to the IIAC calling once again for an extension of the scheme. This time the pressure – supported as it was by hard evidence – was successful, and in January 1953 the Industrial Injuries Act was altered in line with TUC demands. Once again, then, the labour movement had successfully utilised medical knowledge to challenge the inadequacy of the compensation system, although, again, it had been a tough fight.

Trade union pressure regarding dust disease was also apparent in yet another committee set up to decide whether or not to extend the scope of the Industrial Injuries Act to include additional diseases. This committee was chaired by the solicitor F.W. Beney, and thus became known as the Beney Committee. Between 1953 and 1955, the Committee met 21 times and gathered information from 28 organisations, including the NCB, the TUC, the British Medical Association, the British Employers' Federation and relevant government departments. Amongst its 12 members were the doctors Sir E.R. Carling, L.G. Norman and A. Stewart, and three trade unionists, including the titled Sir W. Lawther and Sir A. Roberts. Although the committee's terms of reference were to examine industrial disease provision *per se*, the TUC submitted a proposal to the Committee calling specifically for bronchitis and rheumatism to be included under the industrial injuries system. Consequently, the committee focused significant attention on these conditions.

However, after two years of deliberation the majority of the members of the Beney committee decided that there should be no extension to existing provision. As we noted in Chapter 5, the three trade union members disagreed. Consequently, majority and minority reports were produced. The main stumbling block for the majority of the

102 *Report of the Departmental Committee Appointed to Review the Disease Provision of the National Insurance (Industrial Injuries) Act, 1955*, Cmd. 9548 (hereafter Beney Committee), 'Majority Report', p. 5.

103 TUC, *Congress Report* (1951), p. 153.

104 TUC, *Congress Report* (1953), p. 146.

committee was the necessity and great difficulty of clearly determining that diseases were occupationally caused – a principle which underpinned the whole *raison d être* of the Industrial Injuries system. Clearly, the majority of the Beney Committee fully realised the class-related nature of many diseases not accepted as industrial:

> It is, for instance, an established fact that certain common diseases – notably pneumonia, bronchitis and emphysema – are as causes of death, more common amongst persons whose lives are spent in generally unfavourable conditions than among persons who enjoy a high standard of living. Laboratory work has also shown that certain noxious influences – which include exposure to extreme heat or cold, prolonged immersion in water and the inhaling of heavily contaminated atmospheres – damage living tissues and either render them unduly sensitive to attack by bacteria, viruses etc., or cause premature decay.

The minority of the Beney Committee were also clear on what should be done about bronchitis and rheumatism:

> 1. The aim should be to provide cover for older workers who have spent the greater part of their working lives in jobs carrying a special risk of these diseases involving, e.g., excessive exposure to dust or fume, or wet or cramped working conditions.
> 2. It would be reasonable to limit cover by reference to degree of disability and duration of exposure.
> 3. Claims should be dealt with by a specially qualified medical board, as in the case of pneumoconiosis.

Interestingly, one of the things driving trade union action on this was the knowledge that in 1952, an amendment to South Africa's silicosis compensation scheme had allowed compensation to be paid to miners with a certain type of pulmonary disability, defined as 'impairment of the cardio-respiratory system'. According to the South African Bureau of Mines, this condition could substantially and permanently diminish a miner's capacity to work, and crucially, could result 'from the performance of work in a dusty occupation'.[105]

The decision of the Minister of National Insurance to accept the majority recommendations of the Beney Committee was criticised by the TUC, and its 1954 Congress reaffirmed its determination to secure cover for chronic bronchitis and rheumatism.[106] Moreover, in 1957 at the TUC's annual conference, a NACODS delegate moved that emphysema should be included as a scheduled disease – a motion which was seconded by Abe Moffat of the NUM.[107] The following year, an NUM delegate, J.R.A. Machen, expressed his union's full support for this motion, and also voiced his concern at the lack of progress on the issue of compensation for lung damage to miners other than for pneumoconiosis. He gave a very accurate and

---

105 Beney Committee, 'Minority Report', p. 27. We examined the influence of South Africa in relation to medical knowledge on dust disease in Chapter 3.

106 TUC, *Congress Report* (1956), p. 147.

107 TUC, *Congress Report* (1958), p. 128.

sardonic historical overview of the less than dependable nature of medical science in relation to dust disease in the pits:

> We miners have very great respect for the medical profession, but we cannot ignore the historical facts, and our minds go back to the twenties in connection with dust disease. In the twenties we were told by the medical profession of this country and by scientists too, that not only was coal dust not deleterious, not only was it not a danger, but that in fact it was a prophylactic, that it was one of the reasons why tuberculosis was less prevalent in mining areas than in other areas. We proceed from that time to the thirties and what happened in South Africa ... where they were dealing with silica rock. That led to the basis of what happened in this country, because South Africa recognized the problem arising from silica rock. That led to the basis of what happened in this country ... For another 10 or 13 years until 1943 men puffed their lungs out and died in their thousands from the fact that they had in their lungs this dust which the scientists and the medical men were telling us was not harmful ...[108]

At this time, the NUM was conducting its own inquiry into the assessment and diagnosis of pneumoconiosis.[109] The survey was initiated out of a concern with the different standards of the various Pneumoconiosis Medical Boards regarding disablement, and involved Dr L Howells, Consultant Physician of the United Cardiff Hospitals and the Welsh Regional Hospital Board, who conducted interviews at nine Pneumoconiosis Panels throughout the UK. By 1959, the report was complete and made several recommendations:

> 1. New legislation should be introduced to recognise general emphysema and chronic bronchitis occurring in the presence of pneumoconiosis as industrial hazards.
> 2. New legislation should be introduced to permit the right of an appeal against diagnosis under agreed conditions.

Moreover, as far as death claims were concerned:

> 1. Key centres should be established throughout the country for the performance of post-mortem examinations by a consultant pathologist.
> 2. Post-mortem preparation and examination of the lungs should be by the 'Gough Technique'.
> 3. Members of the Pneumoconiosis Medical Panels should consult with the pathologist who performed the post-mortem in every case.
> 4. New legislation should be introduced to recognise general emphysema and bronchitis as industrial hazards when pneumoconiosis is present as well.[110]

Following the publication of the NUM's report, in May 1959 a TUC deputation – which included Dr Howells – met the Minister of National Insurance to demand the implementation of these proposals. The following year, the Ministry announced that it

---

108 Ibid., p. 344.
109 Ibid., p. 343.
110 TUC, *Congress Report* (1959), pp. 150–51.

was carrying out a large-scale statistical study into the occupational and geographical incidence of a number of diseases, including bronchitis. The arrangements for this survey began in June 1961 when the sickness records of a representative sample of workers in different occupations – covering around 800,000 workers – were analysed, with the main diseases under scrutiny being bronchitis, rheumatism and arthritis, and certain forms of mental illnesses. It was hoped that this would provide a much-needed picture of the distribution of illness in working communities.[111]

Therefore, by the early 1960s the TUC and the NUM were certain there was a clear link between pneumoconiosis and bronchitis, and was pushing strongly for bronchitis and emphysema to be treated as industrial diseases when these conditions were accompanied by pneumoconiosis. The TUC also suggested that too much reliance was being placed on the use of x-rays, which it suggested did not give a true representation of total lung function.[112] The evidence was gathering strength, and was further reinforced in 1961 when the NCB's Pneumoconiosis Field Research found an association between the prevalence rates of pneumoconiosis and other respiratory symptoms at a number of collieries.[113]

The determination to utilise medical expertise to counter inconsistencies in compensation procedure, and sometimes to directly challenge medical orthodoxy, was a recurrent strategy of the miners' trade unions and the TUC. A similar scenario occurred in 1964 when the TUC's General Council suggested to the Minister of Pensions and National Insurance that its Medical Adviser, accompanied by Andrew Meiklejohn (the NUM Medical Adviser), be allowed to visit the Pneumoconiosis Panels to study their standards of diagnosis and assessment. The survey of the nine centres – London, Cardiff, Swansea, Birmingham, Stoke-on-Trent, Sheffield, Newcastle upon Tyne, Edinburgh and Glasgow – was completed in 1964. The two doctors were reasonably satisfied that the panels' investigations were fairly thorough, and that when there were doubtful claims, it was generally the claimant who was favoured. However, despite this, there were still considerable inconsistencies regarding the acceptance and rejection of compensation claims. The main revelations of the study were: there was a lack of uniformity between the panels at the initial stage of scrutiny; there was a shortage of staff, and this was restricting attendance at post-mortems, curtailing field research and hindering communication; also, the panels – according to the investigating medics – were largely certifying bodies with little interest in the *prevention* of lung disease. The outcome of this reconnaissance was that the TUC immediately recommended to the Ministry of National Insurance that it set up a specific unit for pneumoconiosis claims; that Ministry staff make regular visits to the panels to check on standards; that the number of staff at the panels be increased; that the work of the panels be widened out so that staff had the opportunity to act as consultants; that the Ministry publish annual statistical reports

---

111 TUC, *Congress Report* (1961), p. 146.
112 TUC, *Congress Report* (1963), p. 173.
113 TUC, *Congress Report* (1962), p. 137.

on the work of the panels, and that the Ministry publish a pamphlet clearly explaining the law relating to pneumoconiosis.[114]

The NUM and the TUC were also deeply concerned that a system of appeals be set up – similar to those for other industrial injuries – for those men who had been refused certification, and that independent experts needed to be brought in to the system. An NUM delegate at the TUC's 1965 Conference made this point forcibly:

> A man who is about to be hanged does not appeal to the hangman, because he is not likely to get any redress from him. Who are you going to appeal to? You can only appeal to doctors … We should not be appealing to the people who have come to the first decision; we should be appealing to a body which – shall I say – is consultative at least and is not concerned only with the day-to-day running of the establishment.[115]

However, in August 1965 the TUC was told by the Ministry of National Insurance (MNI) that although it was looking into ways of introducing some sort of appeals system, the introduction of a formal statutory appeal procedure would be far too difficult to put into place. In any case, according to the MNI, the Pneumoconiosis Medical Boards were highly expert bodies, and this meant that any appeal specialists would need to have greater knowledge of the disease that the medical board doctors – and this was clearly impractical.[116]

The MNI eventually bowed to labour movement pressure and announced that new arrangements were to be introduced and some changes made to the system. These included the setting up of a special panel consisting of senior pneumoconiosis doctors of the Ministry, together with senior chest specialists. This special panel, though, would only examine sufferers of chest disability whose previous claims had been twice rejected and who could produce a statement from a chest physician that they were indeed suffering from pneumoconiosis. Also, the special panels would examine those death claims in which there was a conflict between findings in life and findings in death. A six-month pilot of the new arrangements was put in place in Cardiff in 1967, and by August of that year, of the 130 men examined by the new central board – men whose claims had already been rejected – 14, around 10% of them, were found to indeed be suffering from pneumoconiosis, and were subsequently assessed at between 10% and 30%. The following year, the government announced that the scheme would be extended to the whole country.[117]

These were certainly moves in the right direction. However, the proposals were criticised by NACODS for not going far enough, and the union demanded that similar Appeal Boards to those already in place for industrial injuries be introduced for dealing with pneumoconiosis. What was driving this demand was the need to prevent the progression of the disease:

---

114 TUC, *Congress Report* (1965), p. 171.

115 Ibid., p. 427.

116 TUC, *Congress Report* (1967), p. 178.

117 TUC, *Congress Report* (1968), pp. 201–2.

What we want is to avoid this disease being progressive, by having an accurate diagnosis in its early stages, and then the workman can change his employment and work in dust-approved conditions. The National Coal Board is doing everything possible regarding dust suppression, but, nevertheless, there are cases on coal faces where it is virtually impossible to suppress the dust ... I was amazed when the medical profession admitted that there was inconsistency in the reading of x-ray plates ... Surely in cases such as I have outlined there is every reason for provision to be made to submit disputed cases to an independent body, and we believe that this independent body ought to be independent all together from the medical panel. By all means let us have expert chest doctors on the panel, and also representatives from the trade union.[118]

Despite the seriousness of the appeals issue, the main gripe of the TUC and the miners' union at this time was the exclusion of bronchitis and emphysema from the compensation legislation. To recap, by the mid-1960s under the Industrial Injuries Act pneumoconiosis medical boards decided whether men were suffering from pneumoconiosis as defined by the act. However, this definition – which was based on fibrosis of the lung – excluded chronic bronchitis and emphysema. Consequently, men suffering from these diseases but who were not judged to have pneumoconiosis were denied industrial injury benefit. Moreover, men who were diagnosed as having pneumoconiosis and who also had bronchitis and emphysema could not be assessed for their total disablement resulting from the combination of the diseases – although some Boards did increase the assessment for pneumoconiosis if its symptoms had been worsened by other respiratory disabilities. For the TUC, this was a sorry state of affairs, and it urged that as a first step, bronchitis and emphysema, when accompanied by pneumoconiosis, should be treated as part of the prescribed disease. As we saw in Chapter 5, in 1966 the government introduced a watered-down version of a Private Member's Bill, the proposals of which were quite similar to that put forward by the TUC's General Council. Consequently, from May 1967, any men diagnosed as being over 50% disabled by pneumoconiosis were allowed to have their accompanying bronchitis and emphysema treated as part of the disease – the number of men falling in to this category of 50% disablement or above at this time was between 3,000 and 4,000 out of a total of around 50,000 assessed with pneumoconiosis.[119] However, although welcoming the changes which the new Act brought about, the TUC did not think that it went far enough:

While fully recognizing the part played by air pollution, cigarette smoking and social conditions not connected with work in the causation and aggravation of bronchitis they have always contended that many men and women in occupations involving excessive exposure to dust and fumes are suffering respiratory problems due to their work and not at present recognized under the Industrial Injuries Act.[120]

118 TUC, *Congress Report* (1967), p. 425.
119 Ibid., p. 183.
120 Ibid.

Clearly, then, once again trade union pressure was acting as a substantial counterweight to intransigent medical and political opinion regarding the non-classification of an industrial disease. Moreover, although we saw in Chapter 6 that the NCB persisted in its adherence to the system of dust approved conditions, the TUC was made fully aware of the shortcomings and dangers of this policy. Indeed, in 1968 the General Council of the TUC expressed its deep dissatisfaction to the Minister of Social Security regarding men suffering from early pneumoconiosis who had been advised by the Pneumoconiosis Panels to work in approved conditions – the standard of which did not guarantee that there would be no risk for these men. Not only that, though, the TUC also recommended that if such men decided to give up work at the coal face, then they should be entitled to claim Special Hardship Allowance.[121] An NUM delegate at the 1969 Congress voiced the union's concern over this, saying that denying men the opportunity of getting off the coal face – without suffering severe financial loss – was tantamount to 'asking them to commit suicide'. He went on to illustrate the financial necessities which many coal face workers faced:

> When a man has 10 per cent pneumoconiosis assessment it all depends on his physical condition whether he can remain at the coalface or go from there ... because when he is a face worker filling coal at the rate of 20 tons a day he can earn anything up to £30 a week. Then he contracts this dreaded disease ... and he is forced to take a light job. A light job on the surface at Cwm Colliery at the moment is about £13 8s a week, half his earnings on the coalface. Yet the Minister denies this man hardship allowance. I think he is entirely wrong.[122]

We saw earlier how in 1958 an NUM delegate at the TUC annual conference utilised historical narrative to hammer home his point that the miners had been short-changed by the medical profession over the issue of coal dust disease. This strategy of using historical knowledge to illustrate the inconsistencies in medical orthodoxy was a powerful one, and was put to good use by the TUC in 1969 when it submitted a detailed memorandum to the IIAC calling for a comprehensive reassessment of chest diseases due to industrial causes. The memorandum traced the development of compensation for industrial lung damage from 1918, and highlighted how a number of factors had been responsible for the snail's pace of development. These included:

> The gradual build up of medical knowledge, the unwillingness of individual employers to accept liability under their workmen's compensation system, excessive concentration on silica dust – which had led the MRC to report in 1934 that they did not regard coal dust as a cause of pneumoconiosis – and restrictions resulting from the legislature's evident concern to exclude possible compensation for non-occupational cases.[123]

---

121 TUC, *Congress Report* (1968), p. 202.
122 TUC, *Congress Report* (1969), pp. 542–3.
123 TUC, *Congress Report* (1970), p. 273.

Therefore, not only did organised labour frequently enlist professional expertise to challenge accepted medical knowledge regarding dust disease, it also demonstrated a sound understanding of the historical development of medical awareness of miners' lung, as well as the stilted evolution of industrial compensation. It could be argued, then, that by acting as a valuable repository for lay knowledge of medical issues, professional expertise and historical knowledge of miners' respiratory disease, organised labour was considerably empowered.

By the early 1970s, the TUC were still pressing the IIAC for 'a comprehensive re-examination of chest diseases due to industrial causes', continuing to argue the case against the restrictive definition of pneumoconiosis, and pressing for a redefinition to encapsulate 'any pulmonary disorder arising from inhalation of industrial contaminants'.[124] They continued to campaign for miners to get Special Hardship Allowance when they left higher-paid face work on diagnosis of pneumoconiosis, for the removal of the 50% pneumoconiosis accompanying bronchitis and emphysema regulation, and more importantly, to amass medical evidence to contest the MRC view (expressed in their report in 1966 – see Chapter 5) that bronchitis could not be attributable directly to occupational dust exposure.[125] The IIAC Majority Report in October 1973 rejected all these claims, however, and went on to recommend to the government the introduction of limitations on benefit in the early stages of pneumoconiosis, reflecting growing medical opinion that diagnoses of up to 10% pneumoconiosis did not necessarily mean any disablement of lung function.[126] Whilst the government rejected any reduction in benefit for early-stage pneumoconiosis and in 1975 finally introduced a statutory right of appeal against Medical Panel decisions of pneumoconiosis diagnosis, it continued to stand firm on the rejection of improved benefits (Income Support) for those pneumoconiotics who left higher-paid face work and to categorically refuse any inclusion of bronchitis and emphysema in the list of prescribed diseases.[127] The unions had to wait a further two decades before this particular breakthrough was achieved.

The Miners' Union in the Workplace

In the workplace, it was the rank-and-file union activists, including those appointed as workmen's inspectors, who ensured a high degree of vigilance over dust control. The discourse here was frequently critical of the union leadership for not going far enough, and quickly enough. For example, Alec Mills, a Communist and Scottish NUM local activist, replied thus in response to a question about how his colleagues felt about union action on dust:

124 Ibid.; TUC, *Congress Report* (1971), p. 127.

125 TUC, *Congress Report* (1970), p. 274. The evidence included a study of foundry workers in 1970.

126 TUC, *Congress Report* (1974), pp.102–4.

127 Ibid., pp. 103–4; TUC, *Congress Report* (1975), pp. 139–40.

Angry. Angry. We never ever went on strike. We never went on strike for masks. But we should have went on strike for masks. A lot of men would be alive today if they had been provided with masks.[128]

He emphasised repeatedly that the miners were relatively powerless to resist the productionist ethos of the NCB in the 1950s and 1960s and also provided much evidence of blatant breaches of dust standards at the coal face. None the less, whilst a certain level of dust was widely considered to be an acceptable and inevitable part of the job, excessively dusty conditions were challenged and miners' officials, and workmen's inspectors like Mills played an important role in protecting miners at the coal face. One colleague of Mills, who was later promoted to pit deputy and oversman, recognised this important role, and the power of the local activists, in response to being questioned about what the unions did on the dust problem:

A lot. A lot. 'Cause they kept shouting. That man kept [pointing to Alec Mills] … He roasted them. I mean, he did it when I was a deputy. Eh, the management would say, 'Alec Mills wants such a thing here and such a thing.' I had to get it done. I mean, if the likes of him hadnae been there, nobody would have bothered.[129]

One Scottish NUM official, R. Farquhar, described in a report how such workplace regulation operated when new technology significantly altered environmental conditions underground:

After a period of over five years' experience on mechanised faces, plus 23 years on conventional hand stripping, I have examined and discovered by complaints from our workmen of excessive dust that every Anderton shearer operating in out face lines required additional adjustments to minimise the dust content in the air current. No later than five weeks ago a new type of machine was introduced into our colliery, the first one and, I believe, the only one in Scotland. This is a Ranger shearer machine, which shears the top half of the seam in one direction along the face and shears the bottom half of the seam 6 feet 9 inches high on the return from the tailgate to the main gate of the face. Within one week from the commencement of cutting operations by this machine I received a series of complaints from my men relative to excessive dust. I immediately made a visit, by permission of the Board, to view the machine operating. Twenty feet from the machine all I could see were clouds and clouds of dust being churned around, and the machine was barely visible. I immediately called a halt, examined the dust suppression equipment on the machine and found it very unsatisfactory. So I told the section oversman and the deputy that my men would not be working under such appalling conditions, and I requested that the speed of the machine when shearing be reduced by 50%. They agreed and there was a very vast improvement in the dust content in the air current. Why the improvement? Because the method of application of the dust suppression equipment comparable with the speed of cutting was way out of proportion and inadequate. One week later this new machine was taken out from the face and replaced by an Anderton shearer.[130]

---

128 Alec Mills, Interview C1 (SOHC).
129 Bobby Strachan, Interview C11 (SOHC).
130 NUM, *Annual Report and Proceedings* (1964), pp. 474–5.

Another Scottish miner articulated the positive role of the union in controlling dust underground:

> JG: The first time I went down and caught people boring without water, I'm talking about bores – see, we also had what we ca' the blast borers which was also water-infused. Now when the water wasnae working, they just bored on because they were on what we ca' piece bonus.
>
> NR: What was their attitude to you when you said to them 'Don't'?
>
> JG: Well, they ken not to argue back because – I caught a lad cutting, I was doing a one, two, three inspection and I went down and he was cutting without water, and I told him then, I says, 'You'll never work on a machine again.' I couldnae do that, but I can go up and report to the manager and say 'I want that man off that machine because I caught him cutting out water.' Now, the men had to back me up, couldnae back the man up, they had to back me up. So that's what happened. So the answer to your question is we didnae get any retaliating because they were frightened to tell us to go and 'F' off if you like [laughs] … because we knew what we were doing was right for their health.[131]

Such rank-and-file vigilance was also evident in South Wales, another militant UK coal field, where pit officials fought to ensure environmental standards were maintained, using the threat of face stoppages and walkouts where dust levels were high. A Welsh miner recalled: 'One or two boys would go on strike, as it were. They wouldn't touch the coal because it was too dusty, and the whole face stopped.'[132]

Another South Wales miner responded to a question about whether anyone cut dry without the water infusion and sprays, recalling the level of peer pressure imposed upon individuals to act responsibly:

> If anybody had done that in Britannia colliery where we spearheaded most mechanisation … we would insist on having him taken off the job, never to go on it again. They wouldn't dare.[133]

Another Welsh miner noted the influence of the union in the workplace:

> Personally, I would never cut without any water. But I've got to be personally honest, anybody who did was a madman. *Was a madman*. 'Cause you wouldn't be able to see a hand in front of you. … I never ever would cut, operate my machine without any water on it. He'd [referring to Tom Bowden – workmen's inspector/union official] soon stop me anyway![134]

Another recalled the walkouts:

---

131 Joseph Goodwin, Interview C43 (SOHC).
132 John Jones, Interview C27 (SOHC).
133 Tom Bowden, Interview C26 (SOHC).
134 Derek Charles, Interview C26 (SOHC).

Well very often we'd come up the road. Very often I had to phone Tom and they'd come up the road because of the dust. They got more educated towards the end, like. Years ago, the colliers just got on with it.[135]

Managers could be hard taskmasters, as one South Wales miner noted: 'some of them were right bloody Nazis, and there's no getting away from it'.[136] His colleague commented on the role of the union in the face of such oppressive work regimes:

If it was not for the union of course insisting and pressing and campaigning for dust suppression, we'd not have any. There's no getting away from it. It was union pressure that was responsible for the improvements.[137]

Therefore, a common theme in oral interviews with miners was the recognition of the positive role of the union on the dust problem. This contrasted sharply with the more trenchant anti-union discourse in interviews of asbestos-related disease victims.[138] One Lanarkshire miner noted of the 1960s:

Things began to get a bit better, due to the miners' union pressing and pressing and pressing – and they've got to be commended on that – they did press hard, but the conditions and the type of mine that we were working, it couldn't be suppressed. [139]

In other cases, miners became frustrated by the same problems recurring again and again. When asked how the colliery management responded to unofficial face stoppages because of dust, one South Wales miner responded:

Slowing down the coal output, but then afterwards they would start speeding again, they would build up ... In the end, you were getting fed up. You finished complaining, y'know. It's like hitting your head against a wall.[140]

Apart from such frustration with the productionist tendencies of some mine managements, there is also evidence that the miners' unions were sensitive to the need to balance job preservation against strict adherence to dust regulations. For example, in 1962 there was serious non-compliance with dust standards at the Penrhiwceiber Colliery in South Wales. Management indicated that the scam would be worked out in twelve months. Rather than taking the option to stop the faces, the union side of the Joint Advisory Committee suggested a time limit for compliance and let the matter drop. The Vice President of the NUM (South Wales Area) commented judiciously: 'the stopping of the faces concerned would have serious repercussions on

---

135 Colin ('Nati') Thomas, Interview C26 (SOHC).
136 Gareth Golier, Interview C25 (SOHC).
137 Howard Jones, Interview C25 (SOHC).
138 See Johnston and McIvor, *Lethal Work*, pp. 160–63.
139 Carl Martin, Interview C8 (SOHC).
140 John Jones, Interview C27 (SOHC).

employment of the men and a great deal of thought had been given to this factor'.[141] Whilst oral evidence shows that unofficial action was taking place on health and safety issues, this form of protest may have been constrained by national policy, especially in the early years after nationalisation when the NUM was most sensitive to demands that it should balance power with responsibility.[142] Like most unions, its rules forbade unofficial strike action.[143]

Compensation Struggles

Where the miners' unions were particularly dynamic was in compensation struggles on behalf of their members. Here the NUM tapped into specialist knowledge accrued by union lawyers, and marshalled evidence (statistical and qualitative) in support of changes in compensation law. At one level, this provided a key support network for workers (and dependents) whose security was threatened by a serious accident or chronic industrial disease. At another level, it has been argued that such financial compensation in theory operated as a deterrent, encouraging improvement in health and safety standards to minimise outlays, and hence having a preventative impact. However, Beaumont has argued that 'there appears to have been relatively little positive spillover from this quite extensive union involvement in the compensatory side of health and safety to the preventative side'.[144] Does the evidence for coal mining support such a pessimistic interpretation?

The coal mining unions were active, both in monitoring and lobbying on compensation legislation and in representing members' interests under both the social insurance schemes and in common law. Indeed, this was a major part of the miners' union business, a reflection of the highly dangerous nature of this work. Of some 50,000 workers in the UK in receipt of benefits under the Workmen's Compensation Act (WCA) in the early 1950s, around 60% were in coal mining, and around 10,000 (or 20%) were coal miners in South Wales.[145] In South Wales, each miner's lodge had a Compensation Secretary, and there were five regional Compensation Agents advising and co-ordinating policy in the late 1940s.[146] Melling and Bufton have examined compensation policies of the MFGB in detail in relation to silicosis and the early years of pneumoconiosis.[147] From the 1940s, the NUM lobbied

141 NUM (South Wales Area), Minutes of Area Executive Council Meeting, 14 August 1962, p. 585.

142 See Taylor, *The NUM and British Politics*, pp. 82–3. In his presidential address in 1947, Will Lawther urged: 'we also have a right to expect that there be an end to unofficial strikes … it is a crime against our own people that unofficial strikes should take place … No stoppage can be justified, having regard to the present dire need for coal.'

143 Taylor, *The NUM and British Politics*, p. 6.

144 Beaumont, *Safety at Work and the Unions*, p. 373.

145 *The Miner* (July/August 1953), p. 5.

146 NUM (South Wales Area), *Annual Conference for 1947–8*, p. 69.

147 See Melling and Bufton, '"A Mere Matter of Rock"'.

hard to improve benefits for pneumoconiotics and to protect the interests of their large benefit-dependent disabled community. This was done both through collective bargaining and supporting individual cases. By the late 1940s, compensation rates were especially inadequate under the WCA. In 1947, at a time when the lowest earner in the industry was on £5 per week, the full benefit under the WCA for a man and non-earning wife was £2 10s.[148] One important early initiative was the negotiation of a Supplementary Benefit Scheme in the coal industry in 1948 which provided additional payments on top of the statutory payments to industrial injury and disease victims, including pneumoconiotics.[149] This helped to ensure payments kept pace with price inflation and address what one union delegate argued was the 'poverty and distress' that characterised the experience of pneumoconiotics under the WCA.[150] The NUM also negotiated with the NCB to get disabled workers included in the House Coal Scheme, whereby they benefited from a free coal allowance every year. The unions were also involved in funding independent medical advice to appeal against what they regarded as unfavourable assessments by the rather conservative Pneumoconiosis Medical Panels. In South Wales, for example, the NUM took 20 cases to the Medical Appeal Tribunals in the year up to mid-1950, winning 15.[151] The unions also campaigned to have the lower threshold raised, so that some compensation was paid for a disability assessment of under 10%. Whilst the NUM conceded that the NCB had a more 'reasonable attitude' than the old coal owners in this respect, this still remained a contested and adversarial terrain.[152]

The union also campaigned, with some success, to widen the scope of the Industrial Injuries Act and to sort out anomalies and injustices. Successes included the passage of the Pneumoconiosis and Byssinosis Benefit Act, 1951, which enabled previously excluded pneumoconiotics to claim benefit, and in 1954 the time bar was removed (previously a miner had to show they had been employed in the industry within five years of certification).[153] However, attempts by the NUM to exert pressure on the Conservative governments in the 1950s to allow those on Workmen's Compensation to transfer in to the Industrial Injuries Act were unsuccessful.[154] Benefit rates for those totally disabled under the WCA were supplemented, though, after NUM pressure in 1956.[155] Whilst it was recognised that the Industrial Injuries Act of 1948 was a marked improvement on the WCA, still the miners' unions worked tirelessly to extend provision and protect members' interests. This included working through the Miners' Parliamentary Group in the House of Commons and through the TUC. None the less, what persisted well into the 1950s was a differential in the experience of those miners certified under the Industrial Injuries Act (1948) and those drawing

---

148 NUM (South Wales Area), *Annual Conference for 1947–8*, p. 61.

149 Ibid., pp. 75–6. The initial supplement was £1 a week for fully disabled men.

150 NUM (South Wales Area), *Annual Conference for 1947–8*, p. 62.

151 NUM (South Wales Area), *Annual Conference, 1949–50*, pp. 89, 93.

152 NUM (South Wales Area) *Annual Conference for 1947–8*, p. 71.

153 *The Miner* (March/April 1954), p. 1.

154 *The Miner* (January/February 1955), p. 20.

155 *The Miner* (September/October 1956), p. 1.

benefits under the less generous WCA. This adverse situation was worsened by price inflation in the early 1950s and by Conservative cuts in public spending, such as the lapsing of Section 62 of the National Insurance Act in 1953, which removed 'extended benefit'. The latter affected pneumoconiotics and other disabled persons (including disabled ex-servicemen) severely, and prompted a massive demonstration by the NUM (South Wales), with up to 50,000 participating in a protest march and rally in Cardiff on 17 October 1953.

Given the high level of trade union activity on behalf of disabled miners at a number of levels, it is perhaps somewhat surprising that the NUM did not pursue claims for damages in the law courts against the NCB on the grounds of negligence or breach of statutory duty in relation to pneumoconiosis through the post-war period. The reasons for this remain rather obscure. Certainly, the records of the NUM show that the union was involved in taking cases to court claiming damages for injuries and trauma, and the case load rose substantially through the 1940s, 1950s and 1960s. Cases were taken by the NUM Areas rather than the national union. The Scottish miners' leader Abe Moffat noted how in Scotland in the 1950s, each common law action pursued by the union produced a larger minimum payment, so that the average pay-out more than doubled in that decade.[156] However, prior to 1970 only two cases were pursued through the courts to obtain damages for pneumoconiotics, and these were very exceptional circumstances and settled out of court, one after a lengthy six-year struggle.[157] The various union Areas routinely refused to take such cases. The main barriers appear to have been a widespread belief that it was too difficult to prove that the contraction of the disease was a result of an employer's negligence, or to prove employers had breached their statutory duties (partly because the wording of the 'dust clause' in the 1956 Mines and Quarries Act was less specific than in the Factory Acts).[158] Furthermore, there was a technical difficulty in that a law (the Statute of Limitations) forbade any claims under common law being made after three years from first knowledge of the disease, and after twelve months from death from the disease. In 1963, the NUM South Wales Area sought the legal advice of two Queens' Counsellors, who indicated that it was inadvisable to proceed with such cases as they were highly unlikely to succeed.[159] In the event, only one case was submitted to the Compensation Department of the NUM South Wales up to 1970, and this was not proceeded with.

In 1970, the NUM was considerably embarrassed when another trade union, the Amalgamated Engineering Union (AEU), successfully fought a case for damages for a pneumoconiotic ex-miner, obtaining an out-of-court settlement of £7,500.[160]

---

156 A. Moffat, *My Life with the Miners* (London, 1965).

157 NUM (South Wales Area), Special Area Conference, 16 March 1960, p. 146. One was in Yorkshire in 1958, the other in Nottinghamshire in 1967. Out-of-court settlements of £2,500 and £800 were accepted respectively in each case.

158 NUM (South Wales Area), Area Executive Council, 10 March 1970, p. 113; NUM (South Wales Area), Area Executive Council, 2 June 1970, pp. 370–72.

159 NUM (South Wales Area), Area Executive Council, 10 February 1970, p. 55.

160 TUC, *Congress Report* (1973), pp. 601–2.

Stanley Pickles had worked at an NCB pit in Durham from 1947 to 1960, then left and became a lathe operator. In 1966 he was certified as suffering from pneumoconiosis (actually silicosis and tuberculosis), and the AEU supported his common law case for damages against the NCB. The pit where he had worked had subsequently closed and the records had been lost, a situation which somewhat undermined the defence of the NCB in the case. The settlement in February 1970 was widely publicised in the press and created a furore within the NUM, with some members bitterly criticising the union for not pursuing similar claims earlier.[161] Albeit belatedly, the NUM encouraged and approved the fighting of such cases by the Areas. What followed was a field day for the lawyers, who reaped substantial fees for issuing writs for damages, and a commensurate draining of union funds. This involved a massive amount of work for the unions and their solicitors. In the North West Division alone, the estimated expenditure by January 1971 had reached £41,000.[162] By mid-1971, around a thousand cases had been submitted or were in the process of submission to the solicitors. The union agreed to pursue 134 of these cases in which certification was after 1 January 1960, in order to maximise the chances of success and build up favourable legal precedent.[163]

However, the legal process in these damages cases was, as the NUM had anticipated, beset with problems. Some of these were made apparent in an internal NUM 'advisory document' in August 1971:

> The basic problem is to prove negligence in respect of a disease which takes a long time to develop and therefore arises over a period during which the technical and medical state of knowledge is changing and in which, therefore, the very yardsticks of what constitute negligence are themselves changing. ... Thus the court will have to satisfy itself in any given case –
> - Of what the general and approved practice was in the mining industry during the relevant period.
> - As to whether that general and approved practice was reasonable having regard to technical and medical knowledge existing at that time, this question to be viewed through contemporary eyes and not through the hindsight of 1971 knowledge.
> - As to whether that general and approved practice was observed at the place of work at which the claimant contracted his disease.[164]

Moreover, a key difficulty in the way of such claims was the defence of *volenti* – 'that the plaintiff cannot sue where his injury resulted from his free and voluntary acceptance of a known risk'.[165] In this regard, the NUM recognised that its formal recognition of the risk, explicit in the negotiation of extra wage payments for

---

161 For example, the Cwm Lodge South Wales. See NUM (South Wales Area), Area Executive Council, 10 February 1970, p. 55.

162 NUM (South Wales Area), Executive Council Meeting, 20 January 1971, p. 42.

163 NUM (South Wales Area), Executive Council Meeting, 8 June 1971, p. 424.

164 NUM (South Wales Area), Executive Council Meeting, 13 September 1971, pp. 568–9.

165 Ibid., p. 570.

working in non-approved dust conditions a decade earlier in 1961, would seriously compromise the chances of winning many categories of claims for damages.[166] Moreover, a proportion of the claims were from miners who had ignored Medical Panel advice on certification to transfer from dusty work. For these reasons, the NUM pressed forward with the cases most likely to be successful, where miners' pneumoconiosis showed medical evidence of deterioration *despite being employed exclusively in dust approved conditions after 1956*. The date was a watershed because the NUM could reasonably claim the NCB was culpable *after* the passage of the 1956 Mines and Quarries Act, when the Board had a more sharply defined statutory duty to maintain a standard of care, rather than the vaguer, more nebulous common law duty which prevailed up until then. The NUM remained divided, however, on the best strategy to pursue. The South Wales Area continued to be deeply sceptical about the chances of success in the courts. The Head of the Social Insurance Department, D.C. Davies, was reported to have commented: 'we may as well collect two million pounds from our members and throw it in the sea, as we had no hope of winning the claims'.[167]

As the volume of claims grew to reach 4,000, the NUM changed tack and approached the government to lobby for a universal lump sum compensation scheme for pneumoconiotics in *lieu* of legal action. Whether this was partly driven by the divisions within the NUM on policy and the divided nature of legal opinion is not apparent. One view was that this was the product of influential right-wing areas, led by Durham, who preferred to negotiate a deal, rather than risk going to the courts.[168] However, South Wales, a left-wing Area, was also sceptical about legal action. In the event, the Conservative government refused to countenance any such scheme unless the NUM accepted its wages policy.[169] This delayed settlement somewhat, until the Conservatives lost the election in February 1974. The new Labour government was much more sympathetic, and a quite unique pneumoconiosis compensation scheme was thrashed out in 1974. The scheme provided tax-free lump sums to almost all categories of certified pneumoconiotics, up to a maximum of £10,000, including a sum for 'pain and suffering', and dependent upon the severity of disability, age at initial certification and the time that had elapsed since initial certification (hence building in a variable element for loss of earnings over the years).[170] Lump sum benefits for 'future' cases were also agreed on a similar basis. Widows of husbands who had died since January 1970 were also able to claim a lump sum of up to £5,000, again dependent upon the age of the miner at first certification and the severity of initial diagnosis. The *quid pro quo* was that the NUM had to agree to drop all the

---

166 Ibid., pp. 569–70.

167 NUM (South Wales Area), Minutes of Special Area Conference, 15 July 1974, p. 563.

168 David Guy, Interview C44 (SOHC).

169 NUM (South Wales), Area Executive Council, 18 June 1974.

170 NUM (South Wales Area), Executive Council, 9 July 1974, pp. 522–3, 562–78; NUM (South Wales Area), Executive Council, 10 September 1974, pp. 652–62.

common law claims, and all individuals in receipt of the new lump sum payments had to agree that this rescinded their rights to pursue any claims for common law damages. The NUM justified this on the grounds that in its estimate some 39,000 pneumoconiotics would benefit, rather than the 4,000 or so cases that the NUM had agreed to support through the courts.[171] In the event, by the end of 1976 over 72,000 claims had been made under the scheme by miners and widows, with an average settled lump sum of almost £2,000, and a cost to the Exchequer of some £123 million.[172] About 150 new applications were also coming in every month for claims by pneumoconiotics and their widows in the mid–late 1970s, indicating the persistence of this problem into the final quarter of the twentieth century. The Scheme was also extended in 1979 to cover those who had been and continued to be employed by private owners.[173]

Undoubtedly, the 1974 Pneumoconiosis Benefit Scheme was a massive victory for the NUM on behalf of pneumoconiotic miners. However, the Scheme was not totally inclusive, and some categories of pneumoconiotics and dependents continued to feel aggrieved, including those under the Workmen's Compensation system who had been 'blackmailed' into commuting their claims and the widows of pneumoconiotic miners who died before January 1970. As Howard Jones – a Pentremawr Lodge official – asked at a branch meeting: 'Are the Union to provide bodyguards for secretaries who have to inform widows that there is nothing for them if their husbands died prior to the 26th of January 1970?'[174] Moreover, some would suggest that claims for damages should have been pursued sooner, and that it may never have happened had not the Pickles case taken by the AEU embarrassed the NUM into action. Furthermore, there were those like David Guy who felt the average payment was too small and that more would have been achieved had the NUM held its nerve and taken the cases through the courts:

> I have to say from a personal point of view, I think the lump sums that are paid out are derisory. They certainly don't reflect the degree of disability or pain and suffering and inconvenience that the condition places upon the individual … I must have serviced hundreds if not thousands of these claims – I've yet to meet anyone who felt as if they'd been adequately compensated.[175]

However, there were real difficulties in the way of claiming damages in common law in the 1950s and 1960s, and conflicting opinions within the NUM and the legal profession. It is also possible that changing public opinion helped alter the battleground. The late 1960s and early 1970s saw dust-induced respiratory disease hit the headlines with the spread of asbestos-related disease and the mesothelioma

---

171 Ibid., pp. 652–3.

172 NUM (South Wales Area), *Annual Report of the Executive Council, 1976–77*, pp. 153–4.

173 David Guy, Interview C44 (SOHC).

174 NUM (South Wales Area) Executive Committee, 9 July 1974, p. 569.

175 David Guy, Interview C44 (SOHC).

panic. There were also TV documentaries which exposed the culpability of the NCB with pneumoconiosis, including the Thames Television production *This Week* screened in July 1973.[176] Whatever the underlying reasons, the NUM congratulated itself on the 1974 no-fault Pneumoconiosis Scheme, with the South Wales General Secretary Dai Francis commenting that this was 'probably one of the greatest achievements that this union has ever attained'.[177] Union members expressed a variety of opinions on the Scheme, but the consensus when reflecting back on it was to see it in a very positive light, as something of a watershed in provision for this particular disabled community.[178] The 1974 Scheme not only provided financial benefits, but also represented an implicit recognition of the failures of NCB policy, especially the inability to protect the workforce against damage caused by dust inhalation, to improve dust control standards and bring an end to the fallacy of 'dust approved' workplaces.

These issues would resurrect again in the 1990s in the political and legal battles over bronchitis and emphysema. The advancing medical knowledge on the occupational etiology of these diseases was reviewed in Chapter 5. The NUM had persistently pressed the claim for bronchitis and emphysema to be scheduled as occupational diseases from the early 1950s, and as we've seen, the TUC had unsuccessfully lobbied the Beney Committee to this end in 1953. Despite the fact that the NUM agreed in 1974 that it would not push for any widening of the 1974 compensation agreement, some argued that the changed circumstances of the 1980s necessitated the inclusion of bronchitis and emphysema in the scheme.[179] What is also evident, however, is the important role played by another of the miners' unions, the National Association of Colliery Overmen and Deputies (NACODS), especially in the final crucial stages of this campaign. It was NACODS which in 1988 initiated a major research project surveying the medical literature which led to the reopening of the scheduling issue and the eventual acceptance by the IIAC of bronchitis and emphysema as certified occupational diseases in 1993. The NACODS General Secretary, Blethyn Hancock, was influential in pursuing this. It was also NACODS which financed the initiation of the eight test cases against British Coal which resulted in the Turner Judgment and Europe's largest single compensation award, affecting over half a million miners, in 1998. One explanation offered for NACODS' higher profile in the later stages of the unions' dust disease campaigns was the financial bankruptcy of the NUM after the year-long miners' strike of 1984–85.[180]

---

176 NUM (South Wales Area), Executive Council, 11 September 1973, pp. 514–15.

177 NUM (South Wales Area) Executive Committee, 9 July 1974, p. 523. After privatisation in the 1990s, the Coal Authority assumed overall responsibility for administering the compensation schemes in regard to former miners' claims for pneumoconiosis.

178 See Tommy Coulter, Interview C21 (SOHC). Tommy provided a copy of the Scheme to us, making the point that this was a great union 'achievement'.

179 *Hansard*, 18 January 1996, part 32, col. 982.

180 'The Price of Coal', *Saga Magazine* (March 1998), consulted at http://www.deadline. demon.co.uk/archive/saga/980301.htm.

Conclusion

In the post-Second World Wars years, some doctors and rank-and-file activists criticised the miners' unions for emphasising the wage packet, compensation and rehabilitation, rather than getting to the root of the causes of the problem and pursuing direct preventative strategies. The Socialist Medical Association (SMA) was one such group. In the 1952 Pneumoconiosis Conference, Dr Frank Tyrer of the SMA took the opportunity to make the point that the miners' unions still devoted more energy to safety than they did to long-term issues of chronic ill health and disease.[181] A couple of years later, the SMA indicted the unions for not initiating systematic epidemiological studies earlier and for placing money (compensation and wages) ahead of effective prevention. In response, the Scottish miners' leader, Abe Moffat worked to develop a closer relationship between the NUM and the SMA, which was campaigning hard to expose the extent of the dust problem in British industry in the 1950s. This included organising and chairing the joint SMA and Scottish Miners' Union conference on 'Dust and Dust Diseases in Industry' in November 1954.

This brings us back to a crucial issue. Just how highly did the NUM *prioritise* occupational health, and was there a tendency to place productivity, job preservation and wage maximisation first? The US literature tends to portray the United Mineworkers' Union (UMW) in an unfavourable light, seeing John L. Lewis and the UMW leadership prioritising production and undermining the fight against black lung, partly because UMW pensions and health benefits were linked to a royalty on the coal produced.[182] Miners' welfare facilities in Britain were funded out of a levy raised on coal tonnage produced, but not so with pensions, and we are aware of no direct evidence that suggests the NUM prioritised productivity over health. However, there were constant tensions within the NUM, reflecting a range of different work and political cultures across the various coal fields. Generally speaking, where the union had less strength and a more 'reformist' politics existed (as in the coal fields of the Midlands), there tended to be less vigilance on health and safety. At times, this could result in pragmatic compromises and strategic decisions by the NUM which were not necessarily popular in all constituent coal fields. The evidence shows that the NUM was part of the broader union consensus which supported the productivity drive of the post-war Labour governments, including, significantly, supporting the *volte-face* in policy which saw pneumoconiotics being re-employed under the so-called 'approved faces' scheme. Francis and Smith were bitterly critical of this policy, arguing that miners' health and well-being was sacrificed to the NUM's support for nationalisation.[183] As we have seen, the 'approved faces' policy was later to be strongly criticised by Justice Turner as ineffective in preventing miners' exposure to

---

181 Minutes of the Pneumoconiosis Conference, 11 October 1952, p. 21, SWCC/MNA/NUM/K17J.

182 A.L. Donovan, 'Health and Safety in Underground Coal Mining, 1900–1969', in R. Bayer (ed.), *The Health and Safety of Workers* (Oxford, 1988). pp. 78–84.

183 Francis and Smith, *The Fed*, p. 441.

damaging levels of dust underground.[184] The NUM also negotiated a supplementary wage scheme in 1961 to provide 'dust money' payments (of 1s. 6d. per shift) to those miners experiencing particularly bad environmental conditions on unapproved faces.[185] Beaumont has argued that such negotiation of 'compensatory wage differentials' was a common enough strategy of trade unions in the dangerous heavy industries, combined with political lobbying to improve 'protective legislation'.[186] The negotiation of such 'compensatory' wage supplements was officially supported by the TUC in the 1960s and early 1970s, but was controversial in the coal fields.[187] Indeed, both the re-employment of pneumoconiotics and 'dust' payments were trenchantly criticised in some coal fields, notably South Wales, on the grounds that such policies legitimised working in dust and failed to prioritise the protection of miners' long-term health. Raising fears that higher levels of mechanisation were increasing dust exposure, Dai Evans (South Wales) commented in 1964: 'to our shame, we have negotiated an allowance payment for working in dust'. He continued: 'as long as we negotiate settlements and accept payment for working in unhealthy conditions, the number of men certified will continue to increase ... This union, in our view, must become more dust conscious.'[188]

Looked at another way, however, these policies placed a financial deterrent upon management and improved the right to work for disabled miners. Moreover, they were the product of a democratic decision-making process within the national union and reflected the views of the majority of miners. In part, they are indicative of the existence of a powerful work culture where job security, the maintenance of the male breadwinner role and wage maximisation were prioritised over the vague and uncertain risks of respiratory damage over the long term. We explore the prevailing work culture and risk in the next chapter. Clearly, there were policy disagreements and internal tensions within the NUM on the issue of dust control, as there were with safety issues in the pits.[189] However, the productivity politics of the UMW were not directly replicated in the UK. The MFGB and the NUM were stronger, more militant and evidently more health-conscious (despite the criticisms of South Wales), as demonstrated in the sustained and eventually effective campaigns to get pneumoconiosis and bronchitis/emphysema recognised, in the ways the unions contested, created and utilised medical evidence, and in the massive efforts the miners' unions put in to extending compensation schemes.

---

184 Judgment of Mr Justice Turner, *The British Coal Respiratory Disease Litigation*, Summary, 23 January 1998, pp. 2–8.

185 NUM, *Annual Conference, Rothesay, 3–6 July 1961*, pp. 274, 507. The extra payments were only paid to day wage men, not to pieceworkers.

186 Beaumont, *Safety at Work and the Unions*, pp. 41–3.

187 Ibid., p. 49.

188 NUM, *Annual Report and Proceedings* (1964), p. 476.

189 See J. Melling, 'Safety, Supervision and the Politics of Productivity in the British Coal Mining Industry, 1900–1960', in J. Melling and A. McKinlay (eds), *Management, Labour and Industrial Politics in Modern Europe* (Cheltenham, 1996), pp. 145–73.

The argument in this chapter, then, is that trade union policy on occupational health and safety is more complex than many commentators have assumed. Our interpretation of the evidence is that the trade unions in British coal mining were divided in response to the dust threat, but were more dynamic in prioritising occupational health issues through creating and contesting medical knowledge, pressing for effective dust control, in compensation struggles and in rehabilitation than many other British trade unions. This was a power struggle in which the miners and their collective organisations were pivotal agents, operating in an environment after nationalisation which was much more conducive to joint regulation and control. Furthermore, from the late 1940s the NUM could rely upon the support of the TUC, which played an important role as a political pressure group campaigning for improvements in dust control and compensation.

The outcomes of occupational health struggles undoubtedly varied across different industries and regions, and depended upon the balance of power and contingent circumstances within workplaces and working communities. A preoccupation in the literature with the asbestos issue in the UK has resulted in a rather skewed picture emphasising corporate power and exploitation, including hegemonic control over knowledge of work-health risks, with workers and their organisations virtually powerless. A more accurate depiction might be to conceptualise workers themselves, and their collective organisations, as more of an agency in this process. Whilst the miners' unions were proactive in the contested terrain of occupational health, they also inevitably reflected and absorbed the highly masculinised pit culture where miners rationalised a high degree of risk. With asbestos, a similar high-risk work culture prevailed, whilst there was a less conducive environment with private enterprise in which to fight health battles, and the capacities of workers to resist were constrained because of lower levels of trade union membership within asbestos manufacturing and the construction industry. In coal mining, there was a more positive application of health knowledge in the workers' interests in a well-unionised sector and, later, a publically owned corporation, which sharply contrasted with the sustained manipulation and conscious distortion of health knowledge in the private sector, where the profit motive dominated.

As far as occupational health struggles in twentieth-century Britain were concerned, power and knowledge were knitted together in a complex symbiotic relationship. Lack of awareness of the asbestos hazard disempowered the labour movement and contributed to the passage of flawed and ineffective regulations in 1931 and thus the persistent exposure of workers through to the 1960s (and beyond). The situation in coal mining, however, was very different. The possibilities and capacity for collective action on health issues was much greater in coal mining. Despite some productionist tendencies, the MFGB and the NUM actively sought to accumulate knowledge of the dust problem, and pressed by their more radical constituents (and especially South Wales), they campaigned aggressively to get reforms – challenging accepted medical knowledge along the way. Vast resources were channelled by the miners' unions into researching and preventing the dust disease epidemic, and into compensation struggles on behalf of members and their dependents. This was one reason why there was no significant separate pressure group activity on respiratory disease in UK coal mining comparable to the US Black Lung Association (or to the Society for the Prevention of Asbestos Industry Diseases and Clydeside Action on Asbestos). The death and disability toll of miners' lung was tragically high in the UK. However, it would have been much worse had the workers and unions not intervened actively and persistently to implement change. Whilst powerless to prevent the pneumoconiosis tragedy and the massive impairment caused by bronchitis and emphysema, the combination of rank-and-file vigilance in the workplace and cumulatively effective pressure group activity at the national level by the miners' unions and the TUC, helped ensure British miners' respiratory health concerns were addressed earlier and more comprehensively than was the case with asbestos in the UK and with coal miners' dust disease in the USA.

PART IV
Miners' Testimonies:
Dust and Disability Narratives

Chapter 8

Workplace Culture:
Risk, Health and Masculinity

Previous chapters have focused on how the issue of dust disease in coal mining was given increasing attention from the 1930s, and undeniably the dust control and improved compensation measures had some ameliorative impact. Nationalisation made a real difference. It is significant that all of our oral interview respondents who expressed a view on this commented that nationalisation brought improved health and safety standards in the pits. The NCB and the Mines Inspectorate were emphatic that such strategies were successful in controlling dust. However, as we will see, the preventative policies of the NCB and the regulators – such as the dust datum and the notion of 'approved faces', together with the employment of a small army of dust suppression officers and medical professionals to monitor respiratory disease and keep mine dust within prescribed legal limits – were only effective to a degree. The degenerative pressures of an intensely productionist managerial regime and a deeply entrenched machismo work culture where miners rationalised (and were inured to) high risk-taking at the point of production circumvented the reformist zeal of the newly established NCB, the regulators and the unions in militant coal fields like South Wales. The acceleration of the colliery closure programme from the mid-1950s introduced further pressures upon the workforce and mine management, influencing tough choices that had to be made between the economic viability of pits and workers' health and well-being. Such economic pressures seeped subtly into miners' consciousness. Customary deeply entrenched ways of working and of managing labour in the pits did not disappear overnight, whilst job security, wage maintenance and protection of the traditional provider role understandably took precedence over uncertain and poorly defined risks of respiratory damage some time in the (relatively distant) future. Moreover, the evidence strongly suggests that a considerable gulf continued to exist between NCB action and statutory controls, and actual workplace practice, especially deep underground, at the coal face, far away from the scrutiny of the regulators. Here, oral evidence is of particular value, helping us to reconstruct a largely lost world of work culture, attitudes and prevailing practice at the point of coal production.

As we will see, such evidence presents a varied and complex picture. However, one thing that does emerge strongly is the divergence between dust control provision and the reality of mining operations. In short, much of what was laid down in law and introduced as policy by the NCB was ignored or subverted as production continued to be prioritised over health by management, and the maximisation of wages and job security dominated miners' thinking. Power relations underground played a part in this, as did gender role-playing, with expressions of masculinity sometimes undermining health and safety. Degenerative as well as ameliorative factors co-existed. Prominent amongst the former, and frequently recalled vividly by miners in their oral testimony, was the deleterious impact of the new phase of mining mechanisation associated with power-loading. Clearly, the imperatives of production and the economics of coal-getting in a shrinking domestic and world market could impinge disastrously upon environmental conditions underground, raising levels of dust inhalation by face workers in particular to unprecedented levels. How this story unfolded at the coal face is the focus of this chapter. It relies heavily upon the oral testimonies of those within the mining community themselves, providing a view on the dust problem in the pits from the point of production. What are privileged here are the discourses of working miners: their perceptions; beliefs, motivations and agency.

Lay Knowledge and the Occupational Landscape of Dust Exposure

Marked variations in the nature of mining work between the different coal fields had a significant bearing on levels of dust exposure. For example, miners in the North East of England and South Wales tended to begin coal face work at an earlier age than their counterparts north of the border, while in Scotland in the mid-1950s there were less distinct occupational groups compared to other parts of the country, where a more clearly defined division of labour was apparent. There were important geological differences too. For example, most of the Scottish pits were known to be fairly wet compared to the drier and dustier pits of South Wales – a fact that was reflected in lower pneumoconiosis rates in most of the Scottish pits selected for the PFR 25-pit survey in the 1950s. Finally, even within coal fields – or NCB Divisions – there were significant variations between areas, with steam coal being got in some South Wales pits, and anthracite in others.

For many British miners, the inhalation of large quantities of dust began at a very early age. In many pits, it was common for young entrants at 14–16 years of age to start at the surface, working at the screens and in the washery (see Chapter 2 for more detail). Dust levels here were usually significantly lower than underground (especially on the coal face), but could be dangerous none the less. One South Wales miner described conditions just prior to Second World War:

> Well, in the coal preparation plant … the coal started coming up … you could not see the man picking on the belt working next to you because of the concentration of dust. And that was …There was one conveyor there which was very wet, and that subdued a little bit of the dust, but ah, generally speaking dust levels were very, very high.[1]

---

1   Howard Jones, Interview C25 (SOHC).

Howard Jones worked with some 'two dozen' or so lads and a couple of older men at the screens for five years from 1937 to 1942, noting that it was the practice to employ infirm and injured miners at the surface in what was regarded to be 'light work'. Despite the existence of some crude exhaust ventilation in the Penrhiwceiber (South Wales) pit washery, conditions were still grim in the late 1930s, as one worker there recalled:

> It was very dusty. You couldn't see your hand in front of you. In them days when the coal come up in the drams you weren't allowed to use water to dampen it, it would drop through into a sieve and a shaker where it was sorted into sizes. Well if you used water to damp the dust all the little holes where the small coal used to drop through would clog up. You'd have got sacked if you used water.[2]

Similarly, in his autobiography Bert Coombes recalled the screens 'working at full speed' in his pit in South Wales in the 1930s, and that 'dust floated in the air around every electric lamp'.[3]

Tommy Coulter recalled surface work as a young miner in the Lothians in the 1940s, and how levels of dust in the work environment were related to the type of coal:

> In the colliery where I worked, one of the picking bands, they were like bars so that the small coal fell down, but one of them was solid plates, it was for bunk [bunker coal]; it was a high quality, a high quality of coal, it was a coking coal. And it was top quality, and this was used for the Navy and the Merchant Navy, for bunker coal. And that yin in particular was very, very dusty because it was plates on the shakers, so you were getting the dust when it fell, you were getting dust when it was jiggin' and then it went down the, there was a floor where you were working, but then at the end of this picking band it obviously tae get in the wagons, there was no floor but there was a fence. And then the wind, if it was going in that direction you got all that dust, eh, and the dust was absolutely appalling. In the morning when the lights were on, you could see the dust. But when you started working there, you just took it for granted that was, that was it. Eh? The procedure was that a' the boys' names were marked on a girder in a turn, so when it came your turn, you got a job in the, up in the pit head, which was not so bad. And then your turn for going underground when you were sixteen. So you had to go through that procedure. Some boys didn't go underground, didn't like it, but that was the procedure. But the dust was absolutely appalling and the noise was horrendous. I mean, you couldn't speak to each other ...[4]

It was the noise and dust at the surface that similarly stuck in the memory of Alec Mills, a post-war Ayrshire miner:

---

2 Tennyson Tipper, cited in 'The Price of Coal', *Saga Magazine* (March 1998), consulted at http://www.deadline.demon.co.uk/archive/saga/980301.htm.

3 Bert Coombes, *These Poor Hands* (London, 1939), p. 262.

4 Tommy Coulter, Interview C21 (SOHC).

I was employed in 1947. Now, the screening plant was a very dusty place. It was a confined area that you worked in. The noise was horrendous. It was steel that was rubbing against steel, and the coal was separated from large right down to the small, to the dross.[5]

Tommy Coulter was relieved to get out of this environment and get underground:

So that was, that was probably the worst job I've ever had, I was glad to get underground to get a rest. Because the boys' jobs underground were out-by mainly, in the haulage ways which were in the fresh air. So that wasnae too bad.[6]

As mentioned earlier, in some regions before the Second World War, miners went straight to the coal face, attached to an experienced miner for on-the-job training. John Evans, who started work in Ferndale pit, Maerdy, South Wales, in 1927 recalled: 'you didn't have a training period, as soon as you started the first day you were on the coal with your buttie, filling with the curling box'.[7] He continued: 'and once you had a little training they expected you to pull your weight'.[8] This is important because it meant that in some coal fields, including South Wales, workers were exposed for longer periods of their working lives to the most dusty working environment at the face. As a consequence, respiratory disability occurred at a younger age. Mostyn Moses, whose father died of pneumoconiosis at 53, went underground to work at the Pentrecalywda pit in South Wales:

I was working with a collier, I was the boy, like. He'd dig the coal out, and I was shovelling all day, filling the dram [rail truck] with the coal, and then they'd bring another one. You couldn't see your hand in front of you. It was terrible, working like that all day.[9]

Elsewhere (as in Scotland), young workers progressed after a year or two from surface work to haulage and/or labouring underground. This could include attending conveyor belts, supplying materials (such as wood for supports), and handling full and empty hutches underground. Some of the haulage tasks could expose miners to large quantities of dust, especially working at the transfer points where coal from the face was being shifted from one conveyor to another, or from a face-line conveyor directly on to hutches (or carriages) for transport to the shaft and hence to the surface. Tommy Coulter described this as the worse experience of dust he had come across in his working life in the pits:

Actually, the worst conditions I ever suffered was, at a loading point there was, I think, about three coal faces operating, and the coal, all their coal was fed out by conveyer belts

---

5   Alec Mills, Interview C1 (SOHC).

6   Tommy Coulter, Interview C21 (SOHC).

7   A large three-sided type of shovel.

8   John Evans, interviewed by Hywel Francis, 13 June 1973, South Wales Coal Miners' Collection (SWCC), Maerdy Community Study, Tape 84, side 1.

9   Cited in 'The Price of Coal', *Saga Magazine* (March 1998). Mostyn had bronchitis, emphysema and pneumoconiosis.

ontae a main conveyer belt, and they filled what we called hutches, wee tubs with wheels on holding about twelve hundredweights ... Now there was a fair force of air coming in and absolutely no dust suppression and it was a very dry colliery and the dust was absolutely appalling, and if you went behind that loading point, you just couldn't see. Again, you see, you became accustomed tae it, and that was part of the job.[10]

A Durham miner working in haulage at the Brandseth pit noted the dusty conditions in the 1950s where he was situated at the end-of-face conveyer:

I was working on what they called the loader end, that was the coal face to the loader end, and the conveyer was bringing the coal from the coal face and leaving it there. Right at the end, filling the tubs, oh it was terrible, terrible dusty, and *oh hell*, it was black, black all day; there was dust, coal dust, stone dust and all sorts just lying about.[11]

All underground workers were exposed to variable levels of dust, though some operations were performed in a relatively clean environment – especially those some distance from the coal face and on the ventilation intake side of the pit. Another Durham miner noted, however, that working in the underground storage bunkers could be difficult:

I was put in charge of a bunker which was designed to hold around about three thousand tonnes of coal, when there was problems with coal clearance; the coal was filled into the bunkers by a means of a conveyor and then extracted when the coal clearance was working again with the use of a coal-cutting machine which I was trained for. It was a power-loading job similar to what I had been doing previously, and again, it was quite a dusty environment because these bunkers were enclosed areas within the pit and it was loose coal that I was flinging onto the conveyors.[12]

It was the coal face workers and those responsible for driving operations such as creating the tunnel and road network and developing new areas – jobs that usually required cutting through rock as opposed to coal – that were exposed to the highest concentrations of dust in the industry. In the 1930s, huge clouds of dust were generated by the processes of drilling and shot-firing (using explosives). One Scottish miner who started work underground in 1930 recalled dry drilling operations in development work, noting: 'even boring in the whin stone there you were like a baker when you came out the pits at night ... there wasnae water. It was stoor.'[13] He went on to comment on how, before nationalisation, it was largely private contractors that were responsible for mine driving, and that health and safety precautions were widely ignored in the push to maximise production:

---

10 Tommy Coulter, Interview C21 (SOHC).
11 Alan Winter, Interview C42 (SOHC).
12 David Guy, Interview C44 (SOHC).
13 Andrew Lyndsay, Interview C4 (SOHC). 'Stoor' is a Scottish word for dust.

They cried them mine drivers … They bored these holes and fired these shots, and then they said that you went down there and swallowed that reek. They maybe had a pound a day more than you. But you were daein' the slavery.[14]

He continued: 'After nationalisation, things seemed to improve.' Mine drivers were more liable to contract silicosis because of the frequency with which they cut through stone rather than coal in their development work. Another Ayrshire miner, who started work in the pits in 1934 and joined a mine-driving contracting team in 1936, also argued vehemently that dust generation was worse in driving operations in the pre-nationalisation period:

In the old days they had a machine called a ricketty, an old hand borer with which you bored shot-holes – laborious, slow, very hard work. And that was superseded by a rotary percussive drill, a rock drill which rotated and percussed at the same time. It was driven by compressed air with the force of roughly a hundred pounds per square inch. It was heavy, cumbersome, and worse of all it drilled quite fast into the rock and it threw out clouds of dust. There was no form of dust suppression of any kind, except that we all carried a big hanky, usually a big, red spotted bandanna, which was soaked with water, and we tied it round our mouth and throat. And at the end of a drilling cycle the front of your handkerchief was as if it had been dipped in concrete. That was the extent of your protection. So, for my money, the periods for the worst dust production was in the 30s to 40s.[15]

This respondent went on to recall the pressure upon production during wartime, and the greater dust concentrations thrown up in some operations, including shot-firing:

They wanted what they called round coal, not smush, not dross. So that was a period when production was high and dust was everywhere … When the shots went off, you couldnae see a hand in front of your face. You had to get back in there because the air vents that were carrying the air in were all loose, torn to shreds by the blast, and the one nearest the face had to be renewed. So you had to do that, choking and gasping. That was very much a contributory factor on the lung damage … Now, what you have to remember is you're under pressure to get progress, so it's no' a matter of saying, 'Well, we'll wait an hour until it clears.' You're no' allowed to do that. You've got to get back in there and get it moving.[16]

For coal hewers in the hand-getting era, the generation of dust at the coal face depended upon a number of variables, including the nature of the coal itself. The geology of the seam was very important. In some seams, the coal was interspersed with veins of crushed fragments, largely carboniferous, though not infrequently with a mixed mineral content, including silica. As miners worked through the coal seam with the pick, awl, chisels and wedges, these 'dirt bands' would be dislodged into the atmosphere. As we noted in previous chapters, mechanisation could make

---

14 Ibid.
15 John Orr, Interview C3 (SOHC).
16 Ibid.

matters worse. The under-cutting machines threw more dust into the vicinity of the face workers, partly because of the pace at which these power-driven machines operated, and partly because they tended to disintegrate the coal into finer particles than working the under-cut with the pick was ever liable to do.[17] One Scottish miner described the machine under-cutting process, using the Anderson Boyce machine, thus:

This machine had a series of ... A chain with picks on it. Small picks about two to three inches long. And the picks revolved at high speed, and when they were starting to cut up the face, which was then usually around two hundred feet, they started the picks moving and they dug in to what they called the stable – which was a wee man-hole they made – and the machine was put in power and it started to walk up a chain, which was right up the coal face and attached to a very stout timber tree [prop.] at the top. So as the machine walked up the chain, the pick was revolving at the base of the coal seam, under-cutting it by about four feet six. The dust ... Because the machinemen, and the men who were putting up trees and removing trees that were in the way of the machine, the only white bits they had were their lips and the whites of their eyes. Because they were always doing ... The dust was so thick that everything was coated thick with dust.[18]

Tommy Coulter described the conditions that had to be endured when clearing out the debris from the under-cutting shift:

Well, when you came in in the morning, that's what you saw, that was a hole about that height [denoting several inches], so and all the cuttings, the chippings of coal were in the track, and that was when you got the worst dust because the first thing you'd to do, you'd to clear up the loose coal first, because after that you've to get the coal off the wall with shot-firing, so when, it meant everybody was, for the first twenty minutes or so, everybody was shovelling this small coal and there was clouds of dust.[19]

Another Scottish miner commented tersely on conditions at the face when using a mechanical cutter: 'and the dust, *you just couldnae see*. Actually, when you were eating your piece, you could actually taste it in your mouth, ken?'[20]

John Evans had experience of machine under-cutting and the transition to mechanical conveyors in the Ferndale pit in South Wales in this period. He recalled:

They opened the two foot eight seam, then they commenced putting in conveyors. From conveyors they went to belt conveyors. That is when the dust started – from conveyors and dry cutting the four feet six cut ... Machinery made you go harder because you was allocated so much to do and you had to do it. The dust was terrible ... Orthodox mining

---

17 Bert Coombes graphically described the worsening environmental conditions that went hand in hand with the transition to mechanical undercutting in a pit in South Wales after the First World War in *These Poor Hands*, pp. 108–18.

18 John Orr, Interview C3 (SOHC).

19 Tommy Coulter, Interview C21 (SOHC).

20 David Carruthers, Interview C23 (SOHC).

was a lot healthier. Apart from that, you had the high seams, and you would never make the dust the machinery would plough'.[21]

Some seams were notoriously dusty, and miners became knowledgeable about the risks associated with particular places. One Durham miner recalled:

> And there was one set of men ... they were good workers, there was five of them died under fifty, with coal dust, pneumoconiosis. There was five in the whole set, team ... when they wanted coal, they used to work six shifts a week, you know ... to get extra coal ... In fact, at that pit I think it was one of the biggest percentages of pneumoconiosis. In fact, the youngest in the county was twenty-three year old.[22]

As we noted in Chapter 2, the transition to power-loading from the mid-1950s – using shearers, ploughs and integrated cutters and conveyors – also generated more dust, and for three main reasons: the machines themselves ground up the coal, producing larger quantities of finer dust in the process; the technology enabled larger quantities of coal to be produced, increasing the dust concentration accordingly; and the new technology necessitated higher roofs, which in turn called for improved, more powerful ventilation systems. David Guy, a miner from the North East of England from 1961, explains:

> Under the previous method of coal production, where people were coal hewing, there would be a very high airborne dust count, but that would probably be affecting the coal hewer himself. I think the big difference between when they moved from the old-type conventional methods of mining coal to the machine operation is that the machine operation had a tendency to affect everybody in the district because of the aggressive way of how the coal was being wrought out of the seam, you know, it was being churned out, churned out by picks, it was high-volume production, so what tended to happen in the circumstances was you had a higher degree of airborne dust which was physically and aggressively pushed into the air, and that would tend to carry.[23]

This spread exposure significantly beyond the face workers, raising levels of dust throughout the pit, affecting other groups of workers underground. As one South Wales miner recalled of the walking required to get to the face: 'when you were walking in like, you were walking in miles, and everybody was walking and the dust was coming up from under your feet, you know, that was in the air all the time'.[24]

This relates to the importance of lay knowledge regarding occupational hazards. British coal miners developed several levels of knowledge about the impact of dust upon the body. Firstly, miners were well aware that it was the volume of dust which caused damage, and that the job inevitably involved the inhalation of such material:

---

21 John Evans, interviewed by Hywel Francis, 13 June 1973 (SWCC).
22 William Clough, Interview C36 (SOHC).
23 David Guy, Interview C44 (SOHC).
24 Malcolm Davies, Interview C29 (SOHC).

Now, before nationalisation and a wee while after it, eh, air borers, blast borers … you had nae dust suppression so you'd tae hold these great big borers up and bore these holes with nae dust suppression. You were swallowing just pure stone dust a' the time.[25]

And this is what an 80-year-old retired Ayrshire miner had to say about mechanical coal cutting:

Now the machineman would be there, and I would be at the back of the machine, you know. And this is true, I couldn't see the machineman's light for the dust. And how could I give men orders with a mask on my face?[26]

Secondly, miners recognised the emergence of characteristic symptoms: persistent cough, spit ranging from black streaks to think inky black expectorant, and a premature deterioration in breathing capacity which usually came on gradually. One miner commented:

You had no man-riding facilities at all, right. You'd to walk most of the road, and it … was long, long walks and I couldnae handle it. You were stopping and you were saying to yourself, 'What the fuck's wrong with me. It's no' me. It's no' me.' You were breaking out in sweat. You were sweating. You were struggling. And you're saying. 'I'm getting old.' But at 53, you werenae old. [27]

Thirdly, this knowledge led to some attempts to neutralise the risk, such as covering the mouth and nose with a wet cloth to reduce dust inhalation. Trial and error produced ingenuous methods to filter out the dust, including miners tying silk stockings and other items of underwear around their mouths. One Ayrshire miner recalled: 'some of them, you got the likes of a brassiere and put that on. But of course the kind of words they got and such like they (laughs) they didnae have it on long (laughs).'[28] Fourthly, like other workers, miners resorted to or depended on lay remedies and 'quack medicine', including decongestants, and the use of stimulants, such as the opium-based laudanum, to ease symptoms. The habit of tobacco chewing was also common, not just because smoking was strictly forbidden underground, but also as a way of assuaging the inhalation of dust. As a Durham miner commented: 'You had to chew baccy, man, to keep the dust down.'[29] The prevalence of this custom and the strong belief amongst the miners in some coal fields of its efficacy as a dust control measure even inspired a research project through the Institute of Occupational Medicine in the early 1970s. This study of miners' sputum from chewers and non-chewers (South Wales was one coal field where tobacco chewing was uncommon) concluded that the practice had no identifiable impact on dust inhalation and

25 Bobby Strachan, Interview C11 (SOHC).
26 William Dunsmore ('Arco'), Interview C16 (SOHC).
27 Carl Martin, Interview C8 (SOHC).
28 John Guthrie, Interview C19 (SOHC).
29 Frederick Hall, Interview C41 (SOHC).

pneumoconiosis incidence.[30] Finally, coal miners could also benefit from especially strong support networks, both within the community and at the workplace, though problems could occur if a miner moved from one area to another:

> When you get older in a pit, the younger men kind of looked after the older ones. They made your work as easy as they could. Now, that was the system in the pit you were reared, but when you go to another pit, they boys werenae going to be as considerate. Oh no, because you were actually shifting to their pit and you were doing their sons out a job.[31]

As we saw in the previous chapters, however, the challenge of dust was met by more aggressive action by the NCB, pressed by the miners' unions, to control the hazard. Just how effective these preventative measures were in the day-to-day working environment underground is addressed in the next section.

The Reality of Dust Control Underground

Improving the quality of the air miners breathed in the pits had been an important aim from the early nineteenth century on. Some of the miners we spoke to could remember working in pits where the air quality was very poor. One extreme example from the 1930s was related to us by a 94-year-old Ayrshire miner who could remember older, less fit miners being used virtually as portable fans to drive away gassy air from the faces:

> I've seen old Howard Ferguson and Louis Ferguson – that was two ex-miners – down the pit on shift work, sitting wafting screen cloth round like this [mimes wind-milling cloth around his head] to clear the gas away from the coal face before the men went in … They were birlin' this screen cloth round about their head, and going in a wee bit further and daein' the same.[32]

Dust and poor ventilation were recurring motifs in Bert Coombes' evocative autobiography. He recalled how statutory controls in one pit in the 1920s in South Wales were subverted:

> One of my duties was to hurry away to where a small auxiliary fan had been placed if I noticed a light approaching that I thought might belong to an Inspector of Mines. I don't think that my turning of the handle of this tiny fan made much of a movement amongst the atmosphere of these workings, but the object was to show that a fan had been put there and that some attempt was being made to improve things.[33]

---

30 We are grateful to Robin Howie, formerly of the IOM, for this information.
31 Harry Steel, Interview C9 (SOHC).
32 Andrew Lyndsay, Interview C4 (SOHC).
33 Coombes, *These Poor Hands*, p. 192.

With advances in mining engineering, air quality did improve throughout the coal fields, and in more and more pits powerful fans were deployed to push air deeper underground.[34] Whilst this had an ameliorative impact, there was a downside, recognised in the previous testimony from David Guy: more powerful and effective ventilation diffused the dust problem throughout the pit. One of the recurring memories often raised without prompting in the oral testimony related to the grim environmental conditions working on the return side of the airway after the dust had been picked up along the whole of the face.

As we saw in Chapter 6, the use of water jets and sprays (and to a lesser extent water infusion of seams) was a central feature of the NCB's campaign to control dust. However, the reality of the workplace frequently diverged from the textbook practice. The application of water underground was extremely problematic. At first, one of the issues was over who should take responsibility at a time in the mid-1940s into the 1950s when there was a nation-wide drive for coal. At the Pneumoconiosis Conference in January 1947, Will Arthur lambasted naïve government officials and complacent colliery engineers, reminding them that actual workplace practice differed significantly from what they thought was happening:

> Disputes arise every week as to whether dust suppression has been carried out during the previous shift. A very large number of coal shifts have been lost, and we believe that a very large number of certifications is the result of some haphazard method of applying dust suppression. We find today one colliery manager will organize his pit as efficiently as we suggest. One man in charge of the pit accepts responsibility for water infusion. He, therefore is the man responsible for that particular class of work and the men so appointed are restricted to do that work. But in a very large number of collieries no one is responsible. Time and time again we find that the reports of the night shift conflict with those of the day shift. ... We have all kinds of grades doing the work. You have the position where a repairer is asked to be responsible for water infusion. If he is asked to do water infusion at the beginning of a shift he hurries because there is an important job to be done in respect of repairs.[35]

Over time, some of these early problems were addressed. However, oral evidence illustrates that production was frequently prioritised by management over dust control at the face. In some cases bonuses were offered where dust was excessive. One South Wales miner noted:

> They'd cut the coal with no water, and they'd be hell to pay then, 'cause there was too much for the miners to go in, see. ... Then they'd decide to go out and phone for the manager. He said, "We'll give you ten bob extra." We'll all go through, then. When he said it's for a bit of money, we'd all go through. So that was going on about once or twice a week. So they said at last that we're not going into the face if there's no water ...[36]

---

34 G. Hutton, *Scotland's Black Diamonds* (Catrine, Scotland, 2001), p. 13.

35 Conference on Pneumoconiosis in Coal Mines, 18 January 1947, Minutes, p. 8, SWCC/MNA/NUM/K17J.

36 Hywel Francis Interview with M. Morris, n.d., SWCC, AUD/389.

Even when water jets and infusion were successfully deployed, problems persisted. A leading hand from Ayrshire acknowledged the impossibility of the task facing the dust suppression experts:

> Mind you, they tried … They introduced water to wet cutting, and they even tried putting soap in the water to make it soapy to stop the dust. It didnae make much difference … If it was very heavy, I took the men this side of the machine. It was not always possible 'cause … the management was on top of me for production. Production, production, production …[37]

Another Ayrshire miner stated:

> They hadnae a chance with yon machines the way they were cutting. It damped it down, certainly, but no' to the extent it was if it was daein' its job right.[38]

And a Lanarkshire miner reacted with some anger when he was asked to comment on the success of water jets on the machines he had to work near:

> No way. Because the minute the stoor hit it, it clogged up, you know … 'Cause the pressure wasnae high enough and wasnae strong enough to keep the stoor out it. You know, it was just fucking dripping out, man. Dripping out the wee holes, out the wee taps, you know … And they had wee nozzles on them. The same wee nozzles … A wee spray, like your shower is … Now, that was supposed to put the water onto the coal so's it done away with the stoor. These things were a' clogged up… I couldnae see you fae here tae there.[39]

This testimony is backed up to some extent by documentary evidence that in 1965 the NCB's Central Engineering Establishment was carrying out an investigation into the problem of water nozzle outlets becoming blocked.[40]

The positioning of hoses and sprays on machines was also important. Some could remember water hoses attached to the machines being too short, which meant faces *had* to be cut dry. A 93-year-old retired miner from Ayrshire remembered quite clearly how the water sprays fitted to the cutters he was working alongside were badly placed:

> When they brought the water in, they put it on the wrong way. Instead of blowing the water into the machine where it was cutting, they blew it into the side. I mean, it was wet on the face. It wasnae wet where the cutting was. And you were still getting the same amount of stoor, and where the water was there, it was hitting the coal face where it was already cut. It wasnae hitting where the machine was cutting, where the jig was birlin'. It should have been fired onto them. Half a dozen jets should have been firing onto that to

37 William Dunsmore ('Arco'), Interview C16 (SOHC).

38 David Hendry, Interview C15 (SOHC).

39 John McKean, Interview C10 (SOHC).

40 NCB Scottish Division, Production Department Dust Suppression – Recent Developments, 15 October 1965, p. 2, NAS/CB 53/10.

keep that stoor down. But it was firing onto the wall, and the stoor was still there, going up the wall.[41]

Some of our interviewees also remembered that many miners were opposed to changing customary work practices to suppress dust. Change could make for a more difficult working environment, reduce productivity and affect the wage packet. Referring to the pre-power-loading era in the 1940s and 1950s, Tommy Coulter recalled:

> When your wages depended on what you produced, that was always, whether you were conscious or no', that was always a spur, I mean, if you didnae get it done, you didn't get paid, you got a minimum wage which was barely breadline stuff, you know. So you had to do it, there was no alternative.[42]

He went on to say that things changed in the 1960s, as dust suppression awareness rose, but before then, the prevailing payment-by-results wage system discouraged safe and healthy working: 'we knew the rules, but if we operated [by] the rules, we didnae get any dough.'

As power-loading developed in the 1960s, an Ayrshire miner recollected that some miners preferred to work dry:

> I can tell you, very often the water manifold was shut off because the men at the machine were like drooket crows, to use a Scot's expression. They got all the water as well as subduing the dust. Very often they shut it off. So there was always a lot of dust. That was in the days of power-loading.[43]

Similarly, a Lanarkshire miner recalled:

> They would turn the water off on the machine 'cause it was making it all into a mess for them to crawl up through. 'Cause you were on your hands and knees, remember, in these faces. … so they would turn the water off and they would cut dry, and that would make it worse. [44]

This testimony was endorsed by the recollections of a miner from the Durham coal field:

> The dust suppression, they would have the water just enough to trickle to keep the juice on because there was pressure valves where you would have enough water to get the juice on etcetera. And there were times once the timer came off, you could keep the juice on. They knew if they had the full water there, they would flood the face, which means that they couldn't get the coal out quick enough, it would bog down the panzer [conveyor] and

41 Andrew Lyndsay, Interview C4 (SOHC).
42 Tommy Coulter, Interview C21 (SOHC).
43 John Orr, Interview C3 (SOHC).
44 Billy Affleck, Interview C2 (SOHC).

they couldn't get it out, so they didn't get their bonus. So they knocked it off so the dust was coming.[45]

Workplace practice in this respect varied considerably across regions, but also diverged across different pits within the same coal fields. The leading hand from Ayrshire noted how, in his working experience:

We werenae allowed to cut without water. These men ... Latterly, they made the machines so that you couldnae switch them on unless the water was going first ... No, if I ever cut without water ... I'll tell you ... I can mind one day in particular. I had only three feet to go into this stable. Now, that's where you re-picked your machine, and I think I had only two or three feet to cut, and I lost the water. So I said to the machineman, 'Just cut that other three feet and I'll go up to see what's ...'. That's the *only* time. Only once did I ever cut without water, and to me it wasnae detrimental to the miners. It was only three feet ...[46]

And the 93-year-old respondent from Ayrshire added:

... they couldnae cut them [the water sprays] off 'cause when the machine started up, they started. They were connected with the machine.[47]

As mentioned earlier, though, a recurrent problem was that of trying to deal with the large amounts of dust that were generated when machines cut through stone – or dirt bands as they were known.[48]

As we have seen, there was a frenzy of activity from the 1950s onwards regarding efforts to suppress dust on the most common coal cutter used in the UK at this time, the Anderton shearer.[49] In 1958, as we have seen, some attempts were also being made to infuse dirt bands with water in Scotland before the machines cut through them, after similar efforts in South Wales had proved to be successful.[50] However, these efforts were disappointing, and the problem persisted.[51]

However, as we noted in Chapter 6, the problem posed by the Anderton shearers was compounded in some instances by operators cranking machine speeds up to increase production rates. One Ayrshire miner had vivid recollections of a particularly difficult face in the early 1970s:

We had a face in Highhouse, and they said it was moon rock ... This thing that came into the face, it was pure white. It was for a' the world like marble, but it wasnae marble, and we used to call it the moon rock, and you couldnae fucking mark it. And we were pumping

45 Alan Napier, Interview C43 (SOHC).

46 William Dunsmore ('Arco'), Interview C16 (SOHC).

47 Andrew Lyndsay, Interview C4 (SOHC).

48 *Colliery Guardian* (March 1970), p. 106.

49 See, for example, Minutes of 13th Meeting of Area Ventilation Engineers, 17 September 1964, in NAS/CB53/4.

50 Scottish NCB, Divisional Dust Prevention and Suppression Advisory Committee (DDPSAC), Minutes of Meeting of 15 April 1958, NAS/CB/099/61/1.

51 Scottish NCB, DDPSAC, 7 July 1960.

this with a machine, and you want to have seen the stoor that was coming off of that. It was no' real.[52]

Once again, then, the problem was trying to balance the drive for production against the need to keep dust levels down. What is evident is that the conveyor belts became a significant source of dust, and and we saw in Chapter 6, were targeted for preventative dust suppression measures. One miner from the Durham coal field who was involved with dust analysis remembered tracing the source of dust in one particular mine to the loading of mining cars at the end of the conveyor belt:

> Now, when they found where the dust was coming from, it was coming from out-by, not off the wall, but out-by on account of the long running of belts going to where there were mining cars, and when the loco were picking the mining cars up they were like juggling them about, you know, just like when you are driving a car, driving about creating its own dust.[53]

What comes across in many of our interviews and in much of the documentary evidence is that efforts to control the dust, no matter how determined, were not keeping up with the increased dust generated by the drive to increase productivity – bearing out Andrew Bryan's comments that dust suppression personnel were having to run faster to stand still.[54] In his autobiography, a Scottish miner reflected back on the impact of new technology and the dust problem:

> It seemed that all improvements in coal getting brought new problems. The new machines which cut and automatically loaded coal in a continuous cycle were extremely noisy and produced masses of dust. Ventilation was never good, and the air always hot and humid. In those conditions men sweated heavily, and the dust settled on them thick and black. Only their eyes and teeth stayed white. The air bags [ventilation tubing] which were supposed to control the ventilation and bring fresh air in to us were often torn by debris or falling coal, and did not really do their job well. We were supplied with masks but at first they were crude and inefficient. Later models were better, but without doubt they did hinder a man's breathing, and a lot of men found they could not wear the masks when doing heavy work. And in spite of all the mechanisation it was still, as always, very heavy work …[55]

---

52 Billy Affleck, Interview C2 (SOHC).

53 Marshall Wylde, Interview C35 (SOHC).

54 Sir A. Bryan, *The Evolution of Health and Safety in Mines* (Letchworth, 1975), p. 112.

55 B. Smith, *Seven Steps in the Dark: A Miner's Life* (Barr, Ayrshire, 1991). For other examples of miners' autobiographies with some focus on occupational health, including dust, see D. Douglass and J. Krieger, *A Miner's Life* (London, 1983); B.L, Coombes, *These Poor Hands: The Autobiography of a Miner Working in South Wales* (London, 1939); A. Moffat, *My Life with the Miners* (London, 1965); For an excellent American example of this *genre*, see R. Armstead, *Black Days, Black Dust: The Memoirs of an African American Coal Miner* (Knoxville, TN, 2002).

Some of our oral history interviewees reported that they were quite impressed by the dust sampling measures taken from the 1970s onwards. Indeed, a Lanarkshire miner could remember the appearance of Dust Suppression Officers around this time:

> They used to come tae the pit every so often and go to every section. But that was in the later stages ... But right up till the 60s you never had much ... You never heard of them.[56]

This is how a Durham miner reflected on dust monitoring:

> Oh the Dust Suppression Officer, he used to come in the tailgate ... They used to get the readings, then they got the readings sent away to the Area and they used to test them and they used to tell us, 'It's getting high' or 'it's getting low' or things like that. If it reached a certain point, the manager was informed and he had to do something about it ... they took a reading every day until it was put right. As I say, they were pretty good, and I was never an NCB man [laughs].[57]

On the other hand, some of our interviewees were convinced that the dust suppression campaign was really window dressing, relatively ineffective in tackling the problem. One South Wales miner noted:

> Well, we had Dust Suppression Officers at each pit, but most of the time they might be down underground once a month. You were lucky to see them .... *cronies of management*.[58]

He continued, in a revealing exchange with another respondent:

> GG: Well, he wasn't doing his job, and I told him, you see, if you don't come down today, that face will be stopped and you'll lose over six hundred tons of coal, I said. The next thing, he was diving to come down. We'd never seem him over a long period of time unless we had a problem and we had to force him to come down.
> AM: Tell us how that worked. Weren't they supposed to regularly check?
> GG: Yes, there was ... it was made up into five districts, and they would go down into every district, one district today, one tomorrow, to check. But they never did.
> HJ: I seem to recall that on the basis of dust counts, there were whole faces which were considered to be dust approved places of work. Yes, that's a fact.[59]

An Ayrshire miner had this to say about the Dust Suppression Officers:

> Coal Board employees. One of these *created* jobs ... So-called Dust Suppression Officers. You had your ain Dust Suppression Officers at the pit, and then you had people come in from District ... The union played at it, and they played up to management.[60]

---

56 Harry Steel, Interview C9 (SOHC).
57 Marshall Wylde, Interview C35 (SOHC).
58 Gareth Golier, Interview C25 (SOHC).
59 Gareth Golier and Howard Jones, Interview C25 (SOHC).
60 Alec Mills, commenting in Interview C2 (SOHC) with Billy Affleck.

In another interview, he stated:

> They would put up on the surface that the dust count in a particular section was lowered. But it was, eh … it was massaged figures. It was massaged figures.[61]

Another Scottish miner noted:

> Believe you me, there were plenty of dodges that they had for getting the dust down. They didnae get it down in the place, but they got the count down in the machine.[62]

Malpractice such as this remained rife for some time to come, and a Yorkshire coal field survey taken in the mid-1970s found incorrect sampling procedures, non-continuous sampling of working faces or full shifts, sampling at incorrect positions, and personnel interfering with sampling equipment, such as removing sealing pads from elutriator nosepieces and replacing them with pieces of card.[63] An occupational hygienist recalled how sometimes the corners of the filter plate would be trimmed to reduce the weight of the sample.[64] Miners recalled how filters in the measuring devices were emptied a couple of times before taking the machine to the surface, and how dust entering the device was restricted, either by positioning the sampler in a relatively non-dusty location (a distance away from the working face) or by covering the machine:

> They had a wee thing like this that men carried for measuring the level of the dust, right. Now the men would come in, and if it was awfully stoorie and there was a danger of the face shutting, they flung their jacket over the top of it, ken. That's the kind of tricks … They put their jacket over the top of these machines so that there was hardly any stoor going into it.[65]

Moreover, as David Guy explained, the system was widely subverted in Durham in order to keep production going:

> If a bad reading was got in a particular district, on a number of occasions the Airborne Dust Sampler would be sent back into the mine to take a further reading, and he would be sent in where the coal production wasn't at its peak, and even in some cases where coal production had stopped, which would have meant an automatic reduction in the amount of airborne dust count. There was a certain amount of a very lax approach, in my opinion, to the working environment as far as coal dust was concerned, and it was endemic, it wasn't just this coal field [Northumberland and Durham], it was every coal field.[66]

---

61 Alec Mills, commenting in Interview C9 (SOHC).

62 John Orr, Interview C3 (SOHC).

63 Judgment of Mr Justice Turner, *The British Coal Respiratory Disease Litigation* (1998), p. 447.

64 We are grateful to Robin Howie for this information.

65 Billy Affleck, Interview C2 (SOHC).

66 David Guy, Interview C44 (SOHC).

Oral evidence thus clearly indicates the limitations of state regulation and NCB dust control efforts in the three decades or so after the Second World War. This kind of testimony can depict workers as victims of a repressive and manipulative regime in which production was placed before health, resulting in considerable bodily damage. Undeniably, management were in control, took the strategic decisions, and power relations in the pit constrained choices. Moreover, the collectively negotiated payment-by-results wage system also constituted a powerful inducement on the men to prioritise production over health. However, it would be wrong to portray the men as helpless victims, lacking any control over their labour process and without some choice and agency in all this. There were cases where the men themselves colluded in cutting dry and allowing the subversion of dust measuring and control equipment because they had a stake in maximising production where wages were tied to output. The pit closure programme and the insecurity and uncertainty it engendered may well have also contributed to this attitude. This is understandable, and the main culprit here wasn't the men themselves, but the wage system that encouraged such cutting of corners, as well as the economic volatility of the industry from the 1920s.

William Clough's father died with 100% silicosis, and he himself was certified with emphysema. He noted how his work ethic exposed him to dust disease:

> Well, I mean, I blame it through working a lot of overtime. I mean, you can imagine, working seven days a week … I mean, I worked a' ma life. I worked till I was sixty-five, you know what I mean? The hours that I put in down the pit is nobody's business, in fact they used to call me 'tattie'; I was down the pit [underground] more than a tattie, you know what I mean, just to make money, you know.
> NR: How many hours were you doing a day?
> WC: *Phoar*, I've seen me work weeks and weeks, five twelve-hour shifts … going back on the Saturday and Sunday.

He continued: 'I was breathing this foul [air] twice as much as what other people were because some wouldn't do it … I was daft, really, but it paid off, because I made more money.'[67]

Two Scottish miners spoke at length about the way management and miners had a tendency to place production and wages before safety and health, and how new wage systems encouraged such behaviour:

> JG: But then again, when the power-loading came along, guaranteed wage, and then the bonus system came along, and that was it, we virtually couldnae control it [dust] because men – they're geared to money, right? The only way we could stop it, if we caught them, and miners will improvise, anyone will improvise when there's money involved, but we had to ensure, we used to have what we call schools, we'd have safety committees at the pit, once a week, safety committee, the manager as the chairman of the committee, in hammering this, but at the end of the day, when they went down that pit and they could

---

67   William Clough, Interview C36 (SOHC).

say, 'Wait a minute, that's going to stop me fae earning a pound or two and I'm going to improvise,' the miner was the greatest improviser you could meet.

NR: Is that why you say he was the worst enemy, because you were trying to stop all that?

JG: I was trying to stop that as a Workmen's Inspector right? The union was trying to stop it because we had to go to big conferences to try and get the safety … imprinted in people's mind, and up to a point we were successful.

GP: Up to a point, aye.

JG: You know, we had men who were very good, but other men who *were so greedy*, and it has *to be said*.[68]

John Gillon added, later in the interview: 'You want it in a nutshell? *The men was the worst enemy* … There are a lot of things I could tell you that the men did that they should not have done.' This testimony is significant at a number of levels. It shows the existence of an individualistic work culture operating even within the renowned collectivist environment of mining communities, and illustrates the gap that existed between health and safety regulations and actual workplace practice. Importantly, however, it also demonstrates the proactive role of the trade union in the workplace in containing tendencies amongst the men to maximise earnings irrespective of the damage such practices could incur to themselves – and fellow miners (see Chapter 7).

The trade-off between higher earnings and the body continued to be evident in mining right through to the end of the twentieth century. This was one reason for the resurgence of pneumoconiosis at the Longannet pit in the late 1990s amongst sub-contractors (discussed in Chapter 5). John Gillon offered this comment:

> Then the late 80s, early 90s, we didn't have a case of that at all, we thought we'd beat it. Then came along Longannet, where they were, what we describe, what I ca' skewing coal, and then we discovered then, then it raised its head again, pneumoconiosis. Six or seven men diagnosed with pneumoconiosis. Now that to me was terrible … Young men, and we says, 'Oh God I thought we'd won that battle,' but then again it was because, when you could hear them talking, you see, safety went – see, they were earning one thousand pounds a week. … and we told them, we said, 'You'll come a cropper.'[69]

The desire to maximise earnings in a relatively insecure economic environment could lead to alliances between management and the miners against the 'interference' of the much-resented Dust Suppression Officers, widely vilified by face workers as unproductive 'oncost men' (that is paid by time, not by results). This clash between the interfering regulator and the working miner was neatly articulated by a Welsh miner when he was asked what the men thought of Dust Suppression Officers:

> Not much. You see, what happened, unfortunately, every man was doing a particular job before nationalisation, well, these were seen as extras living off the backs of the

---

68 John Gillon and George Peebles, Interview C24 (SOHC).

69 Ibid.

nationalisation, and we had this resentful attitude which was wrong in the end, of course … So there was a clear battle, as it were, that they were on your side so long as they didn't delay you from finishing your job. There's a conflict for you![70]

The following recollections of a retired machineman illustrates something of these complex and fluid relationships, as well as the ease with which senior NCB management could undermine preventative action at the face:

> He [the Dust Suppression Officer] come down … 'Arco, stop that machine, there's too much dust, too much dust.' Right, stop the machine. 'You're cutting too much dirt.' I said, 'I'm cutting dirt,' I says, 'I admit I'm cutting dirt, but it's a bad roof and I've got to leave so much coal on the roof. If I lift that up, you'll no' can keep me going in timber.' So I crawled away up to the top road to the phone and I phoned … the manager. 'That's my machine stopped.' 'What's wrong?' 'Oh,' I says 'The Dust Suppression Officer's stopped my machine because there's too much dirt, and *you* know the position, if I bring that machine up, you'll no' can keep me going in wood.' 'Aye. Tell the Dust Suppression Officer to get up to this phone.' I crawled away down. 'You're wanted on the phone.' So he goes up, and I presume the manager gave him hell. So I'm sitting at this machine idle, [the Dust Suppression Officer] comes down, 'Right, Arco, start your machine.' 'Oh *no* … I'm cutting too much dirt.' 'Come on, get it started.' 'No, no, you stopped it. I'm cutting too much dirt.' 'No, eh, eh, start your machine.' (laughs) So, of course, I had to start the machine. So that's nationalisation. Jobs for the boys. Jobs for the boys …[71]

Now, to dissect this testimony a bit, it is probably the case that this account of a worker's triumph over officialdom had been told and retold several times. It may well be, then, that there may be a certain degree of fabrication, or embellishment. However, the fact that the only prompt was the question 'Was there a Dust Suppression Officer in your pit?' suggests that we can – at the very least – accept this as evidence of a generally accepted clash between dust suppression and coal production, in which, in this case, management and miner were in collusion for the sake of production.

Similarly, there existed a sense in some pits that the government-appointed Mines Inspectors were interfering in miners' efforts to make a decent wage. Witness this comment from a Scottish miner:

> One of the big things … was that the fact the way the men seen the government inspectors, you were at the place of work, stripping in your step to lead up, and he would suddenly appear, he was the enemy in your mind, holding you back. You had to change the whole perception of safety in the miners' minds … 'Do it properly.' He was the enemy. They saw him as the enemy.[72]

He added: 'the Mines and Quarries Act were governed very strictly … but, I mean, you managed to get around it'.

---

70 Les Higgon, Interview C30 (SOHC).
71 William Dunsmore, Interview C16 (SOHC).
72 David Carruthers, Interview C23 (SOHC).

NCB policy on respirators was outlined in Chapter 6. What were the men's opinions and attitudes towards such personal protection which should have been an additional line of defence (in conjunction with dust control) in the pits and which the NCB was compelled to make available in 1975? A Welsh miner commented:

> I wore a mask once ... but after ten minutes you just couldn't bear it. It affected your mouth. It affected your breathing. It was no bloody good. ... Generally speaking, the attitude towards masks was similar to mine. Other people tried them, but they were not a success.[73]

Oral evidence largely supports the contention (as we noted earlier, supported by Charles Fletcher of the PRU in 1950) that the masks were ineffective and uncomfortable to wear while working.[74] This situation prevailed until well into the 1970s. A Scottish miner, Robert Clelland, responded to being asked if he ever wore a mask:

> Sometimes aye, sometimes no. But most of the time, no. They were hopeless, and you couldnae breath in them, if you were working hard, if you were on the brushing, on the face, on development, on the advance driveage you had tae physically work hard, shovel away, and you couldnae breath. You wore them for two or three minutes, and they were clogged up, with sweat, moisture, dust, and you had to take them off, they were hopeless.[75]

A 69-year-old Scottish ex-miner reacted angrily when he was asked if he had ever been issued with masks: 'Oh Christ aye, we had masks. Aye ... They wee fucking things that the doctors use ... That's what we had. That's all we had.'[76] This response is borne out by a retired trade union representative who said this about masks: 'Latterly the Board did introduce masks. But it was only a small piece of tin with a gauze inside it. Which you would need to have changed a hundred times.'[77] A 90-year-old Ayrshire miner had similar memories:

> They started bringing these masks in [that] clamped on to your face. A wee bit of gauze. A wee tape went round the back, but you clipped it onto your nose and your mouth, and that was you supposed to be drawing air through this ...[78]

Prior to the introduction of disposable masks, one Scottish miner commented on the unhygienic practice of masks being swapped between the men:

> It was they big, clumsy dust masks that you got, great big rubber things, and you didnae hae your ane personal dust mask, eh? You just put them in at the end of the shift and

---

73 Howard Jones, Interview C25 (SOHC).

74 Charles Fletcher , 'Fighting the "Modern Black Death"', *The Listener* (28 September 1950), p. 407.

75 Robert Clelland, Interview C22 (SOHC).

76 Carl Martin, Interview C8 (SOHC).

77 Alec Mills, Interview C1 (SOHC).

78 Andrew Lyndsay, Interview C4 (SOHC).

they went intae a big basin, so you could maybe hae the one that ah had yesterday or, ah mean, you got some horrors, eh? You wouldn't wear their clothes that they were wearing him doon the pit ... and you think, 'well, ah could maybe get his dust mask the mornin',' eh?[79]

In the Durham coal field, there were similar stories about the ineffectiveness of masks and inadequacy of provision. One Durham miner commented:

The only mask I ever had, ever, was offered, it was like a sponge, just like a triangular sponge. Well, when that used to get wet with the sweat, it used to 'skin' you. And then when you brought them out you had to wash them in the showers as you were getting washed, put it in your locker for the next day. Well, the trouble was, you know what a sponge is like when it gets dried, it's hard, you couldn't wear it, it used to *skin you.* That's the only thing.[80]

Another Durham miner made similar remarks:

Well, that came on later, on but that was o'er late: but you couldn't bloody breathe with them on either. You had the mask on, you're sweating and you were hopeless.[81]

And this lengthy piece of testimony from another Durham miner with experience of using a respirator with a changeable filter illustrates how the supply of masks to workers could be a clumsy and lengthy procedure:

One of the problems with dust masks was that in this particular coal field, particularly on the coastal pits, we would be in production for twenty-four hours a day. They were high-productive collieries with a shift pattern which ensured coal production for twenty-four hours. But the issuing of dust masks or the issuing of the filters that go inside of dust masks are only limited to one person issuing the dust masks between, say, eight o'clock in the morning, four 'o' clock on the afternoon, so any shift that fell outside of that, you wouldn't have access to replacing your filter, or in fact having any replacement to your dust mask if it was damaged or if it was lost ... You had to fill in a form, you had to get someone in to sign it, it then went away for somebody else to countersign, then it went to the stores, and then you went to the stores to see whether or not the chitty had gone through the system and authorisation had been given for the issuing of a dust mask ... There was a dust mask cleansing procedure put in place as well, where you put your dust mask in, and it would be cleaned and returned to your place of allocation between each shift, so there wasn't a problem with that, so they were pretty good with the cleaning of dust masks.[82]

And here's how an Ayrshire miner remembered masks in the Barony pit in the late 1970s:

---

79 Duncan Porterfield, Interview C22 (SOHC).
80 Fredrick Hall, Interview C41 (SOHC).
81 Sam Westhead, Interview C37 (SOHC).
82 David Guy, Interview C44 (SOHC).

In the Barony, if you wanted them, 'Go and get them.' Now, the work was such that if you wanted to make any kind of wage at all, you had to go ahead without the mask. Because these ... A working man has got to breathe. Therefore, maybe *some* people used them, but they maybe werenae daein' much work. So that was that episode with the masks, that you couldnae work and wear them.[83]

Ensuring that masks were available did not mean that the NCB encouraged their use. A Durham miner commented that eventually, the face-cutting machine operators were put under pressure to wear dust masks, whilst 'if you were working ancillary to that, then there didn't seem to be a great deal of pressure placed on anyone to wear them'.[84]

In South Wales, there was a deep-rooted antipathy to wearing the masks. Howard Jones and Gareth Golier commented on their experience up to the 1980s:

HJ: No, I can't remember one single solitary incident where a man, eh, a collier on the coal face had a mask on. The only incidence I can truthfully recollect was the coal-cutting man, and as I said, they were unbearable. After five minutes you just had to take them off, honestly.
AM: But did the coal-cutting men stick it out and wear them?
HJ: I didn't wear them. I tried them. Honestly, if they were comfortable I would not have taken it off. But they were most uncomfortable.
GG: On top of that, when you wore them you were taking deeper breaths more or less, and dust would go in at the sides. They were a blooming nuisance. They boys would wear them for ten minutes and then would throw them into the waste.[85]

Once again, then, the oral history interviews clearly illustrate the complexities of the problem when it came to the practicalities of wearing masks and the significance of the prevailing workplace culture.

Risk, Choice and Masculinity: The Archetypal 'Hard Man'?

Miners performed one of the most dangerous of all jobs, exposing their bodies to the possibility both of traumatic injury and chronic, long-term ill health. As we discussed in Chapter 2, serious disability and death was a daily occurrence in the industry before the Second World War. Miners were constantly reminded of this as men with physical impairments were more evident in mining towns and villages than any other working-class communities. How did miners view this risk? How was this rationalised? Why were such conditions tolerated? And, importantly, to what extent did miners' identities as men, forged in the male-only workplace and in exclusively male social activities up to the mid-twentieth century (such as the pub

---

83 Alec McNeish, Interview C13 (SOHC).
84 David Guy, Interview C44 (SOHC).
85 Howard Jones and Gareth Gower, Interview C25 (SOHC).

and football), affect their behaviour towards their health and their bodies? These are not easy questions to address. However, oral evidence and other personal testimony enables some elucidation of prevailing attitudes and health behaviours within male-dominated high-risk work cultures. What is evident is that views varied considerably within such a diverse community.

Masculinity at its core involves an assumption of power or superiority by men over women. In British working-class culture, at least up until the 1960s, women were widely regarded as inferior and dependent. Historically, the 'essence' of masculinity has been variously located with reference to notions of the man as *provider* (probably the most enduring representation), to male physical prowess, toughness, homophobia, risk-taking, aggression and violent behaviour (including violence against women), a competitive spirit, a lack of emotional display, dispassionate instrumentalism and only limited involvement in fathering.[86] Recently, moreover, masculinity has also become identified with an excess of life-threatening illnesses and premature death.[87] Whilst the home and consumption were designated feminine domains, production was widely regarded historically as a highly masculinised sphere. Closer analysis, however, reveals a more complex and fluid picture. Theorists tend now to see a range of masculinities that can be prevalent at any given moment, and see such masculinities as being socially constructed and subject to significant change over time. There is also disagreement over a precise definition of what masculinity entails, recognition that few men actually 'fit' the norms, and that some of the stereotypical 'core' attributes are not necessarily exclusive to men.[88] Abendstern, Hallett and Wade's recent oral history-based study of female weavers in North West England, for example, shows that risk-taking at work was not just a male phenomenon before 1970, but 'a part of daily life ... tolerated because of peer pressure and managerial expectations'.[89]

None the less, what might be termed 'hegemonic', or dominant, modes of masculinity characterised particular communities and historical periods. A kind of 'hard man' working-class masculinity was nurtured in the tough street culture of the neighbourhood and the recurrent brutality of school life, then forged in arduous, dirty

86 See L. Segal, *Slow Motion: Changing Masculinities, Changing Men* (London, 1997); R.W. Connell, *The Men and the Boys* (Oxford, 2000); P. Willis, 'Shop floor culture, masculinity and the wage form', in J. Clarke, C. Critcher and R. Johnson (eds), *Working Class Culture* (London, 1979); M. Roper, *Masculinity and the British Organization Man since 1945* (Oxford, 1994); D. Wight, *Workers not Wasters: Masculine Respectability, Consumption and Unemployment in Central Scotland* (Edinburgh, 1993); R. Evans, *You questioning my manhood, boy? Masculine Identity, Work Performance and Performativity in a Rural Staples Economy*, Arkleton Research Paper no. 4 (Aberdeen, 2000).

87 See D. Sabo and D.F. Gordon, *Men's Health and Illness: Gender, Power and the Body* (London, 1995); J. Cornwell, *Hard-earned Lives* (London, 1984).

88 J. Watson, *Male Bodies: Health, Culture and Identity* (Buckingham, 2000), pp. 33–5.

89 M. Abendstern, C. Hallett and L. Wade, 'Flouting the Law: Women and the Hazards of Cleaning Moving Machinery in the Cotton Industry, 1930–1970', *Oral History*, vol. 33, no. 2 (Autumn 2005), p. 77.

and often dangerous work in the heavy industries in the first half of the twentieth century.[90] Phillips has commented on how the status of dockers was enhanced within the community by acceptance of risks in what was a highly dangerous occupation, citing the example of the London dock activist Jack Dash, who worked naked from the waist up (nicknamed 'nature boy') and who made light of a death-defying fall fifty feet into a ship's hold.[91] McKinlay has explored the construction of manliness in the inter-war Clydebank shipyards, whilst Ayers has examined the incubation of manly identities amongst Liverpool dockers in the post-Second World War period.[92] The Glasgow shipbuilding union activist Jimmy Reid's famous comment on the 1971 Upper Clyde Shipbuilders' work-in, 'we didn't only build ships on the Clyde, we built men', would equally apply to coal mining.[93] A cult of toughness characterised mining, and young male workers adapted to this and absorbed it through peer pressure. Campbell has noted how Scottish mining communities before the Second World War were 'suffused with a discourse of manliness', with male youths encouraged by older miners to avoid displaying emotion (such as crying) and to play fighting games because, as one said, this was 'the training you got to be hard men'.[94] Dangerous, dirty, dusty and physically exhausting work, with the constant stream of injuries and deaths in the pits, hardened boys up, de-sensitising them to danger and socialising them into a competitive, macho environment.[95] As Bert Coombes noted of his experiences in South Wales before the Second World War, miners were not immune to fear, but daily exposure to risk toughened them up:

> These near escapes make us nervous for a while, especially if we think what might have happened. For some time we see danger in every stone, *then become hardened again*. I remember when a boy of seventeen was killed about twelve yards away from me. More than sixty boys were working there, but not one came to work on the next shift – all were afraid.[96]

Standing up for oneself was also deemed a key attribute within this culture. As one Ayrshire miner noted: 'You found out that men and management in general were

---

90 For a discussion of masculinity and the Glasgow 'hard man', see R. Johnston and A. McIvor, 'Dangerous Work, Hard Men and Broken Bodies: Masculinity in the Clydeside Heavy Industries, c1930–1970s', *Labour History Review*, vol. 69, no. 2 (August 2004).

91 J. Phillips, 'Class and Industrial Relations in Britain: The 'Long' Mid-century and the Case of Port Transport, c1920–1970', *Twentieth Century British History*, vol. 16, no. 1 (2005), pp. 62–3.

92 A. McKinlay, *Making Ships, Making Men* (Clydebank, *c.* 1981); P. Ayers, 'Work Culture and Gender: The Making of Masculinities in Post-war Liverpool', *Labour History Review*, vol. 69, no. 2 (2004), pp. 153–68.

93 Cited in M. Bellamy, *The Shipbuilders* (Edinburgh, 2000), p. 199.

94 A. Campbell, *The Scottish Miners, Volume 1. Industry, Work and Community* (Aldershot, 2000), p. 238.

95 A. Moffat, *My Life with the Miners* (London, 1965), pp. 16–17, 19.

96 Coombes, *These Poor Hands*, p. 121 (our emphasis).

always at loggerheads in the coal mining industry. … If you were a *weak* man, you would have did what the boss said.'[97]

Apart from the harshness and the brutalising nature of the job, though, another important aspect of masculinity was the camaraderie of the workplace.[98] Textile mills and other female-dominated workplaces offered similar opportunities for socialising, but the male bonding aspect was frequently consolidated by contact with work mates out of work hours in the street, on the football field and in the pub or miners' social club. Hard drinking and heavy smoking were symbols of male virility in working-class culture.[99] In his novel *The Kiln*, William McIlvanney depicts this in his portrayal of Tam, a sensitive and intelligent 17-year-old growing up in Ayrshire in 1955:

> You really had to smoke at the dancing, he had decided. It's hard enough trying to camouflage yourself as a tough guy as it is. Go in there without cigarettes and it would be like wearing a blouse.[100]

Within this culture, being able to tolerate the toughest work conditions, take the greatest risks and hold one's alcohol (drinking others 'under the table') were celebrated as praiseworthy male attributes. Moreover, as Wight has shown, even as late as the 1980s, the pub in mining communities operated to confirm masculinity: 'the pubs were at the centre of the men's domain, in contrast to the home which was the women's sphere'.[101] Drinking also reflected a man's earning capacity, with 'big drinkers' being equated with hard workers. One of the last miners in a pit village in Central Scotland proudly told a researcher in the early 1980s: 'I'm the top machine worker in Scotland, put that on your form … aye … you know … status.' He went on to comment on how he welcomed the reverence: 'You know, when you stand at the bar and say "I'll buy yous a round."'[102] The pay packet was the outward symbol of independence, and usually brought with it a certain amount of entitlement and privilege: bringing home a wage invariably meant for the young male worker a quite different treatment in the home, with more respect and preferential treatment, as befitted the transition from dependant to proto-breadwinner.[103]

This type of hegemonic masculinity undoubtedly characterised most mining communities up to the middle of the twentieth century, and perhaps for some time beyond, as the social anthropology of Daniel Wight suggests and the movie *Billy Elliot* nicely caricatures. Wight has shown how miners in central Scotland were

---

97 Alec Mills, Interview C1 (SOHC).

98 David Hendry, Interview C15 (SOHC).

99 K. Mullen, *A Healthy Balance: Glaswegian Men Talk about Health, Tobacco and Alcohol* (Aldershot, 1993), p. 177.

100 W. McIlvanney, *The Kiln* (London, 1996), p. 33.

101 D. Wight, *Workers not Wasters*, pp. 155–6. Wight estimated that in the early 1980s, there was around one woman to every ten men in the Cauldmoss pubs.

102 Wight, *Workers not Wasters*, p. 163.

103 Ibid., pp. 102–3, 138.

expected to be 'strong' and 'tough', both physically and emotionally – expressions of which were protecting female relatives and never crying.[104] Other attributes which enhanced masculinity in the mining village where Wight lived from 1982 to 1984 were ownership of cars and powerful dogs (especially Alsatians and pit bull terriers) and meat-eating (particularly steaks and hot curries). However, not all miners bought into this, and a wide range of identities and relationships existed; other masculinities were on display, and attitudes changed over time. The reality, in other words, was more fluid and complex than the dominant *machismo* discourse implies. As Wight's insightful study of a Scottish mining community shows, something of a divide existed between the rough and respectable – the workers and the 'wasters'.[105] Set against the macho boozing and football were the pit brass bands in the Northern coal fields, the persistence of religion (including strict observance of the Sabbath) in Scotland, and the male voice choirs in the Welsh valleys.

That said, miners – like other workers in the heavy-industry communities – were acculturated to high levels of danger, socialised by their upbringing and daily experience in the pits. Indeed, it may well be the case that the masculinity of coal miners was forged mainly *within* the workplace, rather than outside it – as may well have been the case with urban workers in places like Tyneside and Clydeside, where a kind of 'hard man' working-class culture prevailed. We noted in Chapter 2 how one miner, Tommy Coulter, articulated something of the *machismo* work culture that prevailed in the mining villages, commenting on how miners were 'hardy buggers' and 'strong lads' fully capable of defending themselves with their fists when necessary, 'like soldiers'. In a later comment, this respondent qualified his statement, though again emphasising the masculine element in mining work culture:

> But yes, we were a bit macho, but a' don't think we were nasty, we, you were taught to respect women in particular, and older people, and ah suppose, it was no' only just mine workers, that was the village life. But we were macho, and we thought we were the greatest, and we knew that was the case …[106]

An Ayrshire miner described the transition to manhood associated with the move from haulage work to face work, commenting on the late 1940s:

> That's what you done till once you got a place, eh, on the run, ken, among the men, ken. Eh, and I can mind, sir … I was … I was drawing when I was eighteen year old, nineteen year old, and, eh, that, eh … I was drawing one hundred hutches a day. No kidding you, I was like steel. I was a hard man then. And, eh, I drew off a wee bloke. He was a wee Pole, this wee bloke, and he was a hard man. Arkuski you cried him, ken. Tony Arkuski. He was a hard man, sir. Him and I … Oh, we were down there first go in the morning and last away, ken. Aye, we made good money then, ken …[107]

---

104 Ibid., pp. 42–3.
105 Ibid., pp. 60–86.
106 Tommy Coulter, Interview C21 (SOHC).
107 Thomas McMurdo, Interview C20 (SOHC).

Up to the 1940s, it was the immediate dangers of roof collapse, gas and explosions that dominated miners' thinking, rather than the potential long-term possibility of respiratory problems. Perhaps there was just too much to preoccupy miners in the daily struggle for existence in the depressed 1930s to worry too much about breathlessness twenty or thirty years down the line? Moreover, enduring the risks, dangers and strain of work reinforced masculine values. Taken into the pit at 14 or 15, youths were de-sensitised to the dangers and learned to stoically accept the hot, dusty and vitiated mine environment. As we have seen, for a long time too it was widely believed that it was only stone dust – silica – that was harmful. When asked by Hywel Francis if he realised dust was harmful, John Evans recalled of his working days as a miner from 1927 to the 1940s:

> How can I explain it to you? Brought up in a mining district, you really didn't give it a thought like that in coal dust, because in those days men had to rip their roads, what they call rock. And there was more emphasis on silica than on coal dust. They classed coal dust as if it were nothing, silica was the main concern.[108]

Moreover, well into the 1940s miners believed that they could move from the heaviest work if their breathing worsened after twenty years or so at high-paid work at the face to lighter and less dusty work. This was before the progressive nature of the disease was realised. In other words, it was believed that only if a man was really unlucky would the condition be capable of preventing a man earning a living. As John Evans recalled: 'I always thought, myself, that I could carry on the rest of my days and do a normal day's work until I retired at sixty-five. But it didn't work out that way.'[109] Another South Wales miner commented that he was exposed to dust the whole of his thirty-four years' working underground, but 'Well, when you're a youngster you don't realise, do you? It is later on in life you realise what you've been doing, like.' He added: 'I enjoyed my work.'[110] To some extent, the bodily damage caused by years working underground was accepted because of the very high earnings that were possible from this work and the belief that you would not be so impaired that a living of some kind could not be earned in later years. The 'welfarist' policies of the NCB in providing older, less fit and disabled miners with work in 'approved places' and on the surface, and encouraging transfers to neighbouring pits as the colliery closure programme intensified, would also have contributed to this way of thinking. The responsibilities of family, especially through a miner's twenties, thirties and forties helped to further rationalise such decisions, or constrain choices. As a Yorkshire miner who started work just before the Second World War noted, fulfilling the provider role meant accepting a level of risk: 'You knew there were dangers, of course, but people were ignorant of what to do. But

---

108 John Evans, interviewed by Hywel Francis, 13 June 1973 (SWCC).
109 Ibid.
110 Malcolm Davies, Interview C29 (SOHC).

you had to keep a family, so you had to work whether you liked it or lumped it.'[111] A South Wales miner, John Jones, explained that he left an apprenticeship to work underground in 1950 despite parental opposition and the fact that his father was laid off 'full of pneumoconiosis':

> I was an apprentice toolmaker, but I left that. My father begged me not to leave it, but I left it because my father had to finish work and I was the eldest of three boys and there was more money in the pit than in the factory. I was having £1 17s. 4½d. a week in the factory; my first pay in the colliery was £6.50. It was helping the family along, and that's how I got involved in the pits although my father didn't want me to go down there.[112]

He added later, 'we were struggling in the house', and that he had concealed his reasoning from his parents, telling his father he made the decision because 'all my mates are underground'.

For some, risks were taken to maximise earnings. Within the broader constraints of family responsibilities in a patriarchal culture, lack of alternative job opportunities, a contracting industry and a wage system that paid by results, miners could and did exercise some choice. Hence wage-maximisation and the preservation of jobs could be prioritised over occupational health and well-being. In response to a question about the existence of safety procedures when shot-firing, John Jones noted: 'Yes, well there was, but oh, they were, sometimes we, it's our own fault, we were taking risks. It was our own fault sometimes.' When asked, 'Why were you taking the risks?', he responded: 'To get that stuff out, to get the coal out.'[113] Later in the interview, he reiterated: 'This is the point. We were at fault, our side, by risking it instead of saying, "Oh, I'm leaving it there, I'm not doing it."' John ended up with pneumonconioisis, just like his father, and was one of many miners who continued to work for years at the face after first diagnosis, in his case between 1971 and 1978. He perhaps personified the competitive, work-dominated grafter.

The mine drivers who tended to work for outside contractors such as Cementation and the German firm Tison appear to have had a particularly defined culture of risk-taking. Malcolm Davies recalled that there was never a work stoppage amongst mine drivers in his experience in South Wales as a consequence of excessive working in dust. He recalled:

> You just carried on with your work, you did, you know. What you done, you earned, isn't it? Especially with Tison. If you done like I did, you got good pay, like. If you didn't do like I did, your pay would be down, like, you know. That was a lot to do with it, to tell you the truth.[114]

---

111 'The Price of Coal (Part 2)', *Saga Magazine* (October 1998), consulted at http://www.deadline.demon.co.uk/archive/saga/981001.htm.

112 John Jones, Interview C27 (SOHC).

113 Ibid. However, the interviewer's comment, 'For money? For wages?', might reasonably be construed as a leading question, invalidating the positive response.

114 Malcolm Davies, Interview C29 (SOHC).

But face workers too were capable of prioritising the wage and in some cases the opportunity to get off early, as this exchange between two Scottish miners elucidates:

> DC: But when they were making money, as I said earlier on, and early allowance and money were two of the biggest incentives in the pit. If you were getting away early, you worked harder, and if they were giving you more money, you worked harder because it was money. George might disagree with me, but I reckon that was two of the best incentives or the biggest incentives as far as the men were concerned was money and an early allowance. Ken, if the manager said, 'Right, give me two shears [along the coal face] and you'll go.'
> GB: I couldn't argue with you, because it worked, it worked, but there was a price to pay. There was a price to pay, and we're paying that price now, you have young men with pneumoconiosis now. Of course, when I was working at the coal face, we were taking off three strips a day, sometimes four. Sometimes nine strips in a shift, and the dust, the dust, the dust.
> DC: They've been known to do eleven, they were known to do eleven.[115]

The camaraderie, teamwork and support network underground also perhaps helped to assuage any feelings of danger and insecurity. Miners were all in the same boat, and knew they could rely upon each other to come to assist if they were in trouble. As John Evans noted: 'The best thing underground was the friendship, you'd risk your life for another man, you know, and you stick together.'[116]

There was, then, widespread acceptance within mining communities of a high level of risk, and this was bound up in customary work cultures and attitudes passed down from father to son. That is not to say, however, that this was set in stone. The risk-acceptance threshold was fluid, and subject to change over time. The younger generation of miners after the Second World War were less willing to tolerate the conditions their fathers had accepted. This difference in inter-generational attitudes was evident everywhere, and commented on by the ILO in their 1964 study of the dust problem in coal mining:

> The awareness of the dust danger that young workers may acquire during their vocational training is perhaps more difficult to create in the mind of mature miners, who may be so accustomed to all the dangers of life underground that they tend to forget them.[117]

Moreover, within such a dangerous working environment, long-term health risks tended to take second place to the immediacy of accidents. To some degree, then, although miners became more safety-conscious, they did not become health-conscious at the same pace. This focus on accidents to the detriment of health was

---

115 David Carruthers and George Bolton, Interview C23 (SOHC).

116 John Evans, interviewed by Hywel Francis, 13 June 1973 (SWCC).

117 International Labour Organisation, Coal Mines Committee, 8th Session, *Dust Suppression in Coal Mines* (1964), p. 104, NA/LAB 13 /1836.

neatly summed up in 1964 by L.R. James, who by this time was head of the Safety Department of the NUM:

> How difficult it is to logically associate the careless dragging of a foot through a pile of dust with ultimate disability? ... The same factors are involved in connecting smoking with lung cancer. If people dying as a consequence of smoking did so suddenly whilst actually in the act of smoking, campaigns to reduce smoking would be unnecessary. [118]

Peer group pressure, and to some extent a competitive *machismo* work culture underground, also contributed to a culture of high risk acceptance and stoicism in the face of dusty work environments. Connell in *Men and Boys* reminds us that working-class culture was full of Stakhanovite examples of workers pitting themselves against the accepted effort limits of wage labour – such as the miner who loaded 'sixteen tons of number nine coal'.[119] This was a tough job, and miners were acculturated and hardened to it. Daily exposure to dust de-sensitised miners to its insidious qualities. Moreover, there was friendly rivalry underground, and miners had to be seen to be pulling their weight within the work team – hence the evident embarrassment and sense of encroaching emasculation when breathlessness started to impair their ability to work. To an extent, older and disabled miners would be assisted by their mates, but routinely miners were expected not to shirk hard graft. Bert Coombes commented that in South Wales in the 1930s: 'Men who do not do their share are treated with contempt and are given nicknames, such as "Shonny one tram", by their fellow workmen who are usually too ready to pour out their sweat and their blood.'[120] Mining communities revered their most productive grafters, and fables grew up in many pits around the 'big hewers'.[121] Those who broke production records were looked up to with respect in mining communities – such as the much-celebrated 'Gedlings record breakers'.[122] One Welsh mine driver, Malcolm Davies, described the rivalry as well as the respect and esteem that high producing mineworkers earned from their fellows:

> When I worked with Tison, I was competitive, you know, we tried to beat the other heading and things like. ... We were all good pals, mind, but we would come up, we'd have a chat 'What have you done today?' like, y'know. 'Oh, we put ceilings up or two-way put up,' and things like that. I put five up one day, in one day. Me and three men. Five yards. Five yards travelling, in a twelve-foot heading. ... I don't think anybody else did that, I tell you.

---

118 *The Miner*, vol. 12, no. 5 (September/October 1964), p. 21.

119 Connell, *The Men and the Boys*, p. 188.

120 Coombes, *These Poor Hands*, p. 44.

121 See, for example, the Charles Parker programme for radio produced in 1961, 'The Big Hewer', Aud/580, South Wales Coalfield Collection; Wight, *Workers not Wasters*, p. 163; W.H. Shepherd, *Under the Pulley Wheels: The Memoirs of William Herbert Shepherd (1891– 1972)*, Accessed 12 February 2006 at http://www.wheatleyhill.com/pulley.htm.

122 This group of miners broke a colliery production record in 1979 and became the subject of a prize-winning painting by D. Wharton. See the Coal Industry Social and Welfare Organisation, *Annual Report* (1980).

Not five rings. There was a couple of boys from the Rhondda working it up there. Oh, they were very good workers, like. They could work. And that's how it was back years ago.[123]

Two other Scottish miners noted the pervasiveness of peer pressure in keeping up productivity levels, hinting at the loss of manliness and respect if miners were not seen to pull their weight:

> DP: That was the village culture sort of thing, eh? You knew who the good workers were and who the guisers were. A lot of it was everybody trying tae be better than the next one, eh? Ken, you couldnae … you couldnae have an easy shift, sort of thing, or somebody would tell your father, eh? Or somebody doon the street would be talking about you, or they would be talking about you in the pub, the fingers would be pointing at you.
> RC: Oh, there was a pride aspect.
> DP: Pride, pride, oh aye, aye.
> RC: There's a standard in the pit, and if you didnae set your standard, the shift that followed you would see you the next day, 'Hey, dinnae you leave that like that again,' and then so-and-so would talk to so-and-so.[124]

Duncan Porterfield went on to recount a tale of two members of a particular work squad (described as 'nutters') taking their rivalry so seriously that it led to a fight whilst they were abroad on holiday over who was the best shoveller. He added:

> Oh yes, everybody thought they were top dog, eh? You didnae want anybody, if you thought somebody was that wee bitty better than you, you used to work all the harder. Ken, 'You're no' getting ma mantle.' Ken, there was an awful lot of pride at stake, oh aye. More so in your local pit, sort of thing.

The oral testimony, then, suggests a number of reasons for miners tolerating a high degree of risk in their employment. For some, working underground reflected a lack of power, constrained choices and sense of duty – following in their fathers' footsteps, helping to support the family, doing what all miners' offspring had done for generations. Young miners were acculturated to high levels of danger and risk of bodily damage within this tough and unforgiving work environment. Moreover, it may well have been the case that until at least the middle of the twentieth century, the more immediate possibility of traumatic injury took precedence in miners' minds over the more distant possibility of respiratory damage. There were many other immediate economic concerns, in an insecure world as the coal industry contracted, to preoccupy the men. Compromises had to be made to protect jobs and keep the pit going, and if that meant swallowing the dust, so be it.

The oral evidence also indicates a deeply engrained work ethic, with miners gaining esteem and status within the community for being hard grafters – 'top dogs' capable of producing more than the next man. This competitiveness was an integral element of working-class masculine behaviour. It was also fostered within a work

---

123 Malcolm Davies, Interview C29 (SOHC).
124 Robert Clelland and Duncan Porterfield, Interview C22 (SOHC).

regime in which payment by results played a key role. As a number of respondents noted, the wage packet depended upon the effort put in, and many miners would cut corners, or 'improvise', to maximise wages. In part, this was also tied in with the breadwinner ethos – the deeply engrained notion within working-class communities that it was a man's responsibility to provide for the family. Peer pressure at the point of production to 'act as a man' was significant too. Hence, miners re-entered the dusty environment sooner than they should have after shot-firing, endured cutting dry, because their mates did so and it was expected of them. Not to have done so would have risked being labelled as 'soft' and having one's manly identity challenged. Mining labour frequently involved teamwork, and the earnings of the group (or the next shift) might be affected otherwise, and (a logical progression in thinking) ultimately, the viability of the pit.

Moreover, a different managerial culture could have more stringently enforced health and safety measures and protected miners from much respiratory damage, such as preventing them from cutting dry and ensuring that masks were worn. However, the profit-oriented ethos of most private coal owners and the productionist culture of the NCB prevailed against this, as well as the miner's traditional autonomy at the point of production. It is a complex picture. The very locus of most of the work deep underground made the labour process a very difficult one to regulate and control effectively. Beyond this, however, the oral evidence indicates that miners' bodies were neglected, and health and safety issues ignored or at best regarded as of secondary importance within the converging and overlapping degenerative pressures of a productionist and *machismo* work culture.

Conclusion

Dust impacted upon different mining communities in markedly different ways because it was much more of an insidious problem in some coal fields than others. The epidemiological studies in mining communities in the 1950s and 1960s indicated that pneumoconiosis incidence could be more than four times higher in the worst hit coal fields than those with the lowest incidence, whilst the dustiest pits registered more than ten times the levels of respiratory impairment compared to those where the air was purest. Not surprisingly, in these circumstances the miners developed a range of attitudes towards dust. For most miners prior to the Second World War, a certain level of dust was regarded as inevitable, and miners were long socialised into both dangerous and dusty conditions. The oral evidence indicates a significant degree of lay knowledge about the effects of dust inhalation upon the body, as well as an acceptance by miners of a degree of risk regarding chronic respiratory disease. None the less, miners in areas of high dust concentration underground, notably face workers in South Wales, campaigned to get pneumoconiosis certified as an occupational disease, and to gain compensation and the implementation of dust control measures. Even here, however, traumatic injury was uppermost in miners' consciousness, rather than the longer-term risks of respiratory damage.

Moreover, the miners' oral testimonies indicate not only the prevalence of traditional attitudes and beliefs, of much stoicism in the face of danger and bodily damage, but also the prevailing realities of workplace culture. Here, the expression of provider masculinity played a significant part in miners accepting high levels of risk and prioritising the maximisation of wages over health. At its extreme, this led to some cutting coal dry, ignoring dust suppression measures, subverting monitoring arrangements, not wearing protective masks, and cutting corners in aggressive competition with other men and work teams to maximise wages. Working miners were also squeezed by a productionist managerial ethos in the 1930s, in wartime and in the immediate post-war mining era, where all the emphasis was upon getting the coal out. These dual and related degenerative pressures drove down health and safety standards underground. Within this environment, the oral evidence suggests that statutory control and NCB dust control measures were widely subverted through the 1950s, 1960s and beyond. Miners' traditional autonomy at work and the concealed site of production underground contributed to this. Despite much being done to reform dusty conditions by the state, there remained a wide gap between policy and actual workplace practice. Clearly, many miners continued to be exposed to much greater quantities of dust during their employment than the official figures and statements by the Mines Inspectorate and the Coal Board implied. This supports a more mixed, qualified and more pessimistic appraisal of dust control measures than the official record indicates and some historians, such as Ashworth have concluded.[125]

This reappraisal depends, however, upon giving significant weight to the evidence provided by miners in their oral testimonies. Some historians and some commentators on the dust problem have been sceptical about the veracity of such sources. For example, whilst Justice Turner, in the 1990s bronchitis/emphysema litigation, developed a trenchant critique of the failure of the NCB's dust control policies and indicted the nationalised industry for negligence, he argued that 'it would be unwise … to place too great reliance on such [oral] evidence'. He continued: 'at best it depended on distant recollection, extending in one or two instances for over sixty years'.[126] Conversely, we would argue that the oral history evidence plugs many of the gaps in the 'million-plus' documents which were examined by the lawyers involved with the British Coal case, and that it is wrong to discount such evidence. There are weaknesses in oral history testimony, just as there are weaknesses in almost any type of primary source material. For one thing, many of the miners who spoke to us have had their health damaged by working in the pits. It could well be the case, then, that there would be a tendency to exaggerate the bad working conditions which brought about their ill health. In many cases, these were victims' discourses, diffused with anger directed against 'the system' that had damaged their bodies. It is also the case that oral history evidence, collected decades after the events being remembered, has the potential for distortion through memory lapses,

---

125 W. Ashworth, *The History of the British Coal industry, Volume 5. 1946–1982* (Oxford, 1986), pp. 558–72.

126 Judgment of Mr Justice Turner, Summary, p. 8.

and as the work of Thomson and Summerfield has persuasively demonstrated, the entangling of subsequent events and dominant public discourses into the narrative – in what has been termed a 'cultural circuit'. To be sure, in some of the personal testimonies of mine workers it is possible to detect the working through of a kind of heroic victims' narrative, in which the miner is depicted as struggling against grim coal faces and intolerable conditions, with management and the regulators – and even the trade union in some cases – viewed as the culprits, responsible for the bodily damage exacted by winning the coal. Hence, for example, the recurring motif 'blood on the coal'. The unconscious 'framing', reconstructing or reconfiguring of memory in personal reminiscence in order to reach composure is now well accepted in oral history practice. On the other hand, similar embedded discourses and biases characterise many official written records too. The key point to be made here is that oral testimony is undoubtedly both interpretative and informative, especially in relation to areas of work, culture and life experience that are very poorly documented. Oral evidence, used critically and sensitively, can help not only to evoke a hidden past, but also to assist in developing our understanding of experience and attitudes, including the interwoven degenerative pressures upon health of a productionist and a *machismo* work culture in British coal mining.

Chapter 9

Breathless Men:
Living and Dying with Dust Disease

In this chapter we use personal testimony and other source material to reconstruct what it was like to live with chronic respiratory illness, examining how individuals, families and the mining community were affected by and responded to widespread breathing impairment and progressively encroaching disability. This public health catastrophe is contextualised against a backdrop of fundamental economic transformation as Britain experienced rapid de-industrialisation and employment in underground coal mining sharply contracted, indeed virtually disappeared. We concentrate here on the *lived experience* of occupational diseases, including the personal lifestyle transitions caused by occupational disability. In this respect, our work is influenced by and contributes to a growing stream of experiential-based (including oral history) research on health and well-being that places the focus on the material experience and discourses of the person and/or community directly affected – the disabled, the sick and injured.[1]

Whilst research into the history of occupational health has expanded over the past decade or so, we still know little about what it was like to become disabled in middle and later life as a consequence of chronic illness, such as pneumoconiosis, bronchitis and emphysema. As we noted in Chapter 1, the seminal studies in the field of occupational health history focus on the corporation, the regulators, the medical professionals, and to a lesser extent, the trade unions. These are key areas to investigate. However, with one or two limited exceptions, the voices, discourses and experience of those disabled by work feature surprisingly little in the literature.[2]

We argue here that the experience of disability for miners with respiratory disease shows similarities with others with sensory or physical impairments (such as the partially sighted and paraplegics – both common groups within mining communities), but also important divergences. Within the disabled mining community there was a wide range of experience, based upon markedly differing levels of impairment.

---

1   D. Atkinson, 'Research Interviews with People with Mental Handicaps', in J. Walmsley (ed.), *Making Connections* (London, 1989); J. Walmsley, 'Life History Interviews with People with Learning Disabilities', in R. Perks and A. Thomson (eds), *The Oral History Reader* (London, 1988); M. Deal, 'Disabled People's Attitudes toward Other Impairment Groups', *Disability and Society*, vol. 18, no. 7 (December 2003), pp. 897–910. See also A. Borsay, *Disability and Social Policy in Britain since 1750* (Basingstoke, 2005).

2   See, for example, R. Johnston and A. McIvor, *Lethal Work* (East Linton, 2000), pp. 177–208; T. Nichols, *The Sociology of Industrial Injury* (London, 2000).

However, whilst effects and coping strategies varied significantly across a wide spectrum of personal tragedies, the outcomes invariably involved quite fundamental *mutations* in lifestyles, behaviour and identities. Changes included erosion of physical capacity, loss or change of employment, declining standards of living, a collapse of status and self-esteem, a drift towards social exclusion, marginalisation as citizens and towards dependency. These transitions were more sudden and traumatic in some cases than others, depending on the nature and pathology of the disease(s) and the individuals concerned. Given the male domination of the coal mining industry, our story is largely male-centred. Cumulatively, encroaching disability through 'black lung' had a quite profound impact on identity, so masculinity features significantly in our argument in this chapter. As we saw in the last chapter, most of our respondents were socialised into traditional gender roles in the middle decades of the twentieth century, when men were widely perceived to be the providers and absorbed the dominant 'hard man' discourse of masculinity that prevailed in mining communities and the male-dominated heavy industries up to at least the 1970s. The oral testimonies suggest that the essence of manhood could be deeply shaken by occupational disability and subsequent loss of work, and the drift into varying levels of dependency.

There is also a further and very different identifiable impact of such experience. For some miners, chronic illness was radicalising, energising and politicising. Knowledge of bodily damage, pain and premature death, and perceptions of injustice and exploitation, drew miners into political activism – to punish those responsible, to prevent the same thing happening to others, and to get decent levels of compensation. For some miners this response was especially marked, perhaps because of the relatively militant, class-conscious workplace culture that characterised many (though by no means all) coal fields, including Scotland and South Wales. We have already commented on the role of the miners' trade unions in disability politics in Chapter 7. In this chapter, we focus in more depth upon the impact of encroaching respiratory disease and the attitudes, coping strategies and agency of disabled workers themselves, as well as the community welfare services operating in the mining areas.

Dust and Disability

Recently, disability studies have done much to establish those with impairments in our society as socially oppressed, excluded, marginalised and lacking citizenship, and in turn, have developed persuasive critiques of the state, medical profession and lay policies towards the disabled community in Britain in the nineteenth and twentieth centuries.[3] For much of the twentieth century, a 'personal tragedy' model of disability prevailed, where unfortunate victims were perceived to require

---

3 B. Hughes, 'Bauman's Strangers: Impairment and the Invalidation of Disabled People in Modern and Post-modern Cultures', *Disability and Society*, vol. 17, no. 5 (2003), pp. 571–84; C. Barnes and G. Mercer, *Disability* (Cambridge, 2003); M. Oliver, *The Politics*

care, incarceration and segregation, resulting in heavy dependence upon the state for benefits and treatment, and a subsequent loss of independence and erosion of citizenship. However, much of this portrayal of the disabled has been constructed from studies of the congenitally impaired, such as those with mental illnesses, those with learning difficulties, and those with loss of faculties such as sight, hearing and speech. Occupational injury and disease hardly feature in the literature. To what extent did impairment by chronic respiratory illness caused by the inhalation of dust at work fit the patterns of social exclusion and oppression which dominate the disability literature? Frequently, coal miners have been viewed as a unique community, living 'a life apart'. Was the experience of breathing-impaired miners different? Did a disabling injury or disease acquired from work confer a different status upon the sufferer than, say, blindness from birth or multiple sclerosis?

Firstly, we might briefly recap on the physical effects of miners' respiratory diseases. Coal workers' pneumoconiosis is the clogging up of the lungs with inhaled stone, coal and other mineral dust which, over time and in the worst cases, leads to serious lung tissue damage (fibrosis) and scarring. Pneumoconiotics experienced a wide range of impairment, with lung function resulting from the damage caused by inhaled dust varying, quite literally, from 1% to 100%. At low levels (defined officially at less than 10%, and sometimes referred to as 'simple pneumoconiosis'), the disease is virtually symptomless. After the Second World War, it was widely believed that if a miner was removed from the dusty work conditions that caused the problem, he could live a virtually full life, with no effect upon his life expectancy. However, recent research has shown that deterioration (or progression) can occur even in these early-stage cases after removal from the dusty work conditions.[4] What is certain is that after 'simple' or early-stage pneumoconiosis passed into 'complicated pneumoconiosis' (defined by radiological changes), the lung tissue damage usually progressed even after miners withdrew from the dusty conditions. In many, it resulted in encroaching and progressively worsening breathlessness (the most common symptom), loss of vitality, and inability to work, and was often accompanied by characteristic 'black spit' as miners tried to clear their airways of accumulated coal dust and degenerating tissue. One observer described the physical symptoms in this way:

> He made a sound, which would reach a terrible crescendo later, in the pithead baths. It was a heaving from deep in the throat, followed by a stuttering wheeze and, finally a hacking that went on for a minute or for a night, until the black phlegm was brought up. It is called the 'dust' or pneumoconiosis.[5]

---

of Disablement (Basingstoke, 1990). For a classic study, see M. Blaxter, *The Meaning of Disability: A Sociological Study of Impairment* (London, 1976).

4   M.D. Attfield and E.D. Kuempel, 'Pneumoconiosis, Coal Mine Dust and the PFR', *Annals of Occupational Hygiene*, vol. 47, no. 7 (2003), p. 528.

5   J. Pilger, 'Heartlands to wastelands', *New Statesman and Society* (23 October 1992), pp. 10–11.

A Durham pneumoconiotic, Fred Hall, recalled:

> We used to always have a saying amongst the lads, at the end of the shift you used to, to
> give a bit [of a] cough you know, and they used to say, 'Gan on, get the black uns up,' and
> mind, it used to be black phlegm, it was just dust, man.[6]

The most chronic and disabling form of the disease, Progressive Massive Fibrosis
(PMF), was associated with severe breathlessness, chest pain, wheezing and
coughing, which worsened as the disease progressed. One South Wales doctor
described the disease in 1961 as 'concrete in the lung', causing progressive loss of
respiratory function:

> The air spaces are slowly strangled, and eventually, if enough are strangled, then the man
> himself is strangled and loses his power to expand his chest and he drops from say a two-
> and-a-half-inch expansion down three-quarters of an inch ... and that is the overt sign that
> you have of this process.[7]

Death could ultimately occur through respiratory failure and/or cardiac failure.

There was – and remains – no cure for pneumoconiosis. As Dr T.D. Spencer,
Medical Officer of the North East Division of the NCB, noted in 1955: 'The
conversion of lung tissue into scar tissue cannot be reversed', thus, 'much can be
done for the man, if not for his illness, by ensuring that he is given suitable work.'[8]
Palliative measures, which had some effect on the symptoms, were the use of
oxygen (though up to the 1970s this improvement in breathlessness was traded off
against a shortened life span by using oxygen), breathing exercises and medicines
which exerted some control over bronchial muscle spasms. Chemotherapy was
experimented with, as well as anti-TB drugs, including streptomycin, but both were
found to do 'more harm than good'.[9] Up to the 1970s, the disease was sometimes
mistaken for cancer. Marshall Wylde recalled his father's experience in the 1940s:
'It was horrible, horrible; he actually thought he was dying of cancer.'[10] In some
cases, surgeons cut away the worst-affected areas of the lung, but this appears to
have had little ameliorative effect. Joseph Chattors had two-thirds of one of his lungs
removed:

> So, after a while – I was still in hospital – he [the surgeon] come round, and he says, 'I've
> got some good news for you. I've got some good news, I've got some bad news', I says,
> 'Give it whichever way you like.' He says, 'Well, you haven't got cancer.' I says, 'I told
> you that all along,' so he says, 'You've got pneumoconiosis.' 'Oh,' I says, 'thanks very

---

6   Frederick Hall, Interview C41 (SOHC).
7   Interview with Dr Thomas, Audio/374 (SWCC; South Wales Miners' Library).
8   *Transactions of the Institute of Mining Engineers* (1954–55), p. 1019.
9   J.M. Rogan, *Medicine in the Mining Industries* (London, 1972), p. 88.
10 Marshall Wylde, Interview C35 (SOHC).

much, my father died with that.' 'Well,' he says, 'you know what it is, then.' And that was '68.[11]

Not infrequently, pneumoconiosis was found in miners with other respiratory diseases caused by dust inhalation at work, notably bronchitis and emphysema. As we have seen, the latter obstructive airway diseases were significant in their own right, though medical research did not categorically determine their occupational aetiology until the late 1980s. As one Scottish GP commented, miners took these ailments for granted, and it was unusual for local doctors to relate bronchitis and emphysema to the insidious work environments:

> Middle-aged and older miners accepted the fact that the longer they worked in the pits the more breathless they became and the cough developed, got worse. Not many of them attributed it to their working conditions. Eh not many doctors attributed it to their working conditions. It was just one of the things that they developed was this chronic bronchitis.[12]

As we noted in Chapter 2, the number of miners affected by respiratory disability was massive, though particular coal fields – notably South Wales – had a much higher incidence than elsewhere. Pneumoconiotics were the largest single group of registered disabled in Wales in the 1940s and 1950s – some 14,000 out of 54,000 in 1946.[13] Miners could have differing degrees of several respiratory diseases (including asthma), sometimes referred to as 'multiple disabilities', and some combined these impairments with nystagmus (deteriorating eyesight), vibration white finger and trauma injuries (including broken limbs). There may also have been a greater propensity to contract TB with respiratory organs damaged by pneumoconiosis, especially amongst older miners with PMF.[14] A South Wales miner, Mostyn Moses, suffering from pneumoconiosis, bronchitis and emphysema, commented: 'I have been spitting up dust like black lead from my lungs, like black slurry. Then I started seeing blood and now they tell me I've got tuberculosis as well.'[15] This prompted a fear of infection which influenced policy-making and attitudes towards the disease within the community in the 1930s and 1940s. This dissipated with growing awareness of the nature of pneumoconiosis and the development of effective treatment for TB with streptomycin and other antibiotic-based drugs in the later 1940s.

---

11 Joseph Chattors, Interview C39 (SOHC).

12 Dr George Bell (GP in Bellshill), Oral Interview dated 7 October 1992, Motherwell Museum, Transcript T006/7MDC.

13 NUM, South Wales Area, *Conferences and Reports* (1946–47), p. 79.

14 B.G. Staley, *Colliery Guardian*, vol. 221 (November 1973), p. 411; Rogan, *Medicine in the Mining Industries*, pp. 1–17. This presumed synthesis between TB and pneumoconiosis was never proven conclusively either way, as far as we can see. The Rhondda Fach epidemiological surveys of the 1950s showed no such connection.

15 Cited in *Saga Magazine* (March 1998), consulted at http://www.deadline.demon. co.uk/archive/saga/980301.htm.

Living with Pneumoconiosis

In the inter-war period, the vast majority of pneumoconiotics had to continue to work until they were physically unable to do so. Frequently, this meant continuing their exposure to the dust that was crippling them.[16] One pneumoconiotic Maerdy miner, John Evans (who started work in the pits in 1927), recalled the declining health of his silicotic 'buttie' as he went from a full working week to only being able to cope with two or three shifts a week: 'He was suffering and he had silicosis but he struggled to work until he absolutely failed.'[17] Chris Evans, a South Wales miner from 1926 to 1967, recalled the fate of his first work colleague, Dai Thomas:

> He could hardly breathe. I asked what was wrong and between gasps of air he told me quietly, 'You go on, my old chest is none too good.' I didn't want to leave him but he insisted and I went. I had noticed that he had lost a considerable amount of weight lately; he wasn't an old man, he was only about fifty. Though he certainly didn't look fit enough, he was back at work again the next morning. But then came the morning that he didn't turn up, and I was told to continue working the place on my own. He never came back; soon afterwards I learnt that he had died. There was a big enquiry after his death … in 1931. Several strangers visited the place looking for silica, but they failed to find any; the claim for death benefit under the scheme was turned down and Dai's widow didn't receive a penny.[18]

Louise Morgan's series of articles in the *News Chronicle* in February 1936 painted an evocative picture of mining communities in South Wales and North East England blighted by respiratory disease (see Chapter 7 for more detail). Lay knowledge of 'shortness of breath' (*diffug anal* in South Wales) was widespread: 'this is as familiar among them as the common cold,' Morgan noted, though, that no one referred to silicosis or pneumoconiosis.[19] Premature ageing and death were everywhere in evidence, and indeed, taken for granted, especially in the South Wales anthracite coal mines. 'This is the country', Morgan lamented, 'of premature old men. You see them everywhere – bent, shuffling, panting for breath, at any age between 35 and 50.'[20] Marshall Wylde's father was amongst those who were forced off face work in Murton, County Durham, in the late 1930s due to pneumoconiosis. His son recalled: 'to my knowledge, everyone on that wall got pneumoconiosis'.[21] Particular places, such as Murton in Durham and Shotts in Lanarkshire, went down in mining folklore, developing reputations for being especially dusty and deadly. For their part, the coal owners only wanted the fittest and most productive workers, and could afford to pick

---

16 See MFGB, 'Silicosis among Coal miners: Case submitted to the TUC' (June 1930).

17 Interview with John Evans, AUD84, 13 June 1973 (SWCC; South Wales Miners Library).

18 C. Evans, 'A Miner's Life', in R. Fraser (ed), *Work: Twenty Personal Accounts* (London, 1968), pp. 47–8.

19 *News Chronicle* (24 February 1936).

20 *News Chronicle* (18 February 1936).

21 Marshall Wylde, Interview C35 (SOHC).

and choose in the overstocked labour markets of the inter-war depression. Thus some coal owners in the 1930s refused to employ diagnosed silocitics (partly due to the fear of contagion, as TB was strongly believed to be associated with dust disease), and there were some tragic cases reported by the SWMF of suicides amongst those disabled and unemployed in this period.[22]

As we have outlined in previous chapters, the state responded, albeit belatedly, to accumulating knowledge about dust disease in mining, and developed policies to reduce exposure and medically monitor those diagnosed with pneumoconiosis as well as to compensate, treat and rehabilitate afflicted miners. Of central importance was the system of Medical Panels, established to deal with cases of silicosis from 1918 and asbestosis from 1931, but expanded to diagnose cases of coal workers' pneumoconiosis and pronounce upon the *degree* of disability after coal dust was recognised as a causal agent from 1943. Tweedale and Hansen's work has demonstrated the Panels to be of only limited effectiveness in the period 1931–60 in dealing with asbestosis cases. They criticise the Medical Panels for acting cautiously and conservatively, resulting in a large number of deserving cases failing to be awarded compensation.[23] In relation to silicosis claims in the 1930s and 1940s, Dr R.J. Peters at the Department of Health for Scotland noted:

> The Pneumoconiosis Boards have no doubt difficulty in living down the reputation of the old silicosis boards which were in essence established as a defence for employers. They were tied down very tightly by regulations and definitions and often their decisions appeared to be, and in some cases actually were, rather out of touch with reality.[24]

Unfortunately, few of the Pneumoconiosis Medical Panel papers for coal mining appear to have survived, so a detailed statistical analysis is not possible. What can be posited from the oral testimony and other surviving sources is that there was a deep-rooted *perception* within the mining community that the Boards were too stringent in their assessment of miners' respiratory disability. This assessment was based on lay knowledge of the degree of disability and on the evidence of local GPs and hospitals diagnosing cases which the Medical Panels had not detected, and on post-mortems, where men were found to have pneumoconiosis as a main or contributory cause of death without having been accepted as significantly disabled with the disease at the 'boardings'. One recurring bone of contention with the men was that diagnosis, and hence compensation, was based upon x-ray findings rather than a clinical investigation. If the initial Panel x-ray did not show signs of pneumoconiosis, then the claim was rejected. Dr George Bell, a local GP in a mining community in

---

22 SWMF, *Minutes of Meetings* (1935), pp. 92, 124.

23 G. Tweedale and P. Hansen, 'Protecting the Workers: The Medical Board and the Asbestos Industry, 1930s–1960s', *Medical History*, vol. 42, no. 4 (October 1998), pp. 439–57.

24 Internal minute, Dr Peters to Dr Gooding (NCB, Scotland), 1953, Department of Health for Scotland, NLS/HH 104/1.

Scotland from the 1940s to the 1980s, was one of those who recognised the injustice and the unreliability of this dependence upon radiology:

> It was the person and not the x-ray that mattered that eh you could have had this thing and you had this ludicrous situation where you might have two men who started working in the pits side by side in the same seam drawing coal all their working days. They had an x-ray when they finished up or when the mines finished off ... one man was given a pension because his x-ray showed pneumoconiosis and the other man got nothing, eh, that was it, no redundancy thanks very much chum, you know, you've done 40 years in the pits and ye can hardly walk down the road, you've no breath for anything and one man got several pounds a week as a pension and one got nothing ... It was a terrible illness really.[25]

In the 1960s, the Pneumoconiosis Medical Panels rejected roughly half of all those who applied for assessment.[26] In part, at least, this was a reflection of the high proportion of miners suffering from other non-certifiable respiratory diseases, such as bronchitis, emphysema and asthma. Not surprisingly, however, this high rejection rate was a constant and persistent source of anxiety and frustration within the mining community because the level of benefits depended upon the degree of incapacity assessed (over a pre-set minimum). In this sense – and like those with asbestos-related disease – miners suffering from respiratory disease were victims twice over. They had to struggle with their impairment whilst also having to fight to get decent levels of financial compensation.

From 1931 until 1948, those *found* to have pneumoconiosis and silicosis were released from employment in the mining industry, partly because of fears of contagion given the widespread belief of an association between TB and pneumoconiosis. Reflecting on the 1940s, one Scottish miner, Tommy Coulter, recalled:

> Well, it was a known fact that the guys with pneumoconiosis, they, they stood at the welfare corner because they werenae fit to go the pit any more or maybe they were retired ... In the early days we would just see them at the corner coughing and spitting. And it was *fairly* common.[27]

The war saw the absorption of many disabled suspended miners into war-related industries, and attitudes towards the capacity of those with the disease began to change. The wartime government also took up the issue of rehabilitation and re-employment. A committee was established in 1945 under the chairmanship of D.R. Grenfell, MP for the South Wales constituency of Gower, to make recommendations about how pneumoconiotics could be found alternative work after the war. On this committee were two silicotic miners, Evan Phillips and David Davies, respectively the Chairman and Secretary of the Amalgamated Anthracite Combine Committee.

---

25 Dr George Bell (GP in Bellshill), Oral Interview dated 7 October 1992, Motherwell Museum, Transcript T006/7MDC.

26 *Hansard*, 20 May 1963, Oral Answers, pp. 20–21. Department of Health for Scotland, NLS/HH 104/42.

27 Tommy Coulter, Interview C21 (SOHC).

The Committee reported that 'misconceptions' as to the employment potential of men suffering in early stages pneumoconiosis abounded, and that the provision of suitable work was therapeutic: 'There is abundant evidence of marked physical and mental improvement among partly disabled persons when found any suitable kind of work.'[28] The Committee called for an extension of existing government plans to create more jobs in South Wales, with special attention being directed towards the locating of new factories in the anthracite area to the west of the coal field. These recommendations were later accepted by the government, including the establishment of 10 special factories in South Wales to be let at reduced rents on the condition that the labour force constituted a minimum of 50% registered disabled persons.[29]

Whilst some government ministers were optimistic, Manny Shinwell, the first Minister of Fuel and Power, had his doubts from the outset whether these provisions would adequately address the extent of the pneumoconiosis problem in South Wales, where suspensions were running at over 5,000 miners per year in the mid-1940s. He also expressed his objection to the informal policy of the Ministry of Labour giving preference to non-disabled ex-servicemen for jobs 'at the expense of pneumoconiotics'.[30] Shinwell's scepticism in 1946 proved to be well founded. The 'Grenfell' factories took longer to construct and get up and running than expected, and they employed relatively few workers overall, and lower than expected numbers of pneumoconiotics. In June 1950, the 10 Grenfell factories (including one leased to Hoover in Aberdare) which were expected to employ over 1,200 workers were actually employing just 338 in total. Of these, 179 employees were registered disabled, 111 of which were pneumoconiotics.[31] At the same time, there were still some 4,000 registered unemployed pneumoconiotics in South Wales.[32] Two years later, the National Joint Pneumoconiosis Committee (NJPC) reported that just 561 pneumoconiotics were employed in all the special factories, Remploy workshops (established to provide opportunities for the disabled under the Disability Act 1944) and other places where employers were granted special rent concessions in South Wales.[33] Amongst the largest and most well known of the latter initiatives

---

28 Board of Trade, *Provision of Employment in South Wales for Persons Suspended from the Mining Industry on account of Silicosis and Pneumoconiosis, 1945*, NJPC Paper 4, Cmd. 6719, p. 3, NA/PIN 20/118.

29 *Employment in Grenfell Factories*, NJPC Paper 13D (1948), NA/PIN 20/118.

30 Ministry of Fuel and Power and NUM and Training for Pneumoconiosis, 1946; Ministry of Fuel and Power, Letter to Ministry of Labour, 18 November 1946. NA/LAB 18/280.

31 Note by Board of Trade on Factory Building in South Wales, NJPC Paper 26 (*c.* 1950), NA/PIN 20/118. At the end of 1951, employment in the Grenfell factories had risen to 765 in total, but still only 159 were pneumoconiotics. See NJPC Paper 41, *Work of the Industrial Rehabilitation, Training and Employment Sub-Committee* (January 1952), NA/PIN/20/118.

32 *Unemployment among Pneumoconiosis Cases in South Wales*, NJPC Paper 24 (1950), NA/PIN 20/118.

33 *Employment of Pneumoconiosis Cases by NCB*, NJPC Paper 29 (1950), NA/PIN 20/118.

was the Austin Motors factory at Bargoed, which produced children's pedal cars, and employed 106 pneumoconiotics out of a total workforce of 114.[34] Austin's was something of an exception, however.

Moreover, whilst the numbers affected were considerably lower than South Wales, other areas were experiencing high levels of unemployment amongst pneumoconiotics. In Scotland, for example, the unemployment rate amongst registered disabled pneumoconiotics in early 1949 stood at 50% (163 out of 328), despite the opening of special Remploy factories in Motherwell, Stirling and Cowdenbeath.[35] One pneumoconiosis medical specialist, Dr McCallum, later described the re-employment efforts as 'unsuccessful'.[36] Clearly, Grenfell's vision of providing alternative employment for pneumoconiotics had failed. The root of the problem lay in attracting investment in the areas most affected, even with government incentives. The solution to the problem of the employment of pneumoconiotics in the late 1940s and the 1950s was to rest with the coal industry itself, rather than the creation of alternative jobs outwith the pits.

Some of the earliest reports of the Pneumoconiosis Research Unit (PRU) focused upon the social problems caused by disability and the forced suspension policy.[37] In 1946, the PRU initiated a survey of 2,000 pneumoconiotic miners in South Wales. Fletcher commented on the wide range of impairment within this community, the difficulties of re-training miners, and the reluctance of employers to take on new workers over the age of 45. Fletcher came down strongly on the side of re-employment, and lent his weight to the idea that the coal industry should shoulder this burden:

> Probably the most satisfactory form of employment for a case of early pneumoconiosis would be underground work, to which the man is accustomed, but under conditions where the dust exposure is negligible. At present ignorance of what precisely constitutes a dangerous concentration of dust makes it difficult to make definite recommendations on this score.[38]

Fletcher and Cochrane of the PRU were outspoken and unorthodox medical researchers (see Chapter 4). On one occasion they were both censured by the

---

34 This association with pneumoconiosis was recalled affectionately by one of our respondents, who referred to it as 'the Austin dust factory'; Derek Charles, Interview C26 (SOHC).

35 *Report of the Industrial Rehabilitation, Training and Employment Sub-Committee of the NJPC*, NJPC Paper 21 (25 February 1949), NA/PIN 20/118. The highest rates of unemployed pneumoconiotics in Scotland were found in Larkhall and Shotts.

36 Dr R.I. McCallum, in *Transactions of the Institute of Mining Engineers*, vol. 113 (1953–54), p. 105.

37 P. Hugh-Jones and C.M. Fletcher, 'The Social Consequences of Pneumoconiosis Among Coal miners in South Wales', *Medical Research Council Memorandum no. 25* (London, 1951).

38 *Suitable Work for Pneumoconiotics*, Memorandum by Charles Fletcher, NJPC Paper (5 December 1946), NA/PIN 20/118.

Industrial Pulmonary Diseases Committee because they had breached what was considered to be professional behaviour by personally advising some miners with pneumoconiosis (with risk of further progression) to leave the industry. Fletcher was also sensitive, though, to the considerable economic and social ramifications of loss of employment, commenting in 1950:

> In an area such as South Wales, alternative employment outside the mining industry is not easily found. A man advised to leave mining may find himself unemployed and his physical condition may suffer more deterioration as the result of the consequent lowering of his standard of living and from the knowledge of the hopelessness of his future than it would as the result of continuing to work under conditions of dust exposure.[39]

PRU research by this time had indicated that the disabling stage of the disease was 'complicated pneumoconiosis' (or Progressive Massive Fibrosis), and once this stage was reached, further exposure to dust did not significantly affect the *rate* of progression. Hence it was quite rational in such circumstances for those so affected to stay in work in approved conditions. On the other hand, Fletcher and Cochrane argued that younger miners with early signs of pneumoconiosis (less than 10% loss of lung function) should be advised to leave the industry before their condition reached the level where it caused significant impairment of respiratory ability. As Fletcher commented at the 1952 National Pneumoconiosis Conference: 'as far as possible men with pneumoconiosis should be enabled to return to the mines'.[40] He also claimed from his experience of treating pneumoconiotic miners at Llandough Hospital that most of these wanted to continue working in the pits under controlled conditions.

Despite high demand for labour after the war, a wide gap appeared in the employment rates of the fit and the disabled in mining communities. Some disabled miners found employment in the reconstruction period as general labourers in the building industry. However, it was estimated that around a quarter of these were forced to give up because the work was too strenuous. One PRU survey found 60% of pneumoconiotics unemployed in 1946. In part, this was because of what the Ministry of Labour and National Service described in 1948 as 'current misapprehensions about the degree of disability caused by pneumoconiosis'.[41] Amongst these were fears about infection. The dismissal policy and discrimination against the disabled combined to create massive hardship, as Francis and Smith noted:

---

39 C.M. Fletcher, 'The Control of CWP by Means of Periodical X-ray Exams', 1950, MRC Industrial Pulmonary Disease Committee and PRU (1947–53), NA/FD/12/950. The Chairman of the IPDC, Dr Sutherland, once commented on one of Fletcher's papers on pneumoconiosis thus: 'no!, not so, unsound, no!, why? what disease?' and finally 'nonsense', in that order; notes of Dr Sutherland on meeting of IPDC, 4 July 1950, NA/FD/12/950.

40 Pneumoconiosis Conference, Porthcawl, 11 October 1952, SWCC/MNA/NUM/K17.

41 Ministry of Labour and National Service, *The Disabled Persons Employment Act, 1944: Employment of Ex-Miners affected by Pneumoconiosis or Silicosis*, pamphlet (July 1948).

The effect on individuals, families and communities was devastating. With little or no alternative work, particularly in such Anthracite mining villages as Brynamman, Gwaun-cae-Gurwen and Tumble, life became a nightmare for the disabled pneumoconiotic miner.[42]

Over 1931–48, in total some 22,000 pneumoconiotic miners were dismissed from their work, 85% of whom were in South Wales.[43] John Evans was one such early case, diagnosed at 50% pneumoconiosis in the early 1940s. He had worked at one of the notoriously dusty seams (at Ferndale no. 5 pit, near Maerdy) where there was a high mortality and disability rate, and as he described it, 'you were breathing dust, you were eating dust. It was terrible.' In response to the question 'How did you feel about that then, having to leave the colliery?', he recalled in an interview with Hywel Francis in 1973:

> Well I was a little dumbfounded because we had not been brought up to any other job, it was the only thing we knew, mining. There were no factories like today, and as a married man with one child it was worrying.[44]

Like many others who were unaware that the disease was progressive at the time, John Evans commuted his claim to a lump sum payment (of £320). He worked intermittently thereafter as a handyman, labourer and a watchman, finally having to give up work altogether in 1958. By the late 1960s he was diagnosed as 100% pneumoconiotic. Another South Wales miner, Howard Jones, recalled that some used the lump sum to pay off their houses and others found solace with the money in the local pub. Inevitably though, suspension meant hardship for most:

> Well, if you were earning good money as a collier at the coal face and you suddenly found yourself suspended, then obviously there was no spending power there, was there?[45]

He went on to explain that in the late 1940s, the minimum wage of a collier was around £5 10s., but because of the piecework wage system, 'a good collier could earn double the minimum wage', around £11 a week. Weekly benefit under the Workmen's Compensation Act at this time was set at £2 11s. 6d., with an additional £1 colliery supplement and a further 5s. for each child. Thus an unemployed certified pneumoconiotic miner's income (with three children) would be around £4 6s. – at a conservative estimate perhaps half the income of a decent face worker.

It is hardly surprising, then, that many pneumoconiotics continued to work at the coal face, exposing themselves to dusty conditions, right up to the 1970s, rather than taking the option of a less dusty job. One pneumoconiotic South Wales miner

---

42 H. Francis and D. Smith, *The Fed: A History of the South Wales Miners in the Twentieth Century* (London, 1980), p. 439.

43 Ibid.

44 Interview with John Evans, South Wales Colliery Collection (SWCC) AUD84, 13 June 1973 (South Wales Miners' Library, Swansea).

45 Howard Jones, Interview C25 (SOHC).

from Gorseinon, Les Higgon, noted: 'Some men did not show their dust because they wanted to continue at the face ... Three-quarters of them stayed on until they had to give it in.'[46] Les himself was diagnosed 10% in 1961 and advised to leave face-working. He refused, continuing to work at the face, ignoring the advice of the Medical Panel, in his words, 'for many years ... for the money'. Surface work, he estimated, meant a drop in earnings of up to 50%. He went on to explain that younger boys were put with the older men to assist them, and in some areas disabled miners could continue at the face with the assistance of younger, fitter work mates, though this could be risky and further damage health. A Scottish miner commented:

> That was the bad thing about the pit, you started on a low wage, went to a big wage, and then when you got older or something happened to you and you had an accident, you finished on a low wage. That was the really bad thing, that was, in the pit, unless you were in a team able to soldier on for maybe another couple of year, but you were taking it out of yourself, ken, by forcing yourself to go to face work when you weren't actually fit to do the job.[47]

Another noted:

> You carried lesser men, gie them a hand, wee dig out and that, but you couldn't cover them all, but by and large did a good job covering the weaker elements in society in them days.[48]

As we saw in Chapter 4, the suspension policy was changed in 1948, when new statutory regulations allowed for miners diagnosed with pneumoconiosis after that date to be treated differently according to the severity of the diagnosis. Compulsory suspensions were abandoned, and instead the worst-affected were advised to leave the industry; some were advised to take work at the surface in completely dust-free conditions, and those with the lowest certifications of pneumoconiosis were recommended to transfer to 'approved' jobs underground where dust levels were within the legal threshold limits. This change in policy was interpreted by some as a reflection of the NUM's willingness to place the economic interests of the fledgling NCB (in a period of acute labour shortage and an export drive) above the long-term health of the miners – trading off disability against production.[49] However, in terms of disability policy, this change might be interpreted as a recognition that indiscriminate unemployment unfairly victimised those with low levels of incapacity. As we noted, Fletcher's experience with pneumoconiotics at Llandough Hospital indicated to him that the men wanted to work, rather than be dependent. The 1948 change in policy brought the coal mining industry in line with the 1944 Disability Act, which aimed to improve the chances of those with impairments to get employment. This legislation (passed largely with ex-servicemen in mind) included

---

46 Les Higgon, Interview C30 (SOHC).
47 David Carruthers, Interview C23 (SOHC).
48 George Bolton, Interview C23 (SOHC).
49 Francis and Smith, *The Fed*, p. 441.

for the first time the laying down of a quota for larger employers – who were initially obliged to retain 2% of their places for registered disabled workers (a quota later raised to 3%). The 1948 re-employment policy in the pits was also the product of the failure of initiatives to create alternative employment in the South Wales valleys. The change was largely welcomed, though somewhat controversial in mining communities. For some miners' advocates, it was believed that this was driven by the need to retain labour power, improve the tarnished image of the industry and maximise production in the post-war economic crisis. Others saw it as legitimising the further exposure to dust of already at-risk and partially disabled miners. To the South Wales miners' leader Dai Dan Evans, this 'accelerates the deterioration of the health condition of quite a number of men and the progression of the disease'.[50] The majority, however, appeared to have welcomed the change, and it was followed, in 1951, with new regulations which allowed those previously suspended *before 1948* to be re-employed in the so-called 'approved faces' underground. Tommy Coulter offered this recollection on the processes involved:

> These men [pneumoconiotics] were catered for until it got to the stage where it was no longer possible and we'd to say 'sorry', because the system of payment was what we called a pool system, and, eh, you weren't paid individually, you were paid as a member of that pool, and the amount of coal you produced was your wages. We had x amount a ton, and then if you did extra work, say there was roof problems or that, that was allowances for that. If the conveyer stopped for twenty minutes, you'd tae get paid for it, you'd get a guaranteed wage for that, but then everybody got the same wage, so everybody had to perform. And gradually these guys would be farmed out, but they did get a great deal of sympathy from their fellow workers *and* from management, it's got to be said, and they were usually found reasonable jobs … They were well looked after, ah've got tae say that. But at that time they would find them a job on repairing roadways, y'know, where there was a bit of a crush they would go, and it wasnae a very difficult job, you know.[51]

The outcome was that a large proportion of disabled pneumoconiotics were re-absorbed into the industry that had ejected them. In South Wales, numbers of unemployed pneumoconiotic miners peaked at 4,775 in 1947. In 1954, there were just 655 so unemployed.[52] Concomitantly, the employment of pneumoconiotics by the NCB increased. By 1950, the industry employed 5,140 pneumoconiotics, 1,470 at the surface and 3,670 in the so-called 'approved faces' underground.[53] Ten years later, in 1960, the NCB employed almost 19,000 registered pneumoconiotics, 95% on the surface or in 'approved faces' (see Table 9.1). At this time, some 450 pneumoconiotics were officially continuing to work in *non-approved* faces in the UK, mostly, the NCB claimed, because they refused offers of alternative employment.

---

50 D.D. Evans, *A Survey of the Incidence and Progression of Pneumoconiosis*, NUM (South Wales) (April 1963), p. 11.

51 Tommy Coulter, Interview C21 (SOHC).

52 J.M. Rogan, 'Pneumoconiosis', in *Colliery Guardian* (30 June 1960), p. 731.

53 *Employment of Pneumoconiosis Cases by NCB*, NJPC Paper 29 (1950). NA/PIN 20/118.

Table 9.1   **Pneumoconiotics employed by the NCB, October 1960**

Scotland	1,503
Northern	284
Durham	2,489
North East	2,774
North West	1,929
East Midlands	711
West Midlands	2,452
South West (Wales)	6,391
South East	365
Total GB	**18,898**

Source: NJPC, *Minutes*, 11 May 1960, Appendix, NCB, Employment of Pneumoconiosis Cases, 12 months to October 1960, NA/LAB14/799.

The choices available to pneumoconiotic mineworkers were constrained by economic imperatives, and whatever decisions they made, or were forced upon them, in the decade or so after Second World War, one almost inevitable consequence was an erosion in income. This was of serious proportions in many cases, supporting the view that such disability led to a slide into relative poverty for the worst-affected. The maximum compensation benefit under the Workmen's Compensation Act before the war had been £1 10s. per week. In 1948, benefit under the Industrial Injuries Act was set at £2 5s. for the totally incapacitated man, with an additional 16s. for a dependent wife and 7s. 6d. for the first child. Whilst recognising this as a significant improvement, the NUM South Wales argued: 'these payments … still leave the totally disabled man in poverty and hardship'.[54] Low benefit levels and the lack of alternative employment were amongst a whole raft of economic, social and cultural pressures which forced pneumoconiotic miners to try to stay working at the face, or at least within the mining industry. As one 35-year-old pneumoconiotic miner from Brynamman noted: 'You couldn't get work … As you had no trade it was difficult you see.' This miner's attempt to get his suspension from coal mining rescinded was rejected in 1950 because there was a history of TB in the family, with both his father and brother dying of TB.[55]

In the early 1950s, Dr McCallum noted that the pneumoconiosis problem in North East England was not as severe as in South Wales, but that the economic and social ramifications for victims were just as catastrophic:

---

54 NUM (South Wales), *Minutes of Meetings* (1946–47), p. 79.

55 Cited in Francis and Smith, *The Fed*, pp. 339–40.

In Durham the number affected is smaller but there are few suitable factories other than in the trading estates and in most of these mainly female or skilled male labour is required. The miner with pneumoconiosis is usually too old to learn a new trade and in most mining villages the alternatives are work connected to the colliery or unemployment. This therefore is a problem for the coal industry but there are only a limited number of suitable jobs at a pit for a partially disabled man and even fewer if he is not allowed to work underground.[56]

McCallum went on to counsel that older and middle-aged men 'who can manage their own job underground even though partially disabled should be encouraged to continue at it'. He continued:

In young men with early lung changes and no symptoms, risk of subsequent disability might be avoided altogether if they left the mining industry, but it is just these men who find it most difficult to change their work because of family commitments, the loss of income and lower standard of living and the impossibility of finding accommodation in other parts of the country where they might find work. They are compelled by economic pressure to carry on with their job.[57]

As miners' pneumoconiosis became more debilitating, a downward spiral of falling income frequently occurred. Face-working in the two decades after the Second World War was a relatively well-paid job. The wage erosion of the 1920s and 1930s was reversed during the war and after, and by the 1950s the coal face workers were once again amongst the highest-paid manual workers in the UK. Moving from the face to dust-free work at the surface thus had serious financial implications. 'Resettlement in surface work', as J.J. Jarry noted in 1972, 'may involve permanent reduction in earnings.'[58] Labourers at the surface earned around half the wage of a skilled miner, and the earnings of a craftsman at the surface were around a third lower.[59] What went along with this was a loss of status if a face worker was demoted to haulage or surface work. Tommy Coulter explained:

Aye, aye, it was a stigma. And then it was even worse if they'd to go to the surface. Like my dad, he was bad with his chest, he'd tae go tae the surface and it was a big blow to his prestige ... he made it plain with no' just words, but his general attitude. And then of course the wages were much less too. I mean, if they got a job repairing, you took a reduction, but I mean, they were still reasonably well off. But eh? I don't ever know of anybody who was fired because he had chest problems; I've never known that tae happen. Maybe, eventually they had tae leave, but I personally, I'm no' saying it didn't happen, but I worked in about five different collieries in my working life, and I've never known that tae happen.[60]

---

56 Dr R.I. McCallum, *Transactions of the Institute of Mining Engineers*, vol. 113 (1953–54), p. 105.

57 Ibid.

58 Jarry, cited in Rogan, *Medicine in the Mining Industries*, pp. 357–8.

59 A. Bryan, *The Evolution of Health and Safety in Mines* (Letchworth, 1975), p. 175.

60 Tommy Coulter, Interview C21 (SOHC).

Another medical professional, Dr Leathart, noted in 1972 that many miners in the early stages of pneumoconiosis were unwilling to make the change and tried for as long as possible to hide their encroaching disability because it would 'cause undue financial hardship'.[61] One such case was John Jones in South Wales, who recalled:

> The doctor said, 'You're suffering from pneumoconiosis,' he said, this was before I had the payment for it. ... 1971, and I had a letter to go and see my own doctor, and I went in and he said, 'You're now suffering pneumoconiosis, and I want you to finish underground.' I said, 'I don't know.' And he grabbed me like that, 'Sit down here, sit down.' 'What the hell's happening?' ... He said, 'You know what happened to Dad.' My father died, see, in 1969. Anyway, I went back to the coal, and then, 1978 I think, it was getting worse and worse, so I thought I'd, well this pleurisy come and knocked me all to hell. Then I went in front of six doctors, and for six Coal Board docs to tell you you've finished, there must be something there. And I'd been told by Mr Mallon, the chest specialist, to finish. So I finished 1980.
> SM: So when you were told in 1971 that you had pneumoconiosis, why did you not want to leave the face then?
> JJ: (long pause) Young family. Money. Not greedy, but just, y'know, no money. It was a big drop in the wages, see. Yeh. A minimum wage compared to a coal face worker or a hard heading man. A hell of a big difference.[62]

Another North East miner recalled reluctantly having to eventually finish work aged 47 because of his pneumoconiosis, commenting on his experience before that:

> NF: Were you going to work in the pit with a bad chest?
> FH: Yes, we had to. You had to work because there was nothing else.[63]

The pre-1974 pneumoconiosis compensation schemes continued to include many anomalies, and there persisted a sense within sections of the mining community that the risk of working in mining – and further exposure to dust – was worth it, partly because state support was so meagre. Those who received compensation under the old less generous Workmen's Compensation Act (up to 1948) and those who had commuted their claims to a lump sum payment were amongst the worst off financially in the 1950s and 1960s.[64] Relative poverty was the experience of many in these categories, and despite pleas to the NUM to champion their case, there continued to be a marked difference in experience (right up to the mid-1970s) between those unfortunate enough to be compensated under the old system and those compensated under the new compensation regimes from 1948. As we saw in Chapter 7, policy changed again in 1974, when earnings-related compensation for pneumoconiosis was introduced as a trade-off in return for the NUM dropping the deluge of common

---

61 Rogan, *Medicine in the Mining Industries*, p. 89.
62 John Jones, Interview C27 (SOHC).
63 Frederick Hall, Interview C41 (SOHC).
64 Coal Industry Social and Welfare Organisation (CISWO), *Annual Report* (1960), p. 26; *Colliery Guardian* (5 November 1965), p. 584.

law claims that followed the infamous Pickles' case. Under the new 1974 scheme, compensation was set at 90% of pre-certification earnings (and 60% for widows). Samuel Westhead was amongst those to benefit from this, moving off power-loading immediately in 1980 after he was diagnosed with 10% pneumoconiosis.[65]

In the post-war decades, pneumoconiotic face workers taking surface work and other 'light work' also had to overcome a cultural hurdle. This was widely regarded within mining communities as inferior employment, significantly down the pecking order from winning the coal at the face. In part, this was linked to entrenched notions of masculinity and the traditional status hierarchies in the community. For some, this stigma was hard to stomach: 'There is a marked, even conflicting, difference in character between the communities of underground and surface workers respectively; the underground worker re-employed on the surface is inclined to resent the milieu.'[66] The Miners' Welfare Commission had recognised this during wartime, noting in its report on rehabilitation the relative absence of light work in the mining districts, and 'even where light work can be provided, the man so employed may tend to feel that, as a *compensation man*, he is deprived of full scope for enterprise and has small prospect of becoming fully independent again and of improving his position in the world'.[67]

Choices became constrained further as the industry contracted from the late 1950s. In more overstocked labour markets, disabled miners found it more difficult than younger, fitter miners to retain their jobs, and crucially, to travel farther afield to transfer to other 'viable' local pits as retrenchment gathered pace. Chris Evans noted that it was especially the older and disabled miners who found themselves unemployed in the 1950s and 1960s as pits closed.[68] A differential between the absorption rate of the able-bodied and the impaired community was already widening in the immediate aftermath of the Second World War, when one PRU study found pneumoconiotics 'handicapped in this competition by their disability ... by their age ... and by their living in the remoter mining valleys, away from centres of light industry'.[69] The official figures, cited in Table 9.2, bear this out.

For many serious and chronic sufferers of occupational dust disease, marked deterioration of health resulted in what would now be recognised as social exclusion – being deprived of access to amenities and services widely recognised as the norm within society, increasingly housebound, isolated and unable to operate as independent citizens. For those with complicated pneumoconiosis (PMF), this was invariably a long, drawn-out, incremental process as the lungs become progressively clogged up. Abe Moffat talked of his younger brother, incapacitated with pneumoconiosis and

---

65 Samuel Westhead, Interview C37 (SOHC).

66 Jarry, cited in Rogan, *Medicine in the Mining Industries,* p. 358.

67 *Miners' Welfare in Wartime,* Report of the Miners' Welfare Commission for the six-and-a-half years to June 1946 (n.d., *c.* 1946–47); our emphasis.

68 Evans, 'A Miner's Life', pp. 52–3.

69 Hugh-Jones and Fletcher, 'The Social Consequences of Pneumoconiosis', p. 12.

Table 9.2　**Pneumoconiosis and unemployment in Wales and Great Britain, October 1948**

	Wales	*Rest of GB*
Working population (male)	565,000	10.3m
Male unemployment	28,418	205,985
Unemployment (%)	**5.0**	**2.0**
All registered disabled	64,078	775,427
Registered disabled unemployed	13,879	56,650
Disabled unemployment (%)	**21.6**	**7.3**
All certified pneumoconiotics	11,420	—
Pneumoconiosis unemployed	4,600	—
Pneumoconiotics unemployed (%)	**40.3**	—

Source: P. Hugh-Jones and C.M. Fletcher, 'The Social Consequences of Pneumoconiosis among Coalminers in South Wales', Medical Research Council Memorandum no. 25 (London, 1951), p. 22 (derived from Ministry of Labour figures).

emphysema: 'a physical wreck before he reached the age of fifty'.[70] The harrowing case of James Bishop provides another example. Bishop, who had worked underground in South Wales for thirty-four years and had been bedridden for ten months in the final stages of CWP, was described in an editorial in *The Observer* in 1948 as 'a helpless and destitute invalid' and his caring wife 'almost worn out'. Bishop was noted to be one of 700 or so completely disabled pneumoconiotic miners in South Wales, 80 of whom were receiving no compensation at all. Few pneumoconiotics had access to free coal at this point, further worsening their impoverishment.[71]

It is in the reconstruction of the world of the disabled miner – the perceptions and the lived experience – that oral testimony is particularly illuminating. One Durham miner recalled:

You would see former miners in the village who had maybe retired, who were struggling to be able to walk. Their mobility was very severely restricted, heavy breathing. So we

---

70　A. Moffat, *My Life with the Miners* (London, 1965), p. 232.

71　Pneumoconiosis and Silicosis Newspaper Cuttings; *The Observer* (1 February 1948); *The Observer* (15 February 1948), NA/COAL 26/153; The newspaper subsequently collected over £2,700 in donations for the James Bishop Appeal Fund, including a £100 cheque from an ex-coal owner with a plea, 'do not think too unkindly of us'.

would see quite a lot of that. And the other thing that it tended to do to an individual was that they lost weight very quickly and looked very gaunt and thin ...[72]

Victims, dependants and their families had to deal with the trauma of diagnosis, curtailment and loss of employment, physical deterioration, and invariably, the deeper psychological implications of dependency and loss of self-esteem. Mildred Blaxter described this in her pioneering mid-1970s study of disability as a process of 're-evaluating identity', which could be either a sudden discontinuity or a longer-term process of 'drift'.[73] The latter more aptly describes the experience of pneumoconiotics, where there was such a wide range of impairment and the process of bodily damage was relatively slow and protracted, usually over a number of years. This distinguished those with respiratory diseases from the victims of mining accidents where the loss of function was sudden, such as with paraplegics. Marshall Wylde described his father's condition (70% pneumoconiosis) in the final stages before he died of the disease:

> The horrible thing about it was that my father was a big, strong, stocky man, I'm not the biggest in my family, you know, but when he used to go upstairs, he used to go down on his behind, and when he used to go up, he used to crawl. It was all right medical, but mental, he was such a proud man, and that he had to get things done for him. It was hard seeing my father deteriorate because he was a healthy man and always took an active part in his family life.[74]

Bitterness, frustration and anger were much in evidence in the testimony, directed invariably against 'the system' that cruelly robbed them of their health and/or that of friends and relatives. The experiential testimonies of disabled miners thus illuminate the *transition* from well-respected fit worker, able and willing to do his full share, to a slower unfit worker, increasingly dependent upon others. Varying degrees of social exclusion for those so disabled ensued, the consequence of loss of employment, reduced income and of encroaching physical incapacity.

The Mining Community and the Disabled

We have argued elsewhere that social exclusion is an apt term to describe the position that many asbestos-related disease victims found themselves in during the second half of the twentieth century.[75] For those with advanced asbestosis or mesothelioma, the economic and social ramifications of their impairment were invariably enormous, encompassing a drift into relative poverty, isolation and loss of citizenship, especially prior to the 1980s. As we have argued above, many of those coal miners seriously

---

72 David Guy, Interview C44 (SOHC).

73 Blaxter, *The Meaning of Disability*; Barnes and Mercer, *Disability*, p. 63.

74 Marshall Wylde, Interview C35 (SOHC).

75 See R. Johnston and A. McIvor, 'Pushed into Social Exclusion: Asbestos-related Disability and Relative Poverty on Clydeside', *Scottish Affairs*, no. 32 (Summer 2000).

disabled with pneumoconiosis experienced a similar process. However, the evidence suggests that the picture is more complex in coal mining, and that to some extent the drift towards social exclusion of impaired miners was mitigated by the agency of miners themselves, the role of their trade unions and welfare organisation, and the matrix of support and assistance within the tight-knit mining communities.

In contrast to many occupational groups who worked with asbestos, the coal miners were very well organised, with a virtual trade union closed shop from the Second World War. We have argued in Chapter 7 that the miners' unions played a pivotal role in both *prevention and compensation* struggles. Constant vigilance and pressure from the MFGB and the NUM resulted in progressive improvements in benefits which eased the financial repercussions of disability. The additional £1 per week 'colliery benefit' paid on top of the state disablement benefit (of £2 16s. to a married man) in the 1950s and 1960s would be a tangible example. Another would be the inclusion of the disabled miners, for the first time from 1953, in the House Coal Agreement, which provided cheap, subsidised fuel.[76] The NUM also paid the Medical Panel examination fees of members, and importantly, initiated and financed common law claims for damages for disabled miners, initially for the injured, and later for those with respiratory disease. The union provided a wide range of legal assistance and advice and guidance, not least through the Lodge Compensation Secretaries, who maintained close contact with disabled members. Howard Jones was one such official in the anthracite area to the north and west of Swansea after the Second World War.[77] As the union contracted, moreover, the NUM in South Wales continued to maintain this matrix of support through the creation of a tier of 'voluntary welfare officers', usually ex-lodge officials, many of whom were themselves partially disabled from pneumoconiosis, bronchitis and/or emphysema. From talking to some of these men, it is obvious that they played a key role in helping the impaired community in their districts, in numerous pastoral and practical ways, from assisting with the paperwork for their claims to providing a point of valuable contact in their homes.

The Coal Industry Social and Welfare Organisation (CISWO), created in 1952, also played an important role. This organisation had its origins in 1920 when the Mining Industry Act established the Miners' Welfare Fund (based on a levy of 1d. per ton on coal produced) designed to finance the improvement of health and welfare infrastructure in remote mining communities. Amongst the guiding principles were the discouragement of segregation, and the promotion of 'the integration of all employees in the coal industry in the communities in which they live'.[78] Initiatives included the provision of pithead baths, grants to miners' children to go to university, and the erection of Miners' Welfare Institutes in almost every mining community up and down the country – some with very elaborate facilities, including swimming pools (such as at Bilston, in Scotland, opened in 1958). However, the organisation

---

76 *The Miner* (January/February 1953), p. 6.

77 Howard Jones, Interview C25 (SOHC).

78 CISWO, *First Annual Report* (1953), p. 16.

also played a key role in pioneering what we would now see as social work, as well as the convalescence and rehabilitation of injured and impaired miners. This work was centred around the 19 miners' convalescent homes dotted around the country and several regional miners' rehabilitation centres – such as Uddingston, near Glasgow.[79] In the early 1950s, CISWO claimed to the Committee of Enquiry on the Rehabilitation of the Disabled to be providing 'the most highly developed industrial and social rehabilitation service in the world'.[80]

Initially, the focus of what was then known as the medico-social services of CISWO was directed towards those miners seriously injured in mine accidents, with special attention devoted to paraplegics and those with nystagmus. Pneumoconiosis was also a major concern by the 1940s. By 1951, CISWO had bought property in South Wales and was on the verge of creating a Pneumoconiosis Rehabilitation Centre, with a linked 'comprehensive medico-social service'. This was shelved when rehabilitation was transferred to the NHS in 1951 and the government set up a pneumoconiosis rehabilitation centre at the PRU at Llandough Hospital, Cardiff (and contemplated 15 more such centres up and down the country).[81] None the less, in 1956 CISWO expanded its social work in this field, creating a number of new appointments, including one in South Wales, to service the disabled community, including those with pneumoconiosis, bronchitis and emphysema. This was conceived as an additional tier to the state social services, offering less bureaucracy and a liaison point between the disabled and the local authorities with home visits: 'to serve the special needs of totally disabled mineworkers and to give advice and help to all mineworkers who are sick and disabled'.[82] One of the newly appointed female social workers, R.D. Morris, publicised the service in the SWMF journal, emphasising that the service was inclusive and 'must be built into the social life of the mining community as to be regarded as the right of the disabled mineworker'.[83] By the early 1960s, it was recognised that 'boredom and depression' were real problems for the disabled, and that part of the social worker's role was what was termed 'therapeutic listening' (what now goes partly under the title 'reminiscence therapy').[84] Practical help was also on hand with issues including housing, mobility and form-filling. A tangible example would be the provision through the CISWO social services in the late 1970s of light-weight portable oxygen equipment in South Wales on loan to pneumoconiotics. At this time, this equipment was not available on the NHS, and contributed to the mobility of those most seriously disabled with the disease.[85] These activities pioneered modern-day social work and eased the transitions being undergone in miners' lives as their respiratory disability worsened.

---

79 Note: apart from Uddingston, all the other miners' rehabilitation centres were transferred to the NHS in 1951.

80 CISWO, *Report for 1954* (1955), p. 38.

81 CISWO, *Report for 1953* (1954), pp. 40, 42.

82 CISWO, *Report for 1955* (1956), p. 24.

83 *The Miner*, vol 5, no. 6 (November/December 1957), p 11.

84 CISWO, *Report for 1964* (1965), p. 27.

85 CISWO, *Report for 1978* (1979), p. 20.

This all provided a further layer of personal assistance to the disabled community in the mining areas that was missing in many urban working-class communities.

The value of assisted convalescence for those with pneumoconiosis was also being recognised by the 1950s. The South Wales convalescent home at Court Royal, Bournemouth, was being used through the winter months to provide periods of convalescence specifically for pneumoconiotics from 1956.[86] Twenty years later, this initiative was extended with the provision of a 'recuperative winter holiday in a suitable climate' for mine workers with chronic respiratory disease and their wives. The first group in 1975 went to Bulgaria, followed by a trip to Jersey.[87] By the early 1970s, the winds of change were beginning to blow through CISWO. Resources were becoming strained as the industry contracted, so more and more reliance was being placed on the NHS and state social services. At the same time, CISWO was again pioneering the policy of social inclusion, moving away from the previous policy of segregated activity in welfare, convalescence and sports towards more integrated provision involving the able-bodied and impaired. The 1970s holiday schemes for pneumoconiotics, for example, involved a mix of those in work and partially disabled, and those unemployed. The emphasis was now upon participation of the disabled in areas that had previously been monopolised for the non-disabled person: 'the basic approach to the welfare of the seriously disabled should be based on the simple philosophy of involvement with able-bodied persons'.[88]

The Mabon Club, established by two socio-medical officers attached to the PRU, perhaps epitomised all that was best in the supportive environment of the Welsh mining valleys. This was a social club, providing information, outings and entertainment designed to address the problem of social exclusion amongst pneumoconiotics. It provided an additional and complementary service to the pioneering PRU at Llandough Hospital, which in the 1950s was treating up to 500 pneumoconiotic miners every year, in a specially designated 50-bed unit.[89]

The miners' unions and CISWO were institutionalised elements of the tight-knit mining communities themselves, where much support was organically generated for impaired miners. In the workplace, this was manifest in the oral testimonies which recalled the ways in which the younger, fitter miners would assist the impaired, breathless and older men. Here, in a sense, we have in operation the modern-day equivalent of the Personal Assistant (PA) that some disabled rights' groups are campaigning for in the early twenty-first century. Nor were miners passive recipients of welfare. It would be wrong to claim that the only transformations caused by industrial disability were negative ones – loss of health, work, independence and erosion of masculinity. The growing knowledge of injustice, exploitation, managerial bullying, cutting corners, criminal complacency, corporate crime and the callous

86 CISWO, *Report for 1957* (1958), p.26; *Report for 1958* (1959), p. 26.

87 CISWO, *Report for 1975* (1976), p. 15; *Report for 1978* (1979), p. 20.

88 CISWO, *Report for 1973* (1974), p. 14.

89 Minutes of a meeting on 9 May 1958 between Department of Health, NCB, NUM and NACODS, Scottish Home and Health Department Records, NAS/HH104/29.

treatment of victims could and did spur a growing number of people to protest, resist and organise to change things. For some, this was therapeutic activity which filled empty days and acted as job-replacement. For others, this re-created workmate social contact and interaction, in the Miners' Welfare Institute or union offices (or the offices of voluntary groups like Clydeside Action on Asbestos).

Furthermore, both able-bodied and the impaired combined to fight for extended economic and social security, and humane treatment, for example from the Medical Panels. As one South Wales pneumoconiotic miner put it: 'there was tremendous sympathy; people understood'.[90] This was manifest in 1953, for example, when around 40,000 took to the streets in an NUM-organised demonstration in Cardiff protesting against the removal of extended unemployment benefits and the re-introduction of 'means-tested' benefits by the Conservative government. This was perceived as a direct attack on the living standards of the disabled community, including the ex-servicemen and pneumoconiotics. The resolution from the demonstration urged a change of policy:

> These reductions in income at a time when the cost of living is continually rising, can only result in acute impoverishment and disruption of family life. This Demonstration declares the Government to be guilty of inhuman treatment of the unfortunate victims of Industry and Wars.[91]

The slogan on one of the banners carried by the Great Mountain Lodge of the NUM indicated the depth of community solidarity on the issue:

> Mountain of despair; valley of doom. Hundreds of miners from one village disabled by
> PNEUMOCONIOSIS, THE DEADLY DUST.
> They toiled to dig the nation's coal
> And breathed the deadly dust.
> Betrayed once more, denied the dole
> By those who held their trust
> They are not here amidst the throng
> Their health is too impaired
> We march for them to right the wrong
> So that they may be spared.[92]

Undoubtedly, however, as the pits closed and younger members of the community moved away, this supportive environment eroded. Cumulatively, however, this combination of community and institutional support played a significant role in mitigating the social exclusion and loss of citizenship that was typically associated with disability.

Moreover, pneumoconiotic miners would have found a supportive network in their communities within what was an established disabled contingent, simply because

---

90 Les Higgon, Interview C30 (SOHC).

91 *The Miner* (November/December 1953), p. 9.

92 Ibid., p. 8.

of the sheer numbers involved with respiratory difficulties, or other impairments caused by work injuries and disease, such as nystagmus, vibration white finger, loss of limbs and paraplegia. Mining communities were certainly accustomed to breathing problems and coughing. These impairments were as 'normal' as the blue-streaked scars which Zweig in 1944 had noted criss-crossed most miners' bodies. Indeed, the Socialist Medical Association began a concerted campaign in the mid-1950s to get such communities to recognise that the cough and breathlessness were signs of impairment, and to break down generations of complacency and socialisation.[93] Hence, within these communities, breathing-impaired miners may well have been regarded as 'normal', rather than as 'others' and different. More research is necessary here, but what appears evident at this stage is that miners were clearly an agency in this process (rather than 'helpless' victims), and the mining communities constituted a distinctive and quite unique social space in which such problems were addressed and significantly alleviated. However, neither agency, union nor community could do much about the personal tragedy of impairment, the inevitable mutations in lifestyles and identities that came with serious disability, nor the physical pain, suffering and premature death which persistently characterised the pneumoconiotic community in the mining villages in the middle decades of the twentieth century.

Coping with Breathlessness: Emphysema and Bronchitis

As with pneumoconiosis, chronic bronchitis and emphysema could have a devastating impact on the lifestyles of those who suffered, resulting in serious physical impairment, and in the worst cases, in relative poverty and social exclusion. A Durham mining union official, David Guy, reflected on the restricted opportunities that faced those with lung impairment as the pits closed:

> As long as they were able to work, or get to work in some shape or form, the management were pretty sympathetic to people in poor health, especially if it was caused by the work at the pit, and there was a tendency for the union and the management to work together to try and fix them up in jobs which they could cope with. Once the pit closed and that type of sympathetic approach wasn't there any longer by employers outside the industry – I mean, the first thing they make you do when you apply for a job is to get you medically examined, and in the vast majority of cases people were told, 'You're not fit enough to work for us, how the hell did you manage at the pit?' So that's resulted in a high percentage of people in the mining communities relying upon sickness benefits, industrial injuries benefits. So I think we've been able to monitor that much better than what we would have done had the pits still been operating. I think the pits *masked* a lot of that, whereas now they're out there now, the reality is there isn't any sympathy for you if you've got a form of disablement. Employers want to take on people who they are going to be able to exploit to the maximum, so they don't want anyone who's got a bad chest or

---

93 Socialist Medical Association, *Dust in the Lungs*, pamphlet (n.d., *c.* 1954); *Stop that Cough* (*c.* 1953); *Challenge of the Rhondda Fach Survey* (*c.* 1952–53).

who have spinal injuries or neck injuries or arthritis. There is a reluctance of employers to employ people in that category.[94]

When a lung condition began to have an effect fairly early on in life, the impact could be devastating, as one retired Ayrshire coal miner remembered:

> You say to yourself … 'I used to be really fit,' and, eh, you'd maybe say, 'Och, I'm just getting a wee bit older, maybe no' up to it.' But you don't realise because this thing, when it hits your chest … you don't realise it's insidious. It's coming on all the time, and you're putting it down to, 'Och, I had a bit of a bump there and I'm sore,' or, eh, 'I had a lot of dust there, that's how my chest's too bad.' And it creeps up and creeps up on you until 1988, I had to give the pit up. I was only fifty-two.[95]

Another Ayrshire miner also testified to how it felt to change from being a very fit worker able to withstand the harshness of a very tough working environment to an unfit one who could not:

> I was hurrying one day, and the pain I got in my chest, and I thought I was going tae drop out. But I just steadied myself and, eh, went tae the pit bottom at my leisure. But, says I, 'There's something bloody well wrong.' I just couldnae get a gasp, and I'll tell you, see anything I was doing after that? I had to take it in moderation. I was big enough and strong enough. I could lift anything. I could dae anything, but I couldnae continue it, couldnae continue it.[96]

Rita Moses, the wife of a South Wales miner suffering from multiple respiratory diseases, noted:

> There's no quality of life for him. He loved his garden and to go for a walk and a drink. Now he can hardly do anything … We've got three sons and two daughters. My Mostyn was a fit and healthy man then.[97]

An ex-coal miner from Durham with emphysema also commented on how his condition constrained his independence and confined him to the home:

> Well, for a start, it's stopped us from getting out, and I only get out once, once a week and I've got to be took in a car and brought back. If I walk about twelve yards, I've got to stop. That's how it's affected me. And then I've got to go to bed with that [tube] … stuck up me nose all night [laughs], so I've really – well, that's how it's affected me anyway. Before, I was an active bloke, you know. I worked at the pits, I used to work regular, but the condition has just gradually caught up on us.[98]

---

94 David Guy, Interview C44 (SOHC).

95 Carl Martin, Interview C8 (SOHC).

96 John Guthrie, Interview C19 (SOHC).

97 Cited in *Saga Magazine* (March 1998), consulted at http://www.deadline.demon. co.uk/archive/saga/980301.htm.

98 Frederick Hall, Interview C41 (SOHC).

In a similar way, a leading hand from Ayrshire told us of the impact on his pride at not being able to keep up with the men under his charge:

> Being a leading man, I never ever asked any man to do anything that I couldnae do myself, and I was embarrassed walking in the tailgate in the 1970s, and I tried to get in before the men got in 'cause if they hear me panting, they'd be saying, 'He's done,' which I presume I was, but I was embarrassed.[99]

Another example is that of a retired pit deputy. He remembered being on holiday when he began to notice other men his own age were much more active than he was, even although he was only 40 years old at the time:

> You could see other folk that wasnae in the pits could dae things that I couldnae dae, ken. They could run about … You used to go to the shore … You were down at the shore, playing football and one thing and another. You were puffed out before anybody else. I mean, your chest wasnae just as good as theirs.[100]

The oral history interviews thus aid our understanding of workers' own perceptions of their bodies and personal transitions in health and well-being, from able-bodied to disabled. They illuminate how such changes were rationalised. One of the crucial questions we asked was 'What has been the impact of your lung disease/condition?' One of the most common complaints was the inability to partake in recreational activities, such as dancing. One pneumoconiotic miner (who started work in 1947 and was first diagnosed with 10% pneumoconiosis in 1980) commented:

> Well, I don't go out. I don't go out drinking or nowt. If I'm in the house I'll have a glass of whisky when I go to bed on a night, and that's it. But when there was a club down here, I used to go down and have a drink now and again, but that was it. I couldn't dance or nowt, I can't bloody well walk, never mind dance.[101]

His wife lamented that he slowed up considerably as his condition deteriorated from 10% to 40% pneumoconiosis: 'Oh, he's like a snail. Oh, it takes you ages to do your shopping with him. He's stopping and having a bit of a walk and, but then stopping.' A 58-year-old disabled miner from Ayrshire remarked:

> I swam a lot. I played golf. I wasnae a bad golfer. And, eh, you cannae do them things now. You cannae *compete* in these things any more. You've no' got the capacity to do it. Aye, I can walk round the golf course, aye, but it's only for fun. I used to go and swim for a couple of hours at one time … It's the same with bowls when you're running up and down a bowling green. And it restricts you … Like decorating a house, I cannae hold a machine to take wallpaper off, and you get frustrated.[102]

---

99 William Dunsmore ('Arco'), Interview C16 (SOHC).
100 Bobby Strachan, Interview C11 (SOHC).
101 Samuel Westhead, Interview C37 (SOHC).
102 Carl Martin, Interview C8 (SOHC). Our emphasis.

Moreover, underscoring the fit-to-unfit transition and the young-to-old transition were the related mutations from high wage-earner and independence to low wage-earner, and unemployment and dependency upon the state. A Durham miner with chronic bronchitis responded in this way when asked how his respiratory condition affected his social life:

> Oh, I can't get out any. I can't go out, I can't *go* anywhere. Even if I walk up the stairs I'm jiggered, and coming down, I'm just as bad. And sometimes you get days like you're playing a tune, you know, like, and wheezing, and oh dear. And, as they say, 'We can hear you upstairs.'[103]

Another Durham miner noted the change in his life that serious breathing difficulties entailed:

> Well, to be quite honest it's turned my life completely upside down, this. I never dreamt, because, when you don't have something, you can't realise what the problem is, but as I say, I can't even do any decorating. Hoovering, if I hoover for [my wife], I mean, it takes me so long because I have to stop and sit down, even dusting. And really, it's turned us upside. I mean, we're talking there about holidays, and more to the [?], the case, I dread it. And you know, they look at you and think, 'What's the matter, has something happened?' I just say, 'No, I suffer with a problem of breathing,' and, I mean, I can only lift it up like that up to there, I'm (pants breathlessly). So really, it's completely turned my life upside down. I mean, I'm okay when I'm in bed, I'm okay when I'm sitting like this, it's as soon as I – even putting a screw in – it affects us.[104]

An Easington (Durham) Councillor, and ex-miner, Alan Napier, offered this poignant recollection about how disability affected mining communities:

> The club I drank in, they used to call 'Death Row', when you were going in there was a row, and there was about ten miners used to sit on that. I mean, it's been beefed up and it's a theme pub now, but even in five years ago, you saw it go from ten, to nine, to eight, to seven, and they were all, in the main, mining-related injuries or diseases that killed them off. And you can see the ones who were lucky to be alive, mind, but they can't get the words out, they can't breathe properly. And in the main, the ones who are in their eighties are bent at right angles ... So you can see the legacy, you can see the legacy of the pit. So you can understand the anger we've got.[105]

Whilst the support networks embedded within mining communities went some way to mitigate the isolation of the severely disabled, none the less, serious respiratory disease clearly affected physical capacities and lifestyles, as well as tragically cutting many lives short. A Durham miner with chronic bronchitis commented at length on how he felt as his physical capacity deteriorated:

---

103 Alan Winter, Interview C42 (SOHC).
104 George Burns, Interview C40 (SOHC).
105 Alan Napier, Interview C43 (SOHC).

But I never dreamt that I would be like this. And it's, as I say, I mean it isn't, I know it isn't embarrassing, but it is for me, because when I go over to the village where I used to live and I go to the local club and they haven't seen us for two or three months, they say, 'Oh, by George you're looking well, you're putting a bit weight on this,' you know, and I says, 'Aye, I am, and if I could only breathe,' I said, 'I would be no different.' 'Well, what do you mean, like?' 'Well,' I says, 'I just can't breathe,' I says, 'the least exertion, and', I says, 'I'm knackered.' And, as I say, I mean, I've told Rita and a lot of them round here, they're lovely neighbours, nobody ever says anything, but when I was doing anything outside, I had to stop and sit down on the wall, you know, and just get a minute. And I used to say to [my wife], 'They'll people watching me and saying, "That's all that bloody bloke does, keeps sitting down,"' and you know, but I mean. See, some people are not embarrassed, they say 'I'm knackered,' and that's the end of it, but, even when I told you when I walked up the village, I thought people will be saying, 'Why, he was on his way up when I went up, and me coming back,' oh dear me. I shouldn't feel like that, but that's my nature and I take it badly because I could do it, and when suddenly you can't. I think, 'Well, I'm a bloody write-off here, waste of time, really.'[106]

He continued: 'It's hard to accept, *it's so hard*.'

Emasculation?

We explored in Chapter 8 how masculinity was forged working in the dangerous and tough environment underground. The sharply segmented and gendered nature of work in mining and heavy industry communities helped both to incubate identities and, by assigning the most toxic and dangerous jobs to men, ensured that occupational injury, disease and mortality rates were substantially higher amongst men than women (even accounting for under-recording of female incidence). There were exceptions, of course, but this constitutes one of the more significant health differences between the genders. In this respect, a work culture in which manliness was expressed through exposure to hazards and high levels of tolerance of danger considerably disadvantaged men. Long-term exposure to heavy physical toil, toxins and dust took its toll on the body (as did heavy smoking and drinking) and could ultimately emasculate. Industrial disability drew workers physically away from a male-dominated work environment, re-locating them within the domestic sphere. It removed the ability of male workers to provide for their families in a material sense – to act out the 'breadwinner' role. Further, industrial disability also eroded their own sense of manly self-esteem by taking away their capacity to work, and through physical impairment, their strength and prowess – curtailing their capacity to partake in other 'manly' social activities, such as sport and the pub.[107]

---

106 George Burns, Interview C40 (SOHC).

107 For some discussion of the impact of encroaching disability in the Clydeside industrial conurbation, see R. Johnston and A. McIvor, 'Dangerous Work, Hard Men and Broken Bodies: Masculinity in the Clydeside Heavy Industries, c1930–1970s', *Labour History Review*, vol.

In response to a question about the impact pneumoconiosis had on their lives, two Scottish miners noted the inter-mingling of economic and social effects:

> DP: Aye, you had, you had a lot of auld boys, like, just wouldnae give in tae it, eh? They just thought they could still dae it, and it was pride. Ken, pride that they could …
> RC: Plus there would be a wage loss tae, eh? … And auld boys maybe worked in the pit thirty year or whatever it may be, and his later life, or whatever it is, he's working on the face, he didnae want tae come off the face and get a wage cut as it happened, because he's, what he's suffered in the pit, tae come off it and go on a working job, he'd suffer a large wage loss … It wasnae right on the auld boys, but that's what happened to them.[108]

The loss of manhood and low esteem brought about by not being able to undertake the many duties and roles regarded as 'manly' was felt acutely by many. The 58-year-old disabled miner from Ayrshire cited earlier told us this:

> I worked a' my life … but it was a big blow to me to be told that I'd never work again. Eh, your pride's dented, ken. I mean, when you're out and your wife's to come out and say to you, 'Come on, I'll get that …'. It definitely hurts your pride.[109]

Others recalled how difficult it was adapting to the slow pace of life dictated by an impaired lung condition, of the reversal of breadwinner roles and the drift into varying degree of dependency. Part of this embedded masculine identity was a reluctance to admit physical weakness or impairment, or to seek medical attention.[110]

However – and this brings us back to our methodology again – when interviewing miners with respiratory disability, it is important to understand that they are not only reflecting on their past, but are trying also to make sense of how the past has impacted on their present circumstances. Their testimonies, then, are a constant and complex interplay of the past upon the present and the present upon the past, in which feelings of anger, the need to apportion blame, combined with elements of guilt that the victims may have in some way contributed to their own and others' injuries, inter-mingle and sometimes clash with the need to recount to a researcher as accurately as possible what happened to them many years ago. To some degree, then, dominant discourses are reflected in the testimony of coal miners and other workers in the heavy industries (such as steel workers and shipbuilders), and one such is the erosion of masculinity which went hand in hand with encroaching disability. The loss of manhood was felt acutely by many of our disabled respondents. What is apparent is that the ramifications on the male psyche could be even more damaging where loss of the provider role (common enough with job losses in the contracting heavy industries) was combined with physical deterioration in health as a consequence of industrial disability or disease. Massive adjustments had to be negotiated in this

---

69, no. 2 (August 2004), pp. 135–51; Johnston and McIvor, 'Pushed into Social Exclusion', pp. 95–109.

    108 Robert Clelland and Duncan Porterfield, Interview C22 (SOHC).
    109 Billy Affleck, Interview C2 (SOHC).
    110 See the comment by David Guy, Interview C44 (SOHC).

forced transition from physically fit, independent provider in a male-dominated work environment to disabled dependent, often confined within what was still perceived by members of this generation as the woman's domain in the home.

Harsh Treatment and Frustrated Expectations

Oral history also reveals the considerable void which existed between intention and execution following the British Coal Respiratory Diseases Litigation in 1998. Although thousands of British miners could now claim industrial compensation if they had emphysema and/or bronchitis, they first had to prove that they suffered from these conditions. In 1999, the government announced it was setting up a national programme of spirometry testing, and by October that year over thirty test centres had been opened. Initially, responsibility for assessing the miners was placed in the hands of a part-American private health company called Healthcall – brought in specially by the miners' trade union to handle the sheer number of claimants.

The IIAC stipulated in 1996 that FEV1 (respiratory capacity measured by volume exhaled) should be at least one litre below that expected for a person of the same age, height, and sex to qualify as COAD. This was based on a lung function formula published in the mid-1960s.[111] This was the standard which miners trying to claim compensation for emphysema and/or bronchitis after the 1998 ruling had to prove that they fell below. Although in 1996 consideration was given to several other systems – that used by the European Community Steel and Coal (ECSC), and that recommended by the Institute of Occupational Medicine (IOM) – the IIAC considered the Cotes formula to be clear, straightforward, and appropriate enough for application to the benefit scheme.[112] Since 1996, though, the IIAC received complaints from various sources – including MPs in mining constituencies and the TUC – that the Cotes formula was not appropriate for the circumstances. The main criticism was that the formula was based on too small a sample which was out of date; did not represent the population; did not take into account that smoking was more prevalent when it was devised in the 1960s, and did not reflect the fact that modern environmental conditions had improved, and consequently the lung function of the general population had improved too. In effect, then, before they could qualify for disability payment, claimants were being asked to measure their loss of lung function against – and fall below by at least one litre capacity – a lower standard of respiratory ability prevalent in the population in the 1990s.[113] The IIAC was aware that complete objectivity in determining lung function was difficult:

---

111 J.E. Cotes et al., 'Average Normal Values for the Forced Expiratory Volume in White Caucasian Males', *British Medical Journal* (23 April 1966), vol. 5,494, pp. 1,016–19.

112 IIAC, *Lung Function Assessment, Industrial Injuries Disablement Benefit, Prescribed Disease D12 (Chronic Bronchitis and Emphysema in Underground Coal-miners)*, Position Paper no. 11 (2000), p. 2.

113 Ibid., p. 3.

It is important to bear in mind that measuring lung function is not an exact science and that the use of spirometers will inevitably entail a margin of error reflecting personal, environmental and other factors.[114]

Over and above this, though, for many the long time lag between the legal decision and the eventual paying out of compensation meant the Turner judgment was a hollow victory anyway. Two statements from 2001 illustrate the political dimensions to the issue. Peter Hain, Minister for Energy and Competitiveness in Europe, commented:

> I, too, have visited many retired miners in their homes and seen the tragic circumstances in which they live. They are frequently trapped on the ground floor, unable to climb the stairs and almost unable to make the short journey from living room to bathroom without having to pause to catch their breath and to recover from a walk that the rest of us would not even notice. For them, it is a journey of miles. I pay tribute to those miners. We shall deliver justice. I also pay tribute to their wives, who care for them in the most difficult circumstances. This is about justice and dignity. It is about redeeming the debt that we owe to miners and to their families who sacrificed their most precious asset, their health, to work underground, so that we can live in comfort.[115]

Dave Douglass, an NUM lodge officer until 1984 and a campaigner for miners' rights, made this point:

> Justice like Hell! True to Blair's Tory roots they refused point blank to sit down with the Miners' Union who represent 90% of all miners working or retired and work out a compensation scheme. The NUM is Blair's class enemy and he turned instead to an alliance of Lawyers nation-wide to draw up a scheme, it is fraught with injustice and legal and technical somersaults aimed at robbing the miners of any claim ... Only 1500 men out of 100,000 victims have been paid out. The average I encounter is £5000 with £3000 being a typical sum. Men like my old mate Benny Marks, 46 years a face worker in blinding blizzards of dust shovelling rock and coal, is awarded £1200.[116]

But although delay in receiving compensation was bad enough, for many, the necessity of having to undergo spirometry testing to prove their breathing capacity was significantly reduced was a humiliating and degrading experience. For example, one 76-year-old retired Ayrshire miner remembered:

> Oh, you had tae blow into one of they things. I couldnae blow into it. He telt you tae hold your breath. I couldnae hold my breath. He's telling you tae blow, blow, *blow*. I says, 'If I could dae that, son, I wouldnae be here.' [laughs] And he got angry, ken. And I just got as angry. He says, 'You'll have tae come back.' I says, 'I'm no caring how many times

---

114 Ibid., p. 4.

115 House of Commons, *Hansard*, Debates for 13 March, 2001, pt 42, col. 346.

116 Dave Douglass, http://www.minersadvice.co.uk/overview/-blairsdisaster.htm, accessed 11 March 2005. Douglass was a miner at Hatfield Main Colliery.

I come back, son. I cannae hold my breath. I havnae got breath tae hold.' He was just a young boy, ken.[117]

A 77-year-old retired oversman from the same region told a similar tale:

I went to, for tests … I went to Drongan, eh, and had these tests, eh. And the boy that was doing it kept saying, 'Fill your lungs.' Well, I did that. I did everything he asked me. And he kept saying, 'That's no' good enough. You'll have to blow harder.' I couldae blow harder. I mean, I kept trying and trying. The wife will tell you I was puffed out, sore when I came home.

Here's another example of a miner's perception of the way in which he was being treated after years of exposure to coal dust. This man – who was suffering from emphysema – took two of his older colleagues along to the assessment centre to help them with their claims, and watched as they were given spirometer tests:

I seen him getting done, and this woman shouting, 'Blow, blow, blow blow, blow, blow!' And, see, every time that man blew in, he was red in the face … And, see, the old man fae Kickonnel? He was the very same … I tell you, there's a boy there, and he'd be lucky if he was twenty year old, and I bet you a pound that he never seen a pit. These men don't ken about the things we had tae dae to make a shilling. They've nae idea.[118]

And some of the men were very angry indeed:

It was a load of bloody rubbish. … There was a boy standing, and you had tae put a tube in your bloody mouth, and he's shouting 'Blow, blow, blow!' … I says, 'Here, son, dae you think it's a barrage balloon I've got in my bloody chest?' He hadn't a bloody clue, the pig. And that's a' it was, a charade. A bloody charade.[119]

The bitterness derived, in part, from a sense that the so-called specialists were 'outsiders' who understood nothing about the mining community. Alan Napier recalled an incident with the lung function testing in Durham:

There's a lad I work with who's only got twenty per cent lung capacity, he's *crippled* with rheumatoid arthritis, and he went in, I was sitting in the room, and I could hear the technicians shouting at him, you know, when he was getting the vibration test, when he was getting the heat test, when he was getting the eye test. And there's something inherent about where they want to knock us about here, you know, 'Why do you think you should be a special case, why?' Them people, mind, have never been down a pit in their lives, you know.[120]

Many of the miners were disgruntled about the way Healthcall conducted the tests:

117 Thomas McMurdo, Interview C20 (SOHC).
118 Dick Easterbrook, Interview C17 (SOHC).
119 John Guthrie, Interview C19 (SOHC).
120 Alan Napier, Interview C43 (SOHC).

This is an American company that the union made an awful mistake in employing … It's an American company, and they're absolutely ruthless. Ruthless. And these are employed by the union and the union lawyers. They're not doing us any favours at all. We don't want favours. But everything that they ask you is smoking-related. And they're adamant about that.[121]

A miners' advice website condemned the spirometer tests in this way:

The required spirometer test was supposed to be less severe than the DSS one, in reality it is more harsh. Old miners are bullied and yelled at and told to blow harder, that they are faking, that the test is not being complied with. Doctors at these centres have been described as 'Nazis' by men who have not the physical strength or lung capacity to blow at the fierce rate demanded by the test. Whereas before the scam was to say that the miner didn't have the compensable pneumoconiosis he had the non-compensatable Chronic Bronchitis or Emphysema, now the man is told he doesn't have CB&E which is compensable, he has asthma which isn't. This is despite having 80% or 90% awards from the already stringent DSS FEV test.[122]

By March 2001 in Scotland, out of a total of 9,665 claims, only 649 men (7%) had received full and final payments. However, 656 miners had died since making their claims.[123] Measures were put in place to speed the process up – for example, Healthcall was instructed to stop booking in claimants on a first-come, first-served basis, and to prioritise older, unhealthier miners. However, the problem of miners' claims for compensation being assessed by young, unsympathetic technicians remained, and the process was perceived as humiliating and degrading by many disabled miners. Whilst the COAD compensation scheme was a long-overdue step in the right direction, these negative experiences associated with the process of determining the *degree* of respiratory damage added significantly to the overall impact of this 'new' occupational health disease.

Conclusion

One of the main justifications for oral history lies in the way sparsely documented areas of human experience can be illuminated and our understanding of attitudes, behaviour and processes enhanced. Our contention here is that oral testimony enables us to elucidate the multi-layered impact of contracting occupational disease, and facilitates a reconstruction of the lives of those with respiratory impairments – including the now almost forgotten pneumoconiotics who were so evident in coal mining towns and villages in the middle decades of the twentieth century. This includes the complex changes in identity that encroaching impairment entailed. Paradoxically, perhaps, work in the British heavy industries under such conditions

---

121 Carl Martin, Interview C8 (SOHC).
122 http://www.minersadvice.co.uk/ourview-blairsdisaster.htm.
123 'Retired Miners Compensation (Scotland)', *Hansard* (13 March 2001), col. 220.

as prevailed through to the final quarter of the twentieth century was capable both of *forging* masculinity (and thus providing a basis for masculine power beyond the workplace) and of *corroding* the very basis of manliness by consuming workers' bodies – their human capital – and removing their capacity to provide for dependants. The scenario that unfolded for many was disability, loss of employment, and encroaching dependency, with their lives invariably reoriented to a different pattern, and for many largely relocated within the confines of the home – the sphere traditionally designated for this generation as the terrain of women. Pneumoconiotics and other victims of industrial injury and disease frequently ended up the very antithesis of healthy manhood.

Whilst it has its usefulness, we argue here that the experience of coal miners indicates that the concept of *social exclusion* also has its limitations. For many miners with pneumoconiosis, bronchitis and emphysema, the experience of disability was associated with varying degrees of pain, suffering, withdrawal and social isolation. This corresponds to the dominant portrayal of the disabled in recent literature as oppressed, powerless, dependent and marginalised. Undoubtedly, the ramifications of serious respiratory disease were catastrophic for many victims and their families. However, others were energised and politicised as the knowledge of corporate and state culpability emerged and they struggled to survive on dwindling earnings or meagre benefits. Our contention here is that those coal miners with respiratory disabilities shared many of the characteristics of the disabled community as a whole, including loss of citizenship, power and independence. However, we posit that there was a very wide range of experience amongst those miners with breathing difficulties – based partly on widely differing levels of impairment – and that coal miners themselves were an agency in this process. Rather than being powerless victims, the workers affected and their solidaristic traditions played a key role in mitigating the characteristic social exclusion associated with disability. In this respect, the miners might offer an archetypal case study of the power and agency of the disabled, and one which demonstrates the complexity of lived experience and the limitations of any simplistic model of social exclusion and oppression. This further emphasises the point that understanding the lived experience of those impaired within our society in the past necessitates not only developing a dialogue (as oral historians) with those directly involved, but also locating those impaired within the specific spatial and social spaces they occupied at that time.

Conclusion

This book has attempted a social history of mining from the point of view of the miner's body, placing at centre stage the devastation wreaked upon mining communities by inhaling dust at work. By tracing the history of pneumoconiosis, bronchitis and emphysema in coal mining, we have explored how and why one of the most deadly and disabling of all occupational health disasters in Britain's history occurred. In so doing, we have also investigated prevailing workplace culture, health behaviour and the impact of dust disease upon individuals, families and communities. Although we have tried to address an evident gap in the historiography of coal mining, we hope that our book has also made broader contributions to industrial relations and labour history, medical history, disability studies and to oral history. Whilst engaging with a clutch of hypotheses generated in the literature, it has also left many questions and research avenues unexplored. We aim to summarise our interpretation here and provide some pointers for the way forward towards possible future work in this field.

We have argued that miners' lung disease needs to be contextualised within the dangerous high risk working environment of the pits, as well as within the profit-oriented and productionist managerial culture of coal mining in the private and public ownership eras. By the nineteenth century, coal mining was an extremely hazardous and unhealthy industry, and the workforce was acculturated to high injury and mortality rates in the underground environment. This was a *milieu* in which the body was constantly under threat. Therefore, it is understandable that compared to the countless safety risks faced by miners in their daily employment, long-term chronic health issues, including the risk of respiratory damage caused through exposure to mine dust, were generally marginalised by workers and employers. Safety, then, took precedence over health. By the early years of the twentieth century, it was widely acknowledged that there was a high human cost in producing coal, and for some time measures had been directed at making the mines safer places to work – notably through the Mines Acts and the growth of a Mines Inspectorate. But it was also the case that because of the nature of their employment in what was perhaps the riskiest of the heavy industries in which to work, miners were generally looked upon as being a breed apart, and able to endure the most hazardous of working conditions. Their acceptance of a certain degree of risk, compensated to some degree by relatively high wages, was seen as an integral element of the miner's occupation, and tacitly this applied to the *health* risks posed by underground mining too. Tweedale has postulated that in the British post-war asbestos industry, a certain level of death and disability was tolerated.[1] This appears to have also been the case with coal mining. Certainly, as far as mine dust was concerned, well into the twentieth century, medical professionals, employers, management and the miners themselves accepted that a certain level of dust had to be endured. This was not stoicism or fatalism, but simply pragmatism and realism. Indeed, it was because of the general acceptance of the unforgiving nature of the working environment that maximum exposure levels for mine dust were consistently pegged at a level which would ensure the continuation of the industry. The idea of reducing mine dust *to a minimum* has only been incorporated in the most recent of coal dust regulations proposed in 2004.

It is on to this distinctive attitude taken towards miners' health and safety in general that we need to map the progress of medical knowledge regarding miners' respiratory diseases. Our analysis of the belated recognition and 'scheduling' of CWP in Britain in 1943 and bronchitis and emphysema in 1993 fits well with Dembe's thesis that medical knowledge is an intensely contested terrain and that occupational diseases are socially constructed.[2] As we have illustrated, advances in medical knowledge and state acceptance of industrial diseases frequently took different trajectories. From its first recognition as a distinctive industrial disease in the eighteenth century and its appearance in medical journals in the 1830s, miners' lung had 'disappeared' by the last decades of the nineteenth century, only to be 're-discovered' in the early twentieth century. To some extent, this pattern of acceptance, denial, then re-acceptance was a harbinger of what was to occur in the twentieth century with bronchitis. For, although bronchitis was initially blamed for most miners' respiratory ill health in the early part of the twentieth century, this also disappeared as an industrial disease, and was not fully recognised as such until the 1990s. Therefore, the recognition of miners' lung as an industrial disease was not representative of an upward curve of growing medical knowledge. On the contrary, the increased attention devoted by medical scientists to miners' lung from the 1890s resulted in a prolonged contest over the exact causation of dust disease amongst miners. Within this long-winded medical debate, miners' lung was termed anthracosis, miners' asthma, bronchitis, then silicosis. In the years before the Second World War, the Medical Research Council's (MRC) research led to the official designation of the 'new' disease of coal workers' pneumoconiosis (CWP) in 1943. This resulted in attention being shifted from rock dust to coal dust, and the doggedly persistent fixation with silica as the *sole* agent of lung damage finally discredited.

From the mid-1950s, the importance of coal to the British economy steadily diminished as markets contracted and the labour force sharply declined. Inversely, though, the coal dust problem grew in national importance as the number of pneumoconiotics in regions other than South Wales began to rise, reflecting poor mining practice in these regions compared to South Wales, where serious attention had been devoted to the problem since the late 1930s. By the 1950s, medical

---

1   G. Tweedale, *From Magic Mineral to Killer Dust* (Oxford, 2000), p. 280.

2   A. Dembe, *Occupation and Disease: How Social Factors Affect the Conception of Work-Related Disorders* (New Haven, CT, 1996), pp. 3-21.

professionals were devoting increasing attention to finding out more about the dangers of mine dust. This intense research activity was driven by several factors: the ideology of the social medicine movement, the rise of epidemiology, and a determination to ensure good standards of occupational health in Britain's flagship nationalised industry. The setting up of the Pneumoconiosis Research Unit (PRU) at Cardiff in 1946, the Rhondda Fach studies led by Archie Cochrane in the early 1950s, and the NCB's own large-scale epidemiological study (PFR) initiated in 1953 illustrate the scientific approach taken towards working miners at this time. Certainly, the NCB's 25-pit Scheme became in effect a controlled experiment in which miners' dust exposure was correlated with the opacity of their x-rays. The survey was by all accounts a serious attempt to solve the coal dust problem. However, there were two negative aspects of the scheme. Firstly, the NCB's long delay in adopting a more rigorous dust datum was to a great extent due to the expectation that the 25-pit Scheme would provide the definitive answer to what constituted a dangerous level of dust exposure – as well as what type of dust was doing miners the most harm. Secondly, although dedicated to protecting miners from CWP, underpinning the 25-pit Scheme was the need to ensure high productivity. What was being sought, then, was not how *low* the dust datum should be, but how *high* it could be pitched before miners' lungs were affected. The implementation of a more common-sense strategy in which dust levels were reduced to as low as possible would have been a much better idea. However, this would have necessitated an unrealistic reduction in the pace of production which would not have been tolerated within the economic situation in which the coal industry found itself.

The epidemiological studies of coal miners' respiratory health entailed that medical approaches to the dust problem and engineering approaches were frequently inter-dependent. This was certainly the case with the 25-pit Scheme. However, implicit in both approaches was that coal production would continue unabated while the problem was being investigated by the medical professionals. NCB and state policy of re-employing pneumoconiotics after 1948 is another good example of the inter-twining of the medical and the engineering solutions. Medical scientists employed by the MRC not only identified CWP as coal dust-related, but also, albeit by default, provided the coal industry with a dust datum (set at 850/650/450 p.p.c.c.) within which miners could supposedly work without any danger to their respiratory health. This was seized upon, and we saw in Chapter 5 how Bedford and Warner's scale was adopted, not only as a way of re-employing pneumoconiotics – primarily in South Wales – but as the NCB's national strategy to protect all its miners from dust levels high enough to cause them to contract CWP. The aim, then, was not to eliminate mine dust, or even to reduce it as far as possible, but to ensure that dust levels were kept below a certain level. This act of expediency resulted in the 'approved/non-approved' faces principle, and an adherence to a standard of maximum dustiness which, although stringent enough to make serious inroads into the pneumoconiosis problem, did not protect miners from other respiratory diseases caused by exposure to mine dust. As importantly, the idea of fixing a maximum permissible level of dustiness – rather than going for as dust-free a mine atmosphere as possible – fitted in with the acceptance of a certain degree of risk in underground coal mining.

Thus, when it came to the coal dust problem, the NCB found itself continually attempting to strike a balance between production and protection. This raises the question of whether and to what extent a nationalised public corporation adopted a different strategy towards the health and well-being of their employees than private enterprise? There is much evidence to support the view that the NCB's initial policy reflected a determination to neutralise the dust problem in the pits, and this did represent a marked advance on the attitudes of the private coal owners. Massive resources were directed to the pneumoconiosis problem by the state and the NCB, including the marshalling of medical expertise. Certainly, the NCB's x-ray programme, which took men out of danger when the first signs of dust damage appeared, was admirable, as was its health and safety infrastructure in general. However, economic imperatives in a difficult market environment from the mid-1950s made the balance between production and health increasingly difficult to ensure. Advancing mechanisation of coal production (with shearing and power-loading) and the ever-increasing speed of coal face advance became prioritised to ensure the survival of the industry. Consequently, in far too many cases, attempts to reduce dust levels amounted to tokenism, or at best an unequal contest between dust generation and dust suppression. However, to complicate the picture even more, a further flaw in NCB policy was its long insistence that the fight against dust disease would be won by dust suppression alone, and not by the cultivation of a culture of self-protection amongst the miners. Only from the mid-1970s was there a change of policy and the provision of respirators legalised, leading to the wearing of masks being encouraged. By this time, though, the antipathy towards dust masks was as ingrained as the inhaled dust, and the issuing of disposable paper masks was treated with a general disdain by most of the workers. Our oral history evidence clearly illustrates the wide gulf between NCB policy and implementation of this policy at the coal face. Certainly, as regards accurate dust measurement and properly enforced dust suppression, it was only when statutory regulations appeared on the horizon that a comprehensive effort was made to systematically improve standards.

Therefore, whilst the dominant public discourse of the NCB was that of an 'enlightened manager', there were flaws in its occupational health strategy linked to its prioritisation of production over its duty to protect its labour force from bodily damage. This was especially evident in the 1960s and early 1970s, and led directly to the imposition of statutory controls and a more stringent dust datum, albeit belatedly, in the mid-1970s. That is not to say, however, that the initiatives of the state and the NCB did not have some positive ameliorative impact upon the pneumoconiosis problem. This was indicated in the steady fall from the mid-1950s in new cases of coal workers' pneumoconiosis diagnosed in the UK and the declining rate of CWP (including PMF) within the employed workforce indicated in the PFR surveys from the late 1950s (see Figures 2.1, 2.2 and 4.1). The sharper rate of fall in the pneumoconiosis morbidity statistics from the 1970s undoubtedly reflected improvements in dust control in the pits from the late 1940s – given the 10–25-year time lag in the incubation period of the disease. Only with hindsight does it become apparent that the attention heaped upon CWP had largely camouflaged the fact that other respiratory diseases were clearly linked to coal mining too. The long struggle from the 1950s to have emphysema and bronchitis scheduled as industrial diseases of coal workers echoed the earlier complexities surrounding CWP, although with the added problem that these miners' diseases were prevalent throughout the wider population, and that smoking was heavily implicated in their causation. Therefore, despite a long acceptance by the medical profession that miners suffered from a range of industrially linked respiratory diseases, and not just CWP, the rapid decline of the coal mining industry, coupled with unshakeable medical opinion regarding the impossibility of designating a smoking-related disease as occupational, made this a protracted struggle. Compensation procedures regarding the undisputable occupational causation of scheduled diseases stood as a barrier against the acceptance of bronchitis and emphysema for most of the twentieth century. Only when evidence became available showing that respiratory damage caused by smoking and similar damage due to the inhalation of mine dust had a common causal pathway was it accepted that either or both could be ruled as causing bronchitis and emphysema. Unfortunately, it was only in the 1990s, by which time the coal mining industry had virtually disappeared, that the acceptance of bronchitis and emphysema as diseases specific to miners was eventually conceded, first by the Industrial Injuries Advisory Committee (IIAC), and then by a High Court judge.

As we have seen, the role of trade unions in occupational health is much debated in the literature, with some commentators positing that the unions failed to prioritise the body, and hence that they played their part in the high death and disability toll that subsequently accrued. As with our previous study of asbestos, our analysis of the coal mining trade unions suggests a more complex picture. We argue here that the actions of the miners' unions must be contextualised within the prevailing economic and political circumstances the industry faced, and within the workplace culture of the miners, which itself varied markedly from coal field to coal field. There was a constant tension operating between conflicting interests within a massive federally structured union, where the regions retained much autonomy. The strongest and most militant coal fields – notably South Wales, and to a somewhat lesser extent Scotland – pressed most vigorously for action on black lung, and in the pre-nationalised era were supported by the MFGB, which, as Melling and Bufton have persuasively argued, played a vital role in the coalition of progressive forces which resulted in getting CWP certified as an occupational disease in 1943.[3] We have argued here that the miners' unions were active thereafter, especially through the National Joint

3   J. Melling and M. Bufton, '"A Mere Matter of Rock": Organized Labour, Scientific Evidence and British Government Schemes for Compensation of Silicosis and Pneumoconiosis among Coalminers, 1926–1940', *Medical History*, vol. 49, no. 2 (April 2005), pp. 155–78; M. Bufton and J. Melling, 'Coming Up for Air: Experts, Employers and Workers in Campaigns to Compensate Silicosis Sufferers in Britain, 1918–39', *Social History of Medicine*, vol. 18, no. 1 (2005), pp. 63–86.

Pneumoconiosis Committee (NJPC) and in the workplace, in protecting the interests of their members, not least through the policing of dust control measures at the point of production. The oral evidence suggests a constant tension between the productionist tendencies of management, the wage-maximising proclivities of many of the miners and the protective matrix provided by the union officials, especially the pivotal workmen's inspectors. The NUM and its regional federations were especially active, moreover, regarding compensation and rehabilitation. As well as the recognition and scheduling of CWP in 1943, key victories were the creation of the 1974 Pneumoconiosis Compensation Scheme and the recognition of bronchitis and emphysema as occupational diseases in 1993.

None the less, there is still something in the argument that the mining unions might have pressed forward with a more proactive occupational health policy earlier, focusing more on prevention than compensation. Despite some criticism, the NUM remained wedded to the policy of re-employing pneumoconiotics and to the principle of 'approved faces' – at least up until the 1970s. Further, the unions largely accepted the rationale for mechanisation, and the NUM even negotiated a 'dirty work' agreement (in 1961) with the NCB to provide some workers with extra wage payments to compensate for the 'discomfort' associated with working in excessively dusty conditions, thus adding legitimacy to miners' exposure to dangerous levels of dust at work. In these areas there was a great deal of consensus and collusion between the NCB and the NUM – especially in the two decades or so after nationalisation. Moreover, whilst there were a number of coal face 'walkouts' against dusty conditions (notably in South Wales), we have come across no evidence of any coal field or pit strikes on the issue of dust, nor did the NUM condone any official strike action to exert pressure on the NCB to improve dust control. In part, perhaps, this was because of the evident sensitivity and responsiveness of the NCB on occupational health, especially from 1947 through the 1950s, when a massive amount of NCB resources, as we have seen, were targeted at tackling pneumoconiosis and creating the most extensive occupational health service in British industry. The NUM was evidently keen to play its part in the economic survival of the nationalised industry. As the pit closure programme intensified from the late 1950s and the industry contracted, it was perhaps inevitable that the unions would prioritise wages, jobs and the survival of the industry over health concerns. With the exception of one or two of the more militant coal fields (including South Wales), union policy was undoubtedly reflecting rather than clashing with the views of the majority of the men in the industry.

In the final analysis, on balance the evidence strongly supports a more positive appraisal of the role of the unions in coal mining on occupational health. In this respect, our research adds weight to the revisionist appraisals of the role of trade unions on occupational health by Bloor, Melling and Bufton, and Bowden and Tweedale.[4] The records of the MFGB, the SWMF and the NUM, combined with

---

4   M. Bloor, 'The South Wales Miners' Federation, Miners' Lung and the Instrumental Use of Expertise 1900–1950', *Social Studies of Science*, vol. 30, no. 1 (February 2000), pp.125–40; Melling and Bufton, '"A Mere Matter of Rock"'; Melling and Bufton, 'Coming Up

the experiential testimony, indicates a great deal of dynamism in contesting and creating medical knowledge, in compensation struggles and in rehabilitation. This certainly contrasted sharply with the failure of the trade unions to act as an effective 'countervailing force' in the asbestos tragedy.[5] Unfortunately, we know relatively little as yet about the health strategies of other trade unions in the UK, and more studies would enable us to more fully comprehend the dynamics operating. Research is also desperately needed into the role of the British and Scottish Trades Union Congress on occupational health. What is evident from coal mining is that the powerful mining trade unions were an active agency throughout the twentieth century in the power struggle over health and the body in the pits. At times they were pivotal agents, operating in an environment during wartime and after nationalisation that was much more conducive to joint regulation and control. Cumulatively, the combination of effective pressure group politics by mining trade unions at the national level (including co-opting the support of the TUC) and vigilant rank-and-file action at the workplace level resulted in much earlier and more effective control of the dust problem in the British coal industry compared with asbestos manufacturers and users. This also contrasts sharply with the relative ineffectiveness on health issues of the productivity politics of the United Mine Workers' Association in the USA. What is patently evident, however, is that respiratory disability devastated coal field communities throughout the world through the nineteenth and twentieth centuries and brought great depths of human misery, pain, distress and loss. There remains much potential for more comparative historical studies and for investigation of the international campaign to tackle the occupational dust problem, spearheaded by the International Labour Office.

Whilst the unions battled with the employers and the NCB, they were also faced with the problem of challenging and trying to break down an established and deeply engrained workplace culture where miners were socialised into acceptance of high levels of risk and danger. This is where we believe oral evidence makes a vital contribution to our understanding of the unfolding tragedy of miners' lung, because it takes us deep into the heart of the mining labour process and into the mentalities of the men. Oral testimony and other experiential evidence illuminates the attitudes and behaviour of the men, suggesting a tension between 'heroic' union activists struggling to protect bodies from damage, and miners themselves stoically accepting levels of respiratory damage over time. As with our previous study of the asbestos tragedy, however, what is clearly evident from the oral testimony is that a wide gulf existed between the official health and safety code relating to dust

---

for Air'; S. Bowden and G. Tweedale, 'Mondays without Dread: The Trade Union Response to Byssinosis in the Lancashire Cotton Industry in the Twentieth Century', *Social History of Medicine*, vol. 16, no. 1 (2003), pp. 79–95.

5   For a recent contribution to this debate, see A. Higgison, 'Asbestos and the British Trade Unions, 1960s and 1970s', *Scottish Labour History*, vol. 40 (2005), pp. 70–86. Walker interprets the unions in a more favourable light in relation to occupational chemical hazards; see D. Walker, '"Working in it, through it and among it all day": Chrome dust at J. & J. White of Rutherglen, 1893–1967', *Scottish Labour History*, vol. 40 (2005), pp. 50–69.

control and actual workplace practice. In reality, rules and regulations designed to minimise exposure to health-damaging levels of dust were widely subverted at the point of production. Colliery management must be held primarily responsible for this. However, in turn, as Perchard has argued, this must also be understood within the context of the pressure being applied from above – from the NCB – on to mine managers and professionals, and within the wider context of an industry which was in terminal decline for much of the twentieth century.[6]

Clearly, there also existed a competitive edge to workplace culture underground that is often overlooked in social and labour histories of this renowned solidaristic community, with miners who broke production records and earned the largest wage packets gaining esteem, status and being exalted within the community. Again, the insights provided by the oral testimony have been invaluable here. This study of miners thus provides support for the validity of Cockerman's notion of 'habitus' – that values and behaviour are reproduced from generation to generation in working class communities.[7] Fatalistic stoicism and competitive macho behaviour in the workplace were capable of undermining and even reversing improvements in occupational health and safety standards. A tough, uncompromising, productionist culture was embraced by many miners, and in the process, working in such a way was capable, as Connell has suggested, of consuming men's bodies.[8] There is much debate today about how expressions of 'hard man' styles of masculinity can be inherently unhealthy – not least through heavy drinking and smoking. This study of miners illuminates some of the ways in which a managerial profit and productionist ethos combined with workers' *machismo* acceptance of risk and danger in the workplace undermined health and well-being. The latter, however, again needs to be understood within the realities of working-class life in mining communities. The wage 'fetish' and productionist ethos were themselves the result of a payment-by-results wage system in the industry and of endemic economic insecurity, exacerbated by the accelerating pit closure programme from the mid-1950s. The degenerative pressures impinging upon miners' bodies were intimately inter-connected. More research is required to further explore these relationships and to better understand the impact that gender identities had upon health behaviour and experience. Iron and steel workers would constitute an apposite case study. However, we also require more focus upon the occupational health experience and attitudes of female workers (such as those employed in textile manufacturing) to better comprehend the gendered nature of bodily damage as a consequence of work. Were there stark differences between the health behaviour and attitudes of men and women in employment? Oral history, we would argue, might make an important contribution here also.

---

6   A. Perchard, 'The Mine Management Professions and the Dust Problem in the Scottish Coal Mining Industry, c. 1930–1966', *Scottish Labour History*, vol. 40 (2005), pp. 87–110.

7   W. Cockerman, 'The Sociology of Health Behaviour and Health Lifestyles in Central Asia', in C. Bird et al. (eds), *Handbook of Medical Sociology*, 5th edn (Englewood Cliffs, NJ, 2000).

8   R.W. Connell, *The Men and the Boys* (Oxford, 2000), p. 188.

Whilst the oral testimony utilised in this book elucidates the poorly documented dynamics of workplace culture, such experiential testimony also enables reconstruction of the impact disease had upon miners' lives, taking us closer to what it was like to experience progressively deteriorating respiratory function. In Chapter 9, we argued that the black lung disaster in the UK left a grim legacy of occupation-related death and impairment, with disability more evident in the coal fields than in any other working-class communities in the UK in the first half of the twentieth century. Respiratory impairment impacted upon miners' lives in varied ways, partly depending upon the severity of their breathlessness and loss of lung function. Degrees of social exclusion were the most obvious outcome, as miners with serious respiratory damage found themselves increasingly housebound. This pattern fits closely with the concept of 'creeping disability' developed by Mildred Blaxter, where chronic disease led to slow but cumulatively meaningful transitions in lifestyles.[9] For disabled miners, these mutations were invariably life-changing in that they involved a spatial transition from the male-dominated world of the workplace to the home – a domain deemed to be feminised, at least until the last quarter of the twentieth century. We posit, then, that miners' lung physically incapacitated men, and that this process was invariably *emasculating*. Working in the pits toughened miners up, made them 'hard men', and honed the physically fit and powerful body, whilst also ironically holding the potential to erode and undermine their masculinity.

Whilst useful as an explanatory framework, ultimately, however, we found the 'social exclusion' thesis to be wanting in relation to coal miners and to much more accurately 'fit' the experience of asbestos-disease victims. Borsay's recent history of disability provides a nuanced and persuasive evaluation of the exclusion of those with disabilities in British society from full citizenship because of their prohibition from the labour market.[10] However, the NCB's systematic employment of pneumoconiotics from 1948 provides a somewhat unusual example which goes against the grain. There was a further qualitative difference, given the widespread *organic* support for disabled miners within their tight-knit communities – supported by institutions such as the Coal Industry Social and Welfare Organisation and the miners' trade unions. The historical study of disability is, however, still in its infancy. Our plea here would be for more research on particular disabled communities, to compare the experience of miners against other groups of workers, and for more comparative international studies and – where relevant – for the systematic integration of oral evidence within such research projects. Used carefully and with sensitivity, participants' voices not only enrich our histories with experiential testimony, but enable us to better understand the complex etiology of occupational disease and more effectively comprehend the impact such chronic occupation-related disease had upon people's lives.

---

9   See M. Blaxter, *The Meaning of Disability: A Sociological Study of Impairment* (London, 1976).

10 See A. Borsay, *Disability and Social Policy in Britain since 1750* (Basingstoke, 2005).

Whilst oral history methodology has its pitfalls and such source material has to be used with care, the experiential testimony derived from oral evidence also allows us to engage critically with hypotheses generated within the literature of medical history, labour history and disability studies. We argue here for more sensitivity towards context, historical contingency and agency. Medical history approaches have too often ignored the dynamics of power within the workplace and wider society, and have tended to perceive the accumulation of medical knowledge as if in a vacuum. Business historians have tended, with some notable exceptions (such as Tweedale), to ignore, or have glossed over, corporate crime, whilst for their part, labour historians have sometimes been guilty of a pathological aversion to capital and of uncritically heaping culpability upon exploitative, profit-maximising bosses. The approach we have adopted in this book has involved a synthesis of medical history, business history, labour history and oral history. The narrative that unfolds, therefore, is a complex and multi-layered one. Paradoxically, perhaps, the NCB emerges as both a welfarist employer and a negligent one. On the other hand, whilst the mining trade unions played a positive role in occupational health, the evidence illustrates that they could undoubtedly have prioritised preventative strategies much more than they did. The oral testimony also points to a significant failure of the state regulatory framework at the point of production, and to a workplace culture where there existed a very high acceptance of risk, and where production and the wage packet were invariably prioritised over health. These inter-related paradoxes disabled miners' bodies. Within an autonomous and deeply *machismo* work culture, overlaid with an intensely productionist Fordist managerial ethos, occupational health and safety standards underground came under severe pressure. The miners took the full force of this. The outcome was a respiratory disease epidemic of monumental proportions which decimated British mining communities throughout the twentieth century. Tragically, the legacy of this catastrophe will continue to scar such communities for many years to come.

Appendix:
The Oral History Project

1. Scotland

Alec Mills
Interview C1
Born 1933
Ayrshire miner
Interview date: 19 June 2000
Interviewers: A. McIvor
and R. Johnston

Billy Affleck
Interview C2
Born 1950
Ayrshire miner
Interview date: 19 June 2000
Interviewers: A. McIvor
and R. Johnston

John Orr
Interview C3
Born 1920
Ayrshire mine driver
Interview date: 19 June 2000
Interviewers: A. McIvor and
R. Johnston

Andrew Lyndsay
Interview C4
Born 1916
Ayrshire miner
Interview date: 29 June 2000
Interviewer: R. Johnston

Archie McLaren
Interview C5
Born 1909
Lanarkshire miner
Interview date: 29 June 2000
Interviewer: R. Johnston

George Devenne
Interview C6
Born 1923
Lanarkshire miner
Interview date: 29 June 2000
Interviewer: R. Johnston

David Marshall
Interview C7
Born 1915
Lanarkshire miner
Interview date: 29 June 2000
Interviewer: R. Johnston

Carl Martin
Interview C8
Born 1935
Fife and Lanarkshire miner
Interview date: 29 June 2000
Interviewer: R. Johnston

Harry Steel
Interview C9
Born 1927
Lothians and Lanarkshire miner
Interview date: 29 June 2000
Interviewer: R. Johnston

Bobby Strachan
Interview C11
Born 1923
Ayrshire miner;
pit deputy
Interview date: 5 July 2000
Interviewer: R. Johnston

Alec McNeish
Interview C13
Born 1927
Ayrshire miner
Interview date: 5 July 2000
Interviewer: R. Johnston

David Hendry
Interview C15
Born 1925
Ayrshire miner
Interview date: 5 July 2000
Interviewer: R. Johnston

Dick Easterbrook
Interview C17
Born 1932
Ayrshire miner
Interview date: 11 July 2000
Interviewer: R. Johnston

John Guthrie
Interview C19
Born 1932
Ayrshire miner
Interview date: 11 July 2000
Interviewer: R. Johnston

John McKean
Interview C10
Born 1936
Fife and Lanarkshire miner
Interview date: 29 June 2000
Interviewer: R. Johnston

Pat Ferguson
Interview C12
Born 1921
Dumfriesshire and Ayrshire miner;
pit deputy
Interview date: 5 July 2000
Interviewer: R. Johnston

Bert Smith
Interview C14
Born 1941
Ayrshire miner
Interview date: 5 July 2000
Interviewer: R. Johnston

William Dunsmore ('Arco')
Interview C16
Born 1924
Fife and Ayrshire miner
Interview date: 11 July 2000
Interviewer: R. Johnston

Davy McCulloch
Interview C18
Born 1924
Ayrshire (and Leicestershire) miner
Interview date: 11 July 2000
Interviewer: R. Johnston

Thomas McMurdo
Interview C20
Born 1929
Ayrshire miner
Interview date: 11 July 2000
Interviewer: R. Johnston

Tommy Coulter
Interview C21
Born 1928
Lanarkshire, Stirling and Fife miner
Interview date: 12 January 2005
Interviewers: N. Rafeek
and H. Young

Duncan Porterfield
Interview C22
Born 1959
Fife miner
Interview date: 12 January 2005
Interviewers: N. Rafeek
and H. Young

David Carruthers
Interview C23
Born 1934
Clackmannanshire and Fife miner
Interview date: 12 January 2005
Interviewers: N. Rafeek
and H. Young

John Gillon
Interview C24
Born 1931
Fife miner
Interview date: 15 January 2005
Interviewers: N. Rafeek
and H. Young

Robert Clelland
Interview C22
Born 1953
Fife miner
Interview date: 12 January 2005
Interviewers: N. Rafeek
and H. Young

George Bolton
Interview C23
Born 1934
Clackmannanshire miner
Interview date: 12 January 2005
Interviewers: N. Rafeek
and H. Young

George Peebles
Interview C24
Born 1930
Clackmannanshire miner
Interview date: 15 January 2005
Interviewers: N. Rafeek
and H. Young

Robin Howie
Interview C45
Freelance Occupational Hygienist;
formerly Institute of Occupational
Medicine
Interview date: 20 September 2001
Interviewer: N. Rafeek

2. South Wales

Howard Jones
Interview C25
Born 1923
South Wales miner
Interview date: 11 May 2004
Interviewers: A. McIvor
and R. Johnston

Gareth Gower
Interview C25
Born 1935
South Wales miner
Interview date: 11 May 2004
Interviewers: A. McIvor
and R. Johnston

Tom Bowden
Interview C26
Born 1933
South Wales miner
Interview date: 12 May 2004
Interviewers: A. McIvor
and R. Johnston

Gerald Hawkins
Interview C26
Born 1944
South Wales miner
Interview date: 12 May 2004
Interviewers: A. McIvor
and R. Johnston

John Jones
Interview C27
Born 1934
South Wales miner
Interview date: 15 September 2002
Interviewer: S. Morrison

Malcolm Davies
Interview C29
Born 1934
South Wales miner
Interview date: 11 May 2004
Interviewers: A. McIvor
and R. Johnston

Anonymous
Interview C31
Born 1920
Wife of a South Wales miner
Interview date: 14 May 2004
Interviewer: A. McIvor

Colin ('Nati') Thomas
Interview C26
Born 1940
South Wales miner
Interview date: 12 May 2004
Interviewers: A. McIvor
and R. Johnston

Derek Charles
Interview C26
Born 1932
South Wales miner
Interview date: 12 May 2004
Interviewers: A. McIvor
and R. Johnston

Mick Antoniw
Interview C28
Solicitor, Thompsons, Cardiff;
involved in COAD litigation
Interview date: 13 May 2004
Interviewers: A. McIvor
and R. Johnston

Les Higgon
Interview C30
Born 1920
South Wales miner
Interview date: 10 May 2004
Interviewers: A. McIvor
and R. Johnston

Anonymous
Interview C32
Born 1922
Wife of a South Wales miner;
father pneumoconiotic
Interview date: 14 May 2004
Interviewer: R. Johnston

Jean Davies
Interview C33
Born 1929
Wife of a South Wales miner;
husband bronchitic/pneumoconiotic
Interview date: 14 May 2004
Interviewer: A. McIvor

Anonymous
Interview C34
Born 1921
Wife of a South Wales miner;
father had silicosis
Interview date: 14 May 2004
Interviewer: R. Johnston

3. North East England

Marshall Wylde
Interview C35
Born 1932
Durham miner
Interview date: 10 March 2004
Interviewer: N. Rafeek

William Clough
Interview C36
Born 1936
Durham miner
Interview date: 28 April 2004
Interviewer: N. Rafeek

Samuel Westhead
Interview C37
Durham miner
Interview date: 1 April 2004
Interviewer: N. Rafeek

Roger Maddocks
Interview C38
Solicitor, Thompsons, Newcastle;
involved in COAD litigation
Interview date: 30 March 2004
Interviewer: N. Rafeek

Joseph Chattors
Interview C39
Durham miner
Interview date: 1 April 2004
Interviewer: N. Rafeek

George Burns
Interview C40
Born 1934
Durham miner
Interview date: 28 April 2004
Interviewer: N. Rafeek

Frederick Hall
Interview C41
Born 1926
Durham miner
Interview date: 29 March 2004
Interviewer: N. Rafeek

Alan Winter
Interview C42
Born 1920
Durham miner
Interview date: 27 April 2004
Interviewer: N. Rafeek

Alan Napier
Interview C43
Durham miner
Interview date: 31 March 2004
Interviewer: N. Rafeek

Joseph Goodwin
Interview C43
Durham miner
Interview date: 31 March 2004
Interviewer: N. Rafeek

David Guy
Interview C44
Durham miner
Interview date: 8 March 2004
Interviewer: N. Rafeek

Charles Walker
Interview C43
Durham miner
Interview date: 31 March 2004
Interviewer: N. Rafeek

Peter John Campbell
Interview C43
Durham miner
Interview date: 31 March 2004
Interviewer: N. Rafeek

These interviews are archived for public access in the Scottish Oral History Centre, University of Strathclyde (reference SOHC, Archive, 017).

Bibliography

Primary Sources Arranged by Archive

Andersonian Library, University of Strathclyde

Chief Inspector of Mines, *Annual Reports* (1930–74).
Health and Safety Commission (HSC), *Annual Report, 1992–3* (1993).
H.M. Inspector of Mines, Scottish Division, *Annual Reports*.
HSC, *Annual Report*, Statistical Supplement (1993).
HSC, *Health and Safety Statistics, 1995–6; 1998–9.*
Miners' Federation of Great Britain, *Coal Mines Eight Hours Bill: Transcript of the House of Commons Second Reading,* 22 June 1908 (Manchester, 1908).
Ministry of Power, *Statistical Digest, 1957.*
NCB, *Annual Reports* (1946–70).
NCB, Medical Services, *Annual Reports* (1960–74).
Safety in Mines Research Board, *Annual Reports* (1940–68).
Transactions of the Institute of Mining Engineers (1933–37).

Gallagher Memorial Library, Glasgow Caledonian University

Scottish Trade Union Congress, *Annual Reports* (1945–80).
Trade Union Congress, *Annual Reports* (1943–85).

Motherwell Museum

Oral History Transcripts, Dr George Bell, GP, Bellshill, Interview 7 October 1992, Transcript T006/7MDC.

National Archives, London

Board of Trade, *Employment in Grenfell Factories*, NJPC Paper 13D (1948), NA/PIN 20/118.
Board of Trade, *Employment of Pneumoconiosis Cases by NCB*, NJPC Paper 29 (1950), NA/PIN 20/118.
Board of Trade, *Provision of Employment in South Wales for Persons Suspended from the Mining Industry on account of Silicosis and Pneumoconiosis*, NJPC Paper 4, Cmd 6719 (1945), NA/PIN 20/118.

Board of Trade, *Note on Factory Building in South Wales*, NJPC Paper 26 (*c.* 1950), NA/PIN 20/118.

Fletcher, C.M., 'The Control of CWP by Means of Periodical X–ray Exams', (1950), MRC Industrial Pulmonary Disease Committee and PRU (1947–53), NA/FD/12/950.

International Labour Organization, Coal Mines Committee, 8th Session, *Dust Suppression in Coal Mines* (1964), NA/LAB 13/1836, p. 104.

IPDC, Minutes, Industrial Pulmonary Disease in Coal Mines, 19 March 1936; 28 May 1936; Letter, Home Office to MRC, dated 23 May 1936; MRC to Home Office, 18 June 1936, NA/FD1/2884.

Memorandum by Lord Citrine, 'The Provision of a Mines Medical Service' (1947), NA/COAL43/2 NCB.

Memorandum by Sir Geoffrey Vickers, 'The Mines Medical Service', General Purpose Committee (1948), NA/COAL43/2 NCB.

Ministry of Fuel and Power, 'A Proposal for a Miner's Medical Service', A. Tudor Hart (1946), NA/COAL43/2.

Ministry of Fuel and Power, Letter from M.J. Bentley, Medical Branch of the NCB, to Dr T.D. Spencer, Divisional Medical Officer, North Eastern Division, dated 15 January 1953. NA/POWE10/259.

Ministry of Fuel and Power, NCB General Purpose Committee, 'Mines Medical Service', paper by Dr Capel (1948), NA/COAL43/2.

Ministry of Fuel and Power, *Pneumoconiosis in the Mining and Quarrying Industries, Digest of Statistics (1954)* (London: HMSO, 1955).

Ministry of Fuel and Power, *Report of Inter-Departmental Committee on Mines Medical Service* (31 July 1942), NA/POWE10/259.

——, *Statutory Rules and Orders 1943, no. 1,696, Coal Mines (South Wales) (Pneumoconiosis), Order 1943, Emergency Powers (Defence)*, NA/POWE26/1150.

Ministry of Fuel and Power, *Water Infusion, a Means of Dust Control. By the South Western Committee on Dust Prevention and Suppression* (1955), Dust Prevention and Suppression Instructional Pamphlet no. 1, NA/POWE31420

Ministry of Fuel and Power and NUM, *Training for Pneumoconiosis* (1946), NA/LAB 18/280.

Ministry of Fuel and Power, NJPC, *Report on the Work of the MRC's Epidemiological and Pneumoconiosis Research Units* (1960), NJPC Paper no. 110, NA/PIN 20/325.

MRC, Letter from C. Fletcher to F.E.K. Green (MRC), dated 27 January 1948, NA/PDI/214.

NCB, 'Colliery Medical Services', Circular no. 15, 25 February 1947, NA/COAL43/2.

NCB, General Purpose Committee, 'Future Policy in Regard to NCB Medical Services', Memorandum by Sir Geoffrey Vickers, 13 March 1951, NA/COAL/43/2.

NCB, General Purpose Committee, Memorandum by Sir Geoffrey Vickers on 'Mines Medical Service', 6 July 1948, NA/COAL43/2.

NCB, Letter from C. Fletcher to Sir Edward Mellanby (MRC), dated 14 April 1948, NA/PDI/214.

NCB, Letter from G.C. Gooding to Sir Geoffrey Vickers, NCB, dated 2 October 1950, NCB, Medical and First Aid Services, Extracts from Scottish Divisional Board, 6 May, 1952, NA/POWE10/259.

NCB, Letter from M.J. Bentley (Medical Branch), to Dr T.D. Spencer, Divisional Medical Officer, North Eastern Division, dated 15 January 1953, NA/POWE/10/259.

NCB, Manpower and Welfare Department, 'Mines Medical Service' (September 1948), NA/COAL43/2.

NCB, 'Medical Centres Programme', 1948–51 (15 January 1953), Table 1. NA/POWE10/259.

NCB, Memorandum by Lord Citrine, 'The Provision of a Mines' Medical Service', 4 February 1947, NA/COAL43/2.

NCB, Proposal for a Miners' Medical Service by A. Tudor Hart (1945), NA/COAL43/2.

NCB, Scottish Division Board Meeting, Memorandum from Labour Director, 'Proposed Divisional Medical Services', 20 July 1948, NA/POWE, 10/259.

NCB, Scientific Department, Pneumoconiosis Field Research, *The Study of the Composition of Respirable Dust in the Pneumoconiosis Field Research* (1960).

NCB, 'Summary of Medical Centre Programme', July 1949, NA/Coal/43/2.

NJPC (National Joint Pneumoconiosis Committee), *Annual Report of the Field Research Steering Committee for the Year Ending 31/12/1959*, NJPC Paper no. 101, NA/PIN 20/325.

NJPC, Minutes, 1956–57, NA/POWE8/422.

NJPC, Minutes, 17 May 1961, NA/LAB 14 / 799.

NJPC, Minutes of Meeting held at the Ministry of Power, 17 December 1957, NA/POWE8/422.

NJPC, Minutes of 19th Meeting held at the Ministry of Power on 11 May 1960, NA/LAB 14/799.

NJPC, Minutes of 21st Meeting held at the Ministry of Power on 18 October 1962, NA/LAB 14/799.

NJPC, *Report of the Field Research Sub-Committee*, NJPC Paper no. 39 (1952).

NJPC, *Report of the Industrial Rehabilitation, Training and Employment Sub-Committee of the NJPC*, NJPC Paper no. 21 (25 February 1949), NA/PIN 20/118.

NJPC, *Report of the Work of the PRU Pneumoconiosis Field Research 20 Pit Scheme*, NJOC Paper no. 46 (November 1952).

NJPC, 'Suitable Work for Pneumoconiotics', Memorandum by Charles Fletcher, NJPC Paper (5 December 1946), NA/PIN 20/118.

NJPC, 'Unemployment among Pneumoconiosis Cases in South Wales', NJPC Paper 24 (1950), NA/PIN 20/118.

NJPC, *Work of the Industrial Rehabilitation, Training and Employment Sub-Committee*, NJPC Paper no. 41 (January 1952), NA/PIN/20/118.

NJPC, *17th Report of the Field Research Steering Committee for the Year Ending 1959*, NJPC Paper 107, NA/PIN 20/351.

NJPC, *24th Report of the Field Research Steering Committee for the Year Ending 31/12/1965*, NJPC Paper no. 107, NA/PIN 20/325.

NJPC, *27th Report of the Field Research Steering Committee* (1961), NJPC Paper 116, NA/PIN 20/325

Pneumoconiosis and Silicosis Newspaper Cuttings: *The Observer*, 1 February 1948; *The Observer*, 15 February 1948; NA/COAL26/153.

Safety in Mines Research Board, *Annual Reports: Eighteenth Annual Report* (1939).

National Archives of Scotland, Edinburgh

DHS (Department of Health for Scotland), Advisory Committee on Medical Research, *Report of the Pneumoconiosis Group*, HOS/15/15.

DHS, Fife and County Council Health and Welfare Department, Letter to Dr Kenneth Cowan, Chief Medical Officer DHS, dated 23 December 1955, SNA/HLA/27/13/FF/1.

DHS, Letter from Labour Party Scottish Council to DHS, dated 28 January 1956, no. 19 in file SNA/HH104/46.

DHS, Letter from Minister of Pensions and National Insurance to Dr Ian Macgregor, dated 12 August 1955, SNA/HLB/2Y/15/FF/1.

DHS, Letter to Secretary of Scottish Division of NCB from R.J. Peters, Department DHS, 16 August 1957, SNA/HOS/15/15.

DHS, Note of meeting on Pneumoconiosis at St Andrew's House Edinburgh, 23 March 1956, SNA/HOS/15/15.

DHS, *Specific Diseases: Pneumoconiosis* (1961), SNA/HH104/46.

DHS, Western Regional Hospital Board, Stirling, Clackmannan and Falkirk Area, Letter from Robert D McIntyre, Area Chest Physician, Royal Infirmary, Stirling, to Dr Ian MacGregor, dated 12 April 1956, SNA/HOS/15/15.

Gilson, J.C. and Cochrane, A.L., *Report of Pneumoconiosis Group*, 'Appendix A: Summary of Evidence', Advisory Committee on Medical Research, SNA/HH104/46.

Interviews with miners who worked at Lady Victoria Colliery, Newtongrange and other pits of the Lothian Coal Company, SNA/ACC 10801/37.

Letter from Ministry of Pensions and National Insurance to Dr Ian Macgregor Department of Health for Scotland, 12 August 1955, SNA/HLB/2Y/15/FF/1.

Letter from MRC to Sir David Dale, The Royal Institution, dated 7 June, 1943. SNA/FD 1/2880.

Letter from SMA to Secretary of State for Scotland, 18 November 1954, Department of Health for Scotland, SNA/ HH 104/1.

Medical Research Council, Special Report Series no. 290, SNA/ HH104/46.

NCB, *Digest of Pneumoconiosis Statistics* (1955), SNA/HH 104/1.

NCB, Divisional Dust Suppression Advisory Committee, Minutes of Meetings, 1958–65, SNA/CB/099/61/1.

NCB, Memorandum on Dust Respirators, from F.H. Morgan (Assistant Divisional Safety Engineer) to Mr T.R. Samson, Divisional Safety Engineer, dated 5 September 1962, SNA/CB/099/63/2.

NCB, Scottish Division, 'Circular to All Area Staff Managers/Secretaries', 10 April 1968, SNA/ CB/120/03/3.

NCB, Scottish Division Executive Minutes, SNA/CB 42/16.

NCB, Scottish Division, Medical Services, 'A short account of Pneumoconiosis in Coalminers with Special Reference to Scotland', 26, December 1955, SNA/ HOS/15/15/PTA.

NCB, Scottish Division, Medical Services, Letter to Dr H.K. Cowan, Chief Medical Officer of Health for Scotland, dated 24 April 1956, SNA/HOS/15/15.

NCB, Scottish Division, Production Department, 'Dust Suppression – Recent Developments', 15 October 1965, NAS/CB 53/10, p. 2.

NCB, Scottish Division, Production Department, 'Dust Suppression – Recent Developments', 15 October 1965, Paper no. AMP(65)4/3, SNA/53/10.

NCB, Scottish Division, Production Department, Minutes of Meetings of Area Ventilation Engineers, 1962–64, SNA/CB53/4.

NCB, Scottish Division, Production Department, Safety Branch, Minutes of Meeting of Area Safety Engineers, 1953–59, SNA/CB 53/8.

NCB, Scottish North Area, Area Dust Prevention Committee, Meeting 14 November 1969, SNA/ CB/120/03/4.

NCB, Scottish North Area, 'Progress Report on Dust Suppression for the Year Ended March 1971', SNA/ CB/120/03/4.

NCB, Scottish South Area, 'Airborne Dust Prevention and Suppression, Report, Final Quarter 1971/72', 31 March 1972, SNA/CB/099/03/6.

NCB, Scottish South Area, 'Airborne Dust Prevention and Suppression, Report, Second Quarter 1972/73', 30 September 1972, SNA/CB/099/03/6.

Scottish NCB, Divisional Dust Prevention and Suppression Advisory Committee (DDPSAC), Minutes of Meeting of 15 April, 1958 (and through 1960–61), NAS/ CB/099/61/1.

South Wales Coalfield Collection, Miners' Library, University of Swansea

Oral Interview Collection
Interview with Dr Thomas, n.d., AUD/374.
Interview with John Evans, 13 June 1973, AUD/84.
Interview with M. Morris (by Hywel Francis), n.d., AUD/389.
'The Big Hewer', Aud/580.

Documentary Source Archives

Amalgamated Anthracite Combine, Memorandum, 'The Need for New Industries to Provide Employment for Men Suspended from the Mining Industry on Account of Silicosis and Pneumoconiosis', prepared for Amalgamated Anthracite Combine Committee, 1945–46, SWCC/NWA/PP/127/C19.

Coal Industry Social and Welfare Organisation, *Annual Reports* (c. 1948–80).

Conference on Pneumoconiosis in Coal Mines, 18 January 1947, SWCC/MNA/NUM/K17J.

Correspondence between Louise Morgan and Evan Williams, 22 February 1936 and 24 February 1936, SWCC/MNA/NUM/G20.

Fletcher, C., 'Fighting the Modern Black Death', *The Listener* (28 September 1950).

Gilson, J.C., 'Is Coal Dust Harmful to Man?', PRU, *Collected Papers*, vol. 4 (1954–55), no. 95.

Higgins, I.T.T., 'Bronchitis', PRU, *Collected Papers*, Paper no. 243 (1960), pp. 138–57.

King, E.J., and Fletcher, C.M. (eds), *Industrial Pulmonary Diseases* (London:, J. & A. Churchill, 1960).

Letter from J.R. Felton, Ministry of Fuel and Power, to Mr Carey, South Wales Coalowners' Association, dated 23 July 1943, SWCC/MNA/NUM/K175.

Meeting of the South Wales Pneumoconiosis Sub-Committee, 28 July 1943, SWCC/MNA/NUM/K175.

Memorandum relating to Pneumoconiosis Cases, Prepared by R.W. Williams for the NJPC, 1947, SWCC/MNA/NUM/K17J.

MFGB, *Annual Volume of Proceedings* (1930–45).

MFGB, 'Silicosis among Coalminers: Case Submitted to the TUC' (June 1930).

Miners' Welfare Commission, *Miners' Welfare in Wartime*, report of the six-and-a-half years to June 1946 (n.d., c. 1946–47).

Ministry of Fuel and Power (Coal Division), 'Dust Suppression Measures on Coal Faces in South Wales', 23 July 1943, SWCC/ NWA/NUM/KI17J.

Minutes of the Pneumoconiosis Conference, 11 October 1952, SWCC/MNA/NUM/K17J, p. 21.

MSWCOA (Monmouthshire and South Wales Coal Owners' Association), *Coal Dust Research Committee, 9th Report* (July 1943).

MSWCOA, *Coal Dust Research Committee, 8th Report* (February 1943).

MSWCOA, *Fifth Report of the Coal Dust Research Committee* (September 1942).

MSWCOA, *Seventh Report of the Coal Dust Research Committee* (December 1942).

MRC, *Chronic Pulmonary Disease in South Wales Coalminers, Environmental Studies* (1943).

MRC, *Chronic Pulmonary Disease in South Wales Coalminers, Medical Studies* (London, 1942).

NCB, Confidential Report by A. Hudson, 'The Engineering Aspects of Dust Suppression with Particular Reference to Modern Practice in South Wales'.

NCB, 'Report of the Progress of Dust Suppression in the English and Scottish Coalfields', F.H. Price, Divisional Chief Scientist, South Eastern Division (1950).

NUM, *Annual Reports and Proceedings*.

NUM, *Enquiry into the Incidence of Silicosis* (24 August 1945), SWCC:NUM/ K17J.

NUM (South Wales Area), Area Executive Council.

NUM, South Wales Area Council, *Annual Conference Reports*.

NUM (South Wales Area Council), *Annual Conference and Report for 1947–8*.

NUM, South Wales Area Council, Letter to Lodge Secretaries, 24 August 1945, SWCC/MNA/PP/127/C19 (D.J. Williams Collection).

NUM (South Wales Area) Executive Council Meeting.

NUM (South Wales Area), Minutes of Area Annual Conference, 10–14 May 1965.

SWMF (South Wales Miners' Federation), Anthracite District, The Prevention of Silicosis and Anthracosis, 'Methods of Preventing Miners' Silicosis and some other Lung Diseases in the Anthracite District', J.H. Davies (n.d.).

SWMF, Compensation Department, Memorandum on Pneumoconiosis, 30 June 1944.

SWMF, Compensation Department, Letter to Lodge Secretaries, dated 21 July 1944, SWCC/MNA/NUM/K17J.

SWMF, Minutes.

SWMF, Minutes of Safety Committee, 20 August 1943, SWCC:NWA/NUM/K17j.

Newspapers and Journals

Colliery Engineering.
Colliery Guardian.
Edinburgh Evening News.
Glasgow Herald.
Hansard.
News Chronicle.
Radio Times.
South Wales Evening Post.
The Miner.
The Scotsman.
The Times.
Transactions of the Institute of Mining Engineers.
Western Mail and South Wales News.

Miscellaneous Reports

NCB, *Approved Conditions for Airborne Dust, Standards and Procedures for Sampling* (F4040).

Report of the Departmental Committee Appointed to Review the Disease Provision of the National Insurance (Industrial Injuries) Act, 1955, Cmd 9548, Majority Report, p. 5.

Testimony of Dr Julian Hart, Wellcome Institute for the History of Medicine, Witness Seminar, 'The MRC Epidemiology Unit (South Wales)', vol. 13, November 2002.

Secondary Sources

Abendstern, M., Hallett, C. and Wade, L., 'Flouting the Law: Women and the Hazards of Cleaning Moving Machinery in the Cotton Industry, 1930–1970', *Oral History*, vol. 33, no. 2 (Autumn 2005), pp. 69–78.

Abrams, H.K., 'A Short History of Occupational Health', *Journal of Public Health Policy*, vol. 22, no. 1 (2001), pp. 34–80.

Abrams, L., *The Orphan Country* (Edinburgh: John Donald, 1998).

Afacan, A.S. and Scarisbrick, D.A., 'Respiratory Health Surveillance in the UK Coal Mining Industry', *Transactions of the Institute of Mining and Metallurgy* (February 2001), pp. 3–7.

Aldrich, M., *Safety First: Technology, Labor, and Business in the Building of American Work Safety, 1870–1939* (Baltimore, MD: John Hopkins Press, 1997).

Allen, V.L., *The Militancy of British Miners* (Shipley: The Moor Press, 1981)

Arlidge, J.L., *The Hygiene, Disease and Mortality of Occupations* (London: Percival & Co., 1892).

Armstead, R., *Black Days, Black Dust: The Memoirs of an African American Coal Miner* (Knoxville, TN: University of Tennessee Press, 2002).

Arnot, R. Page, *The Miners: Years of Struggle – A History of the Miners' Federation of Great Britain from 1910* (London: Allen & Unwin, 1953).

Ashworth, W., *The History of the British Coal Industry, Volume 5. 1946–1982: The Nationalised Industry* (Oxford: Clarendon Press, 1986).

Atkinson, D., 'Research Interviews with People with Mental Handicaps', in A. Brechin and J. Walmsley (eds), *Making Connections* (London: Hodder Arnold, 1989).

Attfield, M.D. and Kuempel, E.D., 'Pneumoconiosis, coal mine dust and the PFR', *Annals of Occupational Hygiene*, vol. 47, no. 7 (2003), pp. 525–9.

Attfield, M.D. and Kuempel, E.D., 'Commentary: Pneumoconiosis, coalmine dust and the PFR', *The Annals of Occupational Hygiene*, vol. 47, no. 7 (2003), pp. 525–9.

Austoker, J. and Bryder, L. (eds), *Historical Perspectives on the Role of the MRC* (Oxford: Oxford University Press, 1989).

Ayers, P., 'Work Culture and Gender: The Making of Masculinities in Post-war Liverpool', *Labour History Review*, vol. 69, no. 2 (2004), pp. 153–68.

Barnes, C. and Mercer, G., *Disability* (Cambridge: Polity Press, 2003).

Bartrip, P.W.J., '"Petticoat Pestering": The Women's Trade Union League and Lead Poisoning in the Staffordshire Potteries, 1890–1914', *Historical Studies in Industrial Relations*, vol. 2 (September 1996), pp. 3–26.

——, *The Home Office and the Dangerous Trades: Regulating Occupational Disease in Victorian and Edwardian Britain* (Amsterdam: Rodopi, 2002).

——, *The Way from Dusty Death: Turner and Newall and the Regulation of Occupational Health in the British Asbestos Industry 1890s–1970* (London: Athlone Press, 2001).

——, 'Too Little Too Late': The Home Office and the Asbestos Industry Regulations, 1931', *Medical History*, vol. 42 (1998), pp. 421–38.

——, *Workmen's Compensation in Twentieth Century Britain* (Aldershot: Avebury, 1987).

Bayer, R. (ed.), *The Health and Safety of Workers: Case Studies in the Politics of Professional Responsibility* (New York: Oxford University Press, 1998).

Beaumont, P.B., *Safety at Work and the Unions* (Beckenham: Croom Helm, 1983).

Beck, E., *Risk Society: Towards a New Modernity* (London: Sage, 1992).

Bellaby, P., *Sick From Work: The Body in Employment* (Aldershot: Ashgate, 1999).

Benson, H., *British Coalminers in the Nineteenth Century* (Dublin: Gill and Macmillan, 1980).

Berman, D., *Death on the Job: Occupational Health and Safety Struggles in the United States* (New York: Monthly Review Press, 1978).

Berridge, V., *Health and Society in Britain since 1939* (Cambridge and New York: Cambridge University Press, 1999).

—— and Loughlin, K., 'Smoking and the New Health Education in Britain, 1950s–1970s', *American Journal of Public Health*, vol. 95, no. 6 (June 2005), pp. 958–64.

Berry, J.E. et al., 'A study of the acute and chronic changes in ventilatory capacity of workers in Lancashire cotton mills', *British Journal of Industrial Medicine*, vol. 30 (1973), pp. 25–36.

——, 'Cardiac frequency during sub-maximal exercise in young adults: Relation to lean body mass, total body potassium and amount of leg muscle', *Quarterly Journal of Experimental Physiology*, vol. 58 (1973), pp. 239–50.

Bevin, E., 'The wider issues of health legislation in industry', *British Medical Journal* (25 September 1937).

Bird, C. et al. (eds), *Handbook of Medical Sociology*, 5th edn (Englewood Cliffs, NJ: Prentice-Hall, 2000).

Blaxter, M., *The Meaning of Disability: A Sociological Study of Impairment* (London: Heinemann, 1976).

Bloor, M., 'No Longer Dying for a Living: Collective Responses to Injury Risks in South Wales Mining Communities, 1900–47', *Sociology*, vol. 36, no. 1 (2002), pp. 89–105.

——, 'The South Wales Miners' Federation, Miners' Lung and the Instrumental Use of Expertise, 1900–1950', *Social Studies of Science*, vol. 30, no. 1 (February 2000), pp. 125–40.

Bornat, J. (ed.), *Oral History Health and Welfare* (London: Routledge, 2000).

Borsay, A., *Disability and Social Policy in Britain since 1750* (Basingstoke: Palgrave, 2005).

Bowden, S. and Tweedale, G., 'Mondays without Dread: The Trade Union Response to Byssinosis in the Lancashire Cotton Industry in the Twentieth Century', *Social History of Medicine*, vol. 16, no. 1 (2003), pp. 79–95.

——, 'Poisoned by the Fluff: Compensation and Litigation for Byssinosis in the Lancashire Cotton Industry', *Journal of Law and Society*, vol. 29, no. 4 (December 2002), pp. 560–79.

Brodeur, P., *Expendable Americans* (New York: Viking Press, 1974).

Brown, C., *The Death of Christian Britain* (London: Routledge, 2001).

Brown, P., 'Popular epidemiology, toxic waste and social movements', in J. Gabe (ed.), *Medicine, Health and Risk: Sociological Approaches* (Oxford: Blackwell, 1987).

Bryan, A., *The Evolution of Health and Safety in Mines* (Letchworth: Ashire, 1975).

Bufton, M. and Melling, J., '"A Mere Matter of Rock": Organized Labour, Scientific Evidence and British Government Schemes for Compensation of Silicosis and Pneumoconiosis among Coalminers, 1926–1940', *Medical History*, vol. 49, no. 2 (April 2005): pp. 155–78.

——, '"Coming Up for Air": Experts, Employers and Workers in Campaigns to Compensate Silicosis Sufferers in Britain, 1918–1939', *Social History of Medicine*, vol. 18, no. 1 (2005), pp. 63–86.

Burnett, J. (ed.), *Useful Toil* (Harmondsworth: Penguin, 1974).

Buxton, N.K, *The Economic Development of the British Coal Industry* (London: Batsford, 1978).

Campbell, A., *The Scottish Miners, 1874–1939, Volume 1. Industry, Work and Community* (Aldershot: Ashgate, 2000).

—— et al. (eds), *Miners, Unions and Politics* (Aldershot: Scolar Press, 1996)

Cappelletto, F. and Merler, E., 'Perceptions of health hazards in the narratives of Italian migrant workers at an Australian asbestos mine (1943–1966)', *Social Science and Medicine*, vol. 56, no. 5 (March 2003), pp. 1,047–59.

Caufield, C., *Multiple Exposures: Chronicles of the Radiation Age* (Chicago, IL: University Press, Chicago, 1990).

Church, R. *The History of the British Coal Industry, Volume 3. 1830–1913* (Oxford: Claredon Press, 1986).

—— and Outram, Q., *Strikes and Solidarity: Coalfield Conflict in Britain, 1889–1966* (Cambridge: Cambridge University Press, 1998).

Clark, C., *Radium Girls: Women and Industrial Health Reform, 1910–1935* (Toronto: Stoddart, 1997).

Cockerman, W., 'The Sociology of Health Behaviour and Health Lifestyles in Central Asia', in C. Bird et al. (eds), *Handbook of Medical Sociology*, 5th edn (Englewood Cliffs, NJ: Prentice-Hall, 2000).

Cochrane, A.L., online biography at http://www.cardiff.ac.uk/schoolsanddivisions/insrv/libraryservices/research/cochrane/biography.html.

——, 'Pulmonary Tuberculosis in the Rhonda Fach', *British Medical Journal*, vol. 2 (18 October 1952), p. 8.

——, 'The attack rate of progressive massive fibrosis', *British Journal of Industrial Medicine*, vol. 19 (1962), pp. 52–64.

——, 'The Role of Periodic Examinations in the Prevention of Coalworkers' Pneumoconiosis', *British Journal of Industrial Medicine*, vol. 8 (1951), pp. 53–61.

Cockcroft, A. et al., 'Post-mortem study of emphysema in coal workers and non-coal workers', *Lancet*, vol. 2 (1982), pp. 600–603.

Coggon, A. et al., 'Coal mining and chronic obstructive pulmonary disease: A review of the evidence', *Thorax*, vol. 53 (1998), pp. 398–407.

Coggon, R. et al., *Epidemiology for the Uninitiated*, 3rd edn (London: BMJ Publishing Group, 2003).

Cole, G.D.H., *Labour in the Coal Mining Industry (1914–1921)* (Oxford: Clarendon Press, 1923).

Connell, R.W., *The Men and the Boys* (Oxford: Polity Press, 2000).

Coombes, B.L., *These Poor Hands: The Autobiography of a Miner Working in South Wales* (London: Left Book Club, 1939).

Cooter, R. and Luckin, B. (eds), *Accidents in History: Injuries, Fatalities and Social Relations* (Amsterdam: Rodopi, 1997).

Corn, J.K., Responses to Occupational Health Hazards, a Historical Perspective (New York: Van Nostrand Reinhold, 1992).

Cornwell, J., *Hard Earned Lives* (London: Tavistock, 1984).

Cotes, J.E., 'Average Normal Values for the Forced Expiratory Volume in White Caucasian Males', *British Medical Journal* (23 April 1966), vol. 5,494, pp. 1,016–19.

—— et al., 'Effect of breathing oxygen upon cardiac output, heart rate, ventilation, systemic and pulmonary blood pressure in patients with chronic lung disease', *Clinical Science*, vol. 25 (1963), pp. 305–21.

Dalton, A.J.P., 'Lessons from the United Kingdom: Fightback on Workplace Hazards, 1979–1992', *International Journal of Health Services*, vol. 22, no. 3 (1992), pp. 489–95.

Davidson, C. et al., 'Lay Epidemiology and the Prevention Paradox: The Implication of Coronary Candidacy for Health Education', *Sociology of Health and Illness*, vol. 13 (1991), pp. 1–19.

Deal, M., 'Disabled People's Attitudes toward Other Impairment Groups', *Disability and Society*, vol. 18, no. 7 (December 2003).

Dembe, A., *Occupation and Disease: How Social Factors Affect the Conception of Work-related Disorders* (New Haven, CT: Yale University Press, 1996).

Derickson, A., *Black Lung: Anatomy of a Public Health Disaster* (Ithaca, NY: Cornell University Press, 1998).

——, 'Part of the Yellow Dog: US Coal Miners' Opposition to the Company Doctor System, 1936–1946', *International Journal of Health Services*, vol. 19 (1989), pp. 709–20.

——, *Workers' Health, Workers' Democracy: The Western Miners' Struggle, 1981– 1925* (Ithaca, NY: Cornell University Press, 1988).

Doll, R. et al., 'Mortality in relation to smoking: 50 years' observations on male British doctors', *BMJ*, vol. 328 (26 June 2004), 1,519–33.

Donovan, A.L., 'Health and Safety in Underground Coal Mining, 1900–1969', in R. Bayer (ed.), *The Health and Safety of Workers* (Oxford: Oxford University Press, 1988).

Dormandy, T., *The White Death: A History of Tuberculosis* (London: Hambledon, 1999).

Douglass, D. and Krieger, J., *A Miner's Life* (London: Routledge, 1983).

Dwyer, T., *Life and Work: Industrial Accidents as a Case of Socially Produced Error* (New York: Plenum Press, 1991).

Dyer, C., 'Miners win historic battle for compensation', *British Medical Journal*, vol. 316 (31 January 1998), pp. 316–27.

Emsley, J., *The Shocking History of Phosphorus: A Biography of the Devil's Element* (London: Pan, 2001).

Evans, C., 'A Miner's Life', in R. Fraser (ed.), *Work: Twenty Personal Accounts* (Harmondsworth: Penguin, 1968).

Evans, D.D., 'A Survey of the Incidence and Progression of Pneumoconiosis', (NUM, South Wales Area, April 1963).

Evans, R., *You Questioning My Manhood, Boy? Masculine Identity, Work Performance and Performativity in a Rural Staples Economy*, Arkleton Research Paper no. 4 (University of Aberdeen, 2000).

Fletcher, C.M., 'Epidemiological Studies of Coal Miners' Pneumoconiosis in Great Britain', *American Medical Association, Archives of Industrial Health*, vol. 11 (January 1955), pp. 26–31.

——, 'Fighting the Modern Black Death', *The Listener* (28 September 1950), p. 407

——, 'The Clinical Diagnosis of Pulmonary Emphysema: An Experimental Study', Medical Research Council, Pneumoconiosis Research Unit, Papers 1952–1953, Paper no. 49.

—— and Gough, J., 'Coalminers' Pneumoconiosis', *British Medical Bulletin*, vol. 7 (1950), p. 43.

Francis, H., and Smith, D., *The Fed: A History of the South Wales Miners in the Twentieth Century* (London: Lawrence and Wishart, 1980).

Furlong, A. and Cartmel, F., *Young People and Social Change: Individualism and Risk in Late Modernity* (Buckingham: Open University Press, 1997).

Gabe, J. (ed.), *Challenging Medicine* (Oxford: Blackwell, 1994).

—— (ed.), *Medicine, Health and Risk: Sociological Approaches* (Oxford: Blackwell, 1987).

Gersuny, C., *Work Hazards and Industrial Conflict* (Hanover, NH: University Press of New England, 1981).

Gillespie, R., 'Accounting for Lead Poisoning: The Medical Politics of Occupational Health', *Social History of Medicine*, vol. 15, no 3 (1990), pp. 303–31.

Gilson, J.C., 'Is Coal Dust Harmful to Man?', PRU, *Collected Papers*, vol. 4, 1954–55, Paper no. 95 (1955).

——, 'Pathology, Radiology, and Epidemiology of Coal Workers' Pneumoconiosis in Wales', *American Medical Association, Archives of Industrial Health*, vol. 15 (June 1957), pp. 460–71.

Glucksmann, M., *Women Assemble: Workers in the New Industries in Interwar Britain* (London: Routledge, 1990).

Goodell, J., *Our Story: 77 Hours Underground – by the Outcreek Miners* (London: Ebury Press, 2003).

Gordan, A.I, and Booth, R.T., 'Workers' Participation in Occupational Health and Safety in Britain', *International Labour Review*, vol. 121, no. 4 (July–August 1982), pp. 121–87.

Greenberg, M., 'Knowledge of the Health Hazards of Asbestos Prior to the Merewether and Price Report of 1930', *Social History of Medicine*, vol. 7 (1994), pp. 493–516.

Greenwood, W., *How the Other Man Lives* (London: Labour Book Service, 1939)

Haldane, J.S., 'Silicosis and Coal Mining', *The Colliery Guardian* (16 January 1931), p. 226.

Harrison, B., *'Not Only the 'Dangerous Trades': Women's Work and Health in Britain, 1880–1914* (London: Taylor and Francis, 1996).

——, 'Some of Them Gets Lead Poisoned: Occupational Lead Exposure in Women, 1880–1914', *Social History of Medicine*, vol. 2 (1989), pp. 171–95.

——, 'Women's Health or Social Control? The Role of the Medical Profession in Relation to Factory Legislation in Late 19th Century Britain', *Sociology of Health and Illness*, vol. 13, no. 4 (1991), pp. 469–91.

Hart, P. D'Arcy, 'Chronic Pulmonary Disease in South Wales Coal Mines: An Eyewitness Account of the MRC Surveys (1937–1942)', *Social History of Medicine*, vol. 11 (December 1998), pp. 459–68.

Higgins, I.T.T., 'Bronchitis', Pneumoconiosis Research Unit, Paper no. 243 (1960).

Higgins, I.T.T., 'An Approach to the Problem of Bronchitis in Industry: Studies in Agricultural, Mining and Foundry Communities', in E.J. King and C.M. Fletcher, *Industrial Pulmonary Diseases* (London: Churchill, 1960).

Higgison, A., 'Asbestos and the British Trade Unions, 1960s and 1970s', *Scottish Labour History*, vol. 40 (2005), pp. 70–86.

Holt, P.F., *Pneumoconiosis, Industrial Diseases of the Lung Caused by Dust* (London: Arnold, 1957).

HSE, Safety and Health in Mines Research Advisory Board, *Annual Reviews* (1997–

2004).

Hughes, B., 'Bauman's Strangers: Impairment and the Invalidation of Disabled People in Modern and Post-modern Cultures', *Disability and Society*, vol. 17, no. 5 (2003), pp. 571–84.

Hugh-Jones, P. and Fletcher, C.M., 'The Social Consequences of Pneumoconiosis among Coalminers in South Wales', Medical Research Council Memorandum no. 25 (London, 1951).

Hunt, E.H., *British Labour History 1815–1914* (London: Weidenfeld and Nicolson, 1981).

Hunter, D., *The Diseases of Occupations,* 9th edn (London: Arnold, 1995).

Hurley, J.F. et al., 'Coal workers' pneumoconiosis and exposure to dust at 10 British coalmines', *British Journal of Industrial Medicine*, vol. 39 (1982), pp. 120–27.

Hutter, B.M., *Regulation and Risk: Occupational Health and Safety on the Railways* (Oxford: Oxford University Press, 2001).

Hutton, G., *Lanarkshire's Mining Legacy* (Cumnock, Scotland: Stenlake Publishing, 1997).

——, *Scotland's Black Diamonds:Coal Mining in Scotland* (Cumnock, Scotland: Stenlake Publishing, 2001).

IIAC, 'Lung Function Assessment, Industrial Injuries Disablement Benefit, Prescribed Disease D12 (Chronic Bronchitis and Emphysema in Underground Coal-miners)', Position Paper no. 11 (2000).

Jackson, M.P., *The Price of Coal* (London: Croom Helm, 1974).

Jacobsen, M. et al, 'The relation between pneumoconiosis and dust exposure in British coal mines', in W.H. Walton and J.M. Rogan, *Inhaled Particles III*, vol. 2 (Old Woking: Unwin Brothers), pp. 903–16.

Jacobsen, M., 'Reply to WRK Moran and NL Lapp', *American Review of Respiratory Disease*, vol. 138 (1998), pp. 1,643–6.

—— and Maclaren, W.M., 'Unusual pulmonary observations and exposure to coalmine dust: A case-control study', *Annals of Occupational Hygiene*, vol. 26 (1982), pp. 753–65.

—— et al., 'New Dust Standards for British Coal Mines', *Nature*, vol. 227 (1970), pp. 445–7.

James, L.R., *The Control of Dust in Mines* (Cardiff: South Wales NUM, 1959).

James, P. and Walters, D., *Regulating Safety and Health at Work* (London: Institute of Employment Rights, 1999).

Jeremy, D.J., 'Corporate Responses to the Emergent Recognition of a Health Hazard in the UK Asbestos Industry: The Case of Turner and Newall, 1920–1960', *Business and Economic History*, vol. 24 (1995), pp. 254–65.

John, A., *By the Sweat of their Brow* (London: Routledge and Kegan, Paul 1984)

Johnston, R. and McIvor, A., 'Dangerous Work, Hard Men and Broken Bodies: Masculinity in the Clydeside Heavy Industries', *Labour History Review*, vol. 69, no. 2 (August 2004), pp. 135–53.

——, 'Dust to Dust: Oral Testimonies of Asbestos-related Disease on Clydeside, c.

1930–the Present', *Oral History*, vol. 29, no. 2 (Autumn 2001), pp. 38–62.

——, 'Incubating Death: Working with Asbestos in Clydeside Shipbuilding and Engineering, 1945–1990', *Scottish Labour History*, vol. 34 (1999), pp. 74–93.

——, *Lethal Work: A History of the Asbestos Tragedy in Scotland* (East Linton: Tuckwell Press, 2000).

——, 'Oral History in Asbestos Investigations', in G.A. Peters and B.J. Peters (eds), *The Asbestos Legacy: The Sourcebook of Asbestos Diseases*, vol. 23 (New York, STPM Press, December 2001), pp. 1–43.

——, 'Oral History, Subjectivity and Environmental Reality: Occupational Health Histories in Twentieth Century Scotland', in G. Mitman et al. (eds), *Landscapes of Exposure, Osiris*, vol 19 (2004), pp. 234–50.

——, 'The War and the Body at Work: Occupational Health and Safety in Scottish Industry, 1939–1945', *Journal of Scottish Historical Studies*, vol. 24, no. 2 (2005), pp. 113–36.

——, 'Whatever Happened to the *Occupational* Health Service?', in C. Nottingham (ed.), *The NHS in Scotland* (Aldershot: Ashgate, 2000).

Jones, H., 'Employers' Welfare Schemes and Industrial Relations in Inter-war Britain', *Business History* (1983), pp. 61–73.

——, *Health and Society in Twentieth Century Britain* (London: Longman, 1994).

Judkins, B.M., *We Offer Ourselves as Evidence: Toward Workers' Control of Occupational Health* (New York: Greenwood Press, 1986).

Kenny, L.C. et al., 'Evaluation of instruments for dust monitoring in United Kingdom coal mines', *Mining Technology*, vol. 110 (August 2001), pp. 97–106.

King, E.J. and Fletcher, C.M., *Industrial Pulmonary Diseases* (London: Churchill, 1960).

King, M. et al., 'Treatment of Homosexuality in Britain since the 1950s – an Oral History: The Experience of Professionals', *British Medical Journal*, vol. 328, no. 429 (21 February 2004), http://bmj.bmjjournals.com/cgi/reprint/bmj.37984.496725.EE.

Landsbergis, P. and Cahill, J., 'Labor Union Programs to Reduce or Prevent Occupational Stress in the United States', *International Journal of Health Services*, vol. 24, no. 1 (1994), pp. 105–29.

Lane, J., *A Social History of Medicine: Health, Healing and Disease in England 1750–1950* (London: Routledge, 2001).

Levenstein, C. et al. (eds), *Work, Health and Environment: Old Problems, New Solutions* (New York: Guilford Press, 1997).

Liddell, F.D.K., 'Mortality of British Coal Miners in 1961', *British Journal of Industrial Medicine*, vol. 30 (1973), pp. 15–24.

Louis, H., 'Mining', in T. Oliver (ed.), *Dangerous Trades* (London: John Murray, 1902).

M. Bellamy, *The Shipbuilders* (Edinburgh: Birlinn, 2000).

MacDougall, I., *Mungo McKay and the Green Table* (East Linton: Tuckwell Press, 1995).

——, *Voices from Work and Home* (Edinburgh: Merkat Press, 2000)

Maurice, W., *A Pitman's Anthology* (London: James, 2004).

McCallum, R.I., 'Pneumoconiosis and the Coalfields of Durham and Northumberland', *Transactions of the Institution of Mining Engineers*, vol. 113 (1953–54).

McCormack, B.J., *Industrial Relations in the Coal Industry* (London: Macmillan, 1979).

McCulloch, J., *Asbestos Blues: Labour, Capital, Physicians and the State in South Africa* (Oxford: James Currey, 2002).

McEvoy, A.F., 'Working Environments: an Ecological Approach to Industrial Health and Safety', in R. Cooter and B. Luckin (eds), *Accidents in History: Injuries, Fatalities and Social Relations* (Amsterdam: Rodopi, 1997).

McIlvanney, W., *The Kiln* (London: Sceptre, 1996).

McIvor, A.J., *A History of Work in Britain* (London: Palgrave, 2001).

——, 'Employers, the Government and Industrial Fatigue in Britain, 1890–1918', *British Journal of Industrial Medicine*, vol. 44 (1987), pp. 724–32.

——, 'Manual Work, Technology and Health 1918–39', *Medical History*, vol. 31 (1987), pp. 160–89.

——, 'Work and Health, 1880–1914: A note on a neglected interaction', *Scottish Labour History Journal*, vol. 24 (1989), pp. 14–32.

—— and Johnston, R., 'Medical Knowledge and the Worker: Occupational Lung Disease in the United Kingdom, c. 1920–1975', *Labor: Studies in the Working Class History of the Americas*, vol. 2, no. 4 (Winter 2005), pp. 46–72.

——, 'Voices from the Pits: Health and Safety in Scottish Coal Mining since 1945', *Scottish Economic and Social History*, vol. 22, part 2 (2002), p. 111–33.

McKinlay, A., *Making Ships, Making Men: Working for John Brown's between the Wars* (Alexandria, Scotland: Lomond Print, 1981).

Medical Research Council, *Chronic Pulmonary Disease in South Wales Coalminers, Volume 1. Medical Studies* (London: HMSO, 1942).

——, 'Definitions and Classification of Chronic Bronchitis for Clinical and Epidemiological Purposes, a Report to the Medical Research Council by their Committee on the Aetiology of Chronic Bronchitis', *The Lancet*, vol. 1 (10 April 1965), pp. 775–9

Melling, J., 'From Sandstone Dust to Black Lung: The Origins of Pneumoconiosis Regulation in the UK and its Impact on Miners' Compensation c. 1935–1945', unpublished paper delivered to Dust at Work Conference, Glasgow Caledonian University, 28 May, 2004.

——, 'The Risks of Working versus the Risks of Not Working: Trade Unions, Employers and Responses to the Risk of Occupational Illness in British industry, c. 1890–1940s', ESRC Centre for Analysis of risk and Regulation, Discussion Paper no. 12, December 2003.

Messing, K., *One Eyed Science: Occupational Health and Women Workers* (Philadelphia, PA: Temple University Press, 1998).

—— et al., 'Prostitutes and Chimney Sweeps Both Have Problems: Towards Full Integration of Both Sexes in the Study of Occupational Health', *Social Science and Medicine*, vol. 36, no. 1 (1993), pp. 47–55.

—— et al., 'Sugar and Spice and Everything Nice: Health Effects of the Sexual Division of Labor Among Train Cleaners', *International Journal of Health Services*, vol. 23, no. 1 (1993), pp. 133–46.

Miall, W.E. et al., 'An epidemiological study of rheumatoid arthritis associated with characteristic chest x–ray appearances in coal-workers', *British Medical Journal*, vol. 4,848 (5 December 1953), p. 1,231–6.

—— and Oldham, P.D., 'The hereditary factor in arterial blood–pressure', *British Medical Journal*, vol. 1 (1963), pp. 75–80.

—— et al., 'Factors influencing arterial pressure in the general population in Jamaica', *British Medical Journal*, vol. 2 (1962), pp. 497–506.

Miller, B.G. et al., 'Risks of silicosis in coal workers exposed to unusual concentrations of respirable quartz', *Occupational and Environmental Medicine*, vol. 55 (1998), pp. 52–8.

Mills, C., 'A Hazardous Bargain: Occupational Risk in Cornish Mining 1875–1914', *Labour History Review*, vol. 70, no. 1 (April 2005), pp. 53–73.

——, 'The Kinnaird Commission: Siliceous Dust, the Pitfalls of Cause and Effect Correlations and the Case of the Cornish Miners in the Mid-nineteenth Century', *Scottish Labour History*, vol. 40 (2005), pp. 13–30.

Ministry of Labour and National Service, *The Disabled Persons Employment Act, 1944: Employment of Ex-miners Affected by Pneumoconiosis or Silicosis*, pamphlet (July 1948).

Ministry of National Service, 1917–19, *Report upon the Physical Examination of Men of Military Age by National Service Medical Boards*, vol. 1 (1919).

Moffat, A., *My Life with the Miners* (London: Lawrence and Wishart, 1965).

Morrison, S., 'The Factory Inspectorate and the Silica Dust Problem in the UK Foundries, 1930–1970', *Scottish Labour History*, vol. 40 (2005), pp. 31–50.

MRC, 'Streptomycin the treatment of pulmonary tuberculosis: and MRC investigation', *British Medical Journal*, vol. 2 (1948), pp. 769–82.

Mullen, K., *A Healthy Balance: Glaswegian Men Talk about Health, Tobacco and Alcohol* (Aldershot: Ashgate, 1993).

Murphy, S., 'The Early Days of the MRC Social Medicine Research Unit', *Society for the Social History of Medicine*, vol. 12, no. 3 (1999), pp. 389–406.

Navarro V. and Berman, D. (eds), *Health and Work Under Capitalism: An International Perspective* (Farmington, NY, Baywood Publishing, 1983).

NCB, *A Short History of the Scottish Coal-mining Industry* (Edinburgh: National Coal Board, Scottish Division, 1958).

——, South Western Division, *Observations on Dust Suppression* (n.d.).

Nichols, T., *The Sociology of Industrial Injury* (London: Mansell, 1997).

Nott-Bower, G. and Walkerdine, R.H., *The NCB: The First Ten Years* (London: Colliery Guardian, 1958).

O'Neil, R., 'When it Comes to Health and Safety, Your Life Should be in Union Hands', *Labour Education*, no. 126 (2002/1), ILO Bureau for Workers' Activities, http://www.ilo.org/public/english/dialogue/actrav/new/april28/index/htm.

Oldham, P.D., 'The Nature of the Variability of Dust Concentrations at the Coal Face', *British Journal of Industrial Medicine*, vol. 10 (1953), p. 227.

Oliver, M., *The Politics of Disablement* (Basingstoke: Macmillan, 1990).

Orwell, G., *The Road to Wigan Pier* (London: Penguin, 2001).

Outram, Q., 'The Stupidest Men in England? The Industrial Relations Strategy of the Coalowners between the Lockouts, 1923–1924', *Historical Studies in Industrial Relations*, vol. 4 (September 1997).

Page Arnot, R., *The Miners in Crisis and War: A History of the Miners' Federation of Great Britain from 1930 Onwards* (London: George Allen & Unwin, 1961).

——, *The Miners: Years of Struggle – A History of the Miners' Federation of Great Britain (from 1910 Onwards)* (London: George Allen & Unwin, 1953).

Perchard, A., 'The Mine Management Professionals and the Dust Problem in the Scottish Coal Mining Industry, c. 1930–1966', *Scottish Labour History*, vol. 40 (2005), pp. 87–110.

——, 'The Mine Management Professions in the Scottish Coal Industry, 1930–1966' (PhD thesis, University of Strathclyde, 2005).

Phillips, J., 'Class and Industrial Relations in Britain: The 'Long' Mid-century and the Case of Port Transport, c1920–1970', *Twentieth Century British History*, vol. 16, no. 1 (2005).

Pilger, J., 'Heartlands to wastelands', *New Statesman and Society* (23 October 1992).

Porter, D., 'John Ryle and the Making of Social Medicine in Britain in the 1940s', *History of Science*, vol. 30 (88, part 2) (June 1992), pp. 137–64.

Queen's University Belfast, *Alumni Magazine* (Autumn 2004), p. 3.

Renfrew, A., 'Mechanisation and the Miner: Work, Safety and Labour Relations in the Scottish Coal Industry, 1890–1939' (unpublished PhD thesis, University of Strathclyde, 1997).

Roach, A.S., 'A Method of Relating the Incidence of Pneumoconiosis to Airborne Dust Exposure', *British Journal of Industrial Medicine*, vol. 10 (1953), pp. 220–24.

Rodmell, S. and Watt, A. (eds), *The Politics of Health Education* (London: Routledge and Kegan Paul, 1986).

Rogan, J.M., 'Chest Disease in coalminers, with special reference to the Pneumoconiosis Field Research', *The Mining Engineer* (November 1960), pp. 108–9.

——, *Medicine in the Mining Industries* (London: Heinemann Medical Books, 1972)

Roper, M., *Masculinity and the British Organisation Man Since 1945* (Oxford: Oxford University Press, 1994).

Rosen, G., *A History of Public Health* (Baltimore, MD: Johns Hopkins Press, 1993).

Rosner, D. and Markowitz, J., *Deadly Dust: Silicosis and the Politics of Occupational Disease in Twentieth-century America* (Princeton, NJ: Princeton University Press, 1994).

—— (eds), *Dying for Work: Workers' Safety and Health in 20th Century America* (Bloomington, IN: Indiana University Press, 1987).

—— 'Labor Day and the War on Workers', *American Journal of Public Health*, vol. 89, no. 9 (September 1999), pp. 1,319–21.

Rudd, R., 'Coalminers' respiratory disease litigation', *Thorax*, vol. 53 (1998), pp. 337–40.

Sabo, D. and Gordon, D.F., *Men's Health and Illness: Gender, Power and the Body* (Thousand Oaks, CA, Sage, 1995).

Saracci, R., *The History of Epidemiology*, http://www.oup.co.uk/pdf/0-19-263066-0.pdf.

Schilling, R., *A Challenging Life: Sixty Years in Occupational Health* (London: Canning Press, 1988).

Scott, W.H., *Coal and Conflict: A Study of Industrial Relations at Collieries* (Liverpool: Liverpool University Press, 1963).

Seaton, A., 'The new prescription: industrial injuries benefits for smokers?', *Thorax*, vol. 53 (1998), p. 1.

——, 'Quartz and pneumoconiosis in coal miners', *Lancet*, vol. 2 (1981), pp. 1,272–5.

Segal, L., *Slow Motion: Changing Masculinities, Changing Men* (London: Virago, 1990).

Sellers, C., *Hazards of the Job: From Industrial Science to Environmental Health Science* (Chapel Hill, NC: University of North Carolina Press, 1997).

Shepherd, W.H., *Under the Pulley Wheels: The Memoirs of William Herbert Shepherd (1891–1972)*, accessed 12 February 2006 at http//www.wheatleyhill.com/pulley.htm.

Shrivastava, P., *Bhopal, Anatomy of a Crisis* (London: Paul Chapman Publishing, 1992).

Skidmore, J.W. et al., 'The retention of high and low rank coals in rats' lung', *Annuls of Occupational Hygiene*, vol. 8 (1965), p. 183.

Smart, A., 'Note on Anthracosis', *British Medical Journal*, vol. 2 (5 September 1885), p. 493.

Smith, B., *Seven Steps in the Dark: A Miner's Life* (Barr, Scotland: Luath Press, 1991).

Smith, B.E., *Digging Our Own Graves: Coal Miners and the Struggle Over Black Lung Disease* (Philadelphia, PA: Temple University Press, 1987).

Smith, G. et al., 'Treatment of Homosexuality in Britain since the 1950s – an Oral History: The Experience of Patients', *British Medical Journal*, vol. 328, no. 427 (21 February 2004), http://bmj.bmjjournals.com/cgi/reprint/bmj.37984.442419.EEv1.

Smither, W.J. et al., 'Diffuse pleural mesotheliomas and exposure to asbestos dust', *Lancet*, vol. 2 (1962), p. 1,228.

Stewart, J., *'The Battle for Health': A Political History of the Socialist Medical Association* (Aldershot: Ashgate, 1999).

Summerfield, P., *Reconstructing Women's Wartime Lives* (London: Routledge, 1998).

Supple, B., *The History of the British Coal Industry, Volume 4. 1913–1946: The Political Economy of Decline* (Oxford: Oxford University Press, 1987).

Tatham, T., 'Dust-producing Occupations', in T. Oliver (ed.), *Dangerous Trades* (London: John Murray, 1902).

Taylor, A., *The NUM and British Politics, Volume 1. 1944–1968* (Aldershot: Ashgate, 2003).

——, *The NUM and British Politics, Volume 2. 1969–1995* (Aldershot: Ashgate, 2005).

Tweedale, G., *From Magic Mineral to Killer Dust: Turner and Newall and the Asbestos Hazard* (Oxford: Oxford University Press, 1999).

—— and Hanson, P., 'Protecting the Workers: The Medical Board and the Asbestos Industry, 1930s–1960s', *Medical History*, vol. 42 (1998), pp. 439–57.

Wagner, J.C. et al., 'Mesothelioma in rats after inoculation with asbestos and other materials', *British Journal of Cancer*, vol. 28 (1973), pp. 173–85.

Walby, S., *Patriarchy at Work* (Oxford: Blackwell, 1986).

Waldron, H.A., 'Occupational Health during the Second World War: Hope Deferred or Hope Abandoned?', *Medical History*, vol. 41 (1997), pp. 197–212.

Walker, D., ' "Working in it, through it and among it all day": Chrome dust at J. & J. White of Rutherglen, 1893–1967', *Scottish Labour History*, vol. 40 (2005), pp. 50–69.

Wallace, A.F.C., *St Clair: A Nineteenth Century Coal Town's Experience with a Disaster-prone Industry* (Ithaca, NY: Cornell University Press, 1987).

Walmsley, J., 'Life History Interviews with People with Learning Disabilities', in R. Perks and A. Thomson (eds), *The Oral History Reader* (London: Routledge, 1988).

Walters, D., 'Trade Unions and the Effectiveness of Worker Representation in Health and Safety in Britain', *International Journal of Health Services*, vol. 25 (1996), pp. 625–41.

Warren, C., *Brush with Death: A Social History of Lead Poisoning* (Baltimore, MD: Johns Hopkins Press, 2001).

Waterson, A., 'Occupational Health and Illness: The Politics of Hazard Education', in S. Rodmell and A. Watt (eds), *The Politics of Health Education* (London: Routledge and Kegan Paul, 1986).

Watson, J., *Male Bodies: Health, Culture and Identity* (Buckingham: Open University Press, 2000).

Weber, M., *Economy and Society* (Berkeley, CA: University of California Press, 1978).

Weindling, P. (ed.), *International Health Organisation and Movements, 1918–1939* (New York: Cambridge University Pres, 1995).

—— (ed.), *The Social History of Occupational Health* (London: Croom Helm, 1985).

Wellcome Witness Seminar, 23 March 1999, *Population-based Research in South Wales: The MRC Pneumoconiosis Research Unit and the MRC Epidemiology Unit*, vol. 13 (November 2002).

Welshman, J., *Municipal Medicine: Public Health in Twentieth Century Britain* (Oxford: Peter Lang, 2000).

Wight, D., *Workers not Wasters: Masculinity, Respectability, Consumption and Employment in Central Scotland* (Edinburgh: Edinburgh University Press, 1993).

Williams, C., *Capitalism, Community and Conflict: The South Wales Coalfields, 1897–1947* (Cardiff: Cardiff University Press, 1998).

——, 'Is a Working Man Any Greater Value than the Dust?' Lung Disease in the Writings of B. L. Coombes', unpublished paper delivered at the 'Dust at Work' Conference, Glasgow Caledonian University, 28–29 May 2004.

Williams, G. and Popay, J., 'Lay knowledge and the privilege of experience', in J. Gabe (ed.), *Challenging Medicine* (London: Routledge, 1994).

Willis, P., 'Shop Floor Culture, Masculinity and the Wage Form', in J. Clarke, C. Critcher and R. Johnson (eds), *Working Class Culture* (London: Hutchison, 1979).

Wilson, G.K., *The Politics of Safety and Health: Occupational Safety and Health in the United States and Britain* (Oxford: Clarendon Press, 1985).

Wohl, A.S., *Endangered Lives: Public Health in Victorian Britain* (London: Dent, 1983).

Woolfson, C., Foster, J. and Beck, M., *Paying for the Piper: Capital and Labour in Britain's Offshore Oil Industry* (London: Mansell, 1997).

Wyke, T., 'Spinners' Cancer', in A. Fowler and T. Wyke (eds), *The Barefoot Aristocrats* (Littleborough: George Kelsall, 1987).

Young, H., 'New Men, Hard Men: An Oral History of Masculinity in Glasgow, from 1950–2000' (Honours Dissertation, History Department, University of Strathclyde, 2001).

Zinn, J., 'The Biographical Approach: A Better Way to Understand Behaviour in Health and Illness', *Health Risk and Society*, vol. 7 (2005), pp. 1–9.

Zweig, F., *Men in the Pits* (London: Victor Gollancz, 1948).

Index